ADVANCES IN

Anesthesia

Editor-in-Chief
Thomas M. McLoughlin, MD

ELSEVIER

An Imprint of Elsevier, Inc.

PHILADELPHIA   LONDON   TORONTO   MONTREAL   SYDNEY   TOKYO

Vice President, Continuity Publishing: John A. Schrefer
Associate Developmental Editor: Yonah Korngold

Editorial Office:
Elsevier
1600 John F. Kennedy Blvd,
Suite 1800
Philadelphia, PA 19103-2899

International Standard Serial Number: 0737-6146
International Standard Book Number-13: 978-0-323-06820-8

ADVANCES IN
Anesthesia

Editor-in-Chief

THOMAS M. MCLOUGHLIN, MD, Associate Chief Medical Officer, Chair, Department of Anesthesiology, Lehigh Valley Health Network, Allentown; and Professor of Surgery, Division of Surgical Anesthesiology, University of South Florida College of Medicine, Tampa, Florida

Associate Editors

JOEL O. JOHNSON, MD, PhD, Professor, Department of Anesthesiology, University of Wisconsin, Madison, Wisconsin

FRANCIS V. SALINAS, MD, Staff Anesthesiologist; Section Head of Orthopedic Anesthesia; and Coordinator of Ultrasound-Guided Regional Anesthesia Education, Virginia Mason Medical Center, Seattle, Washington

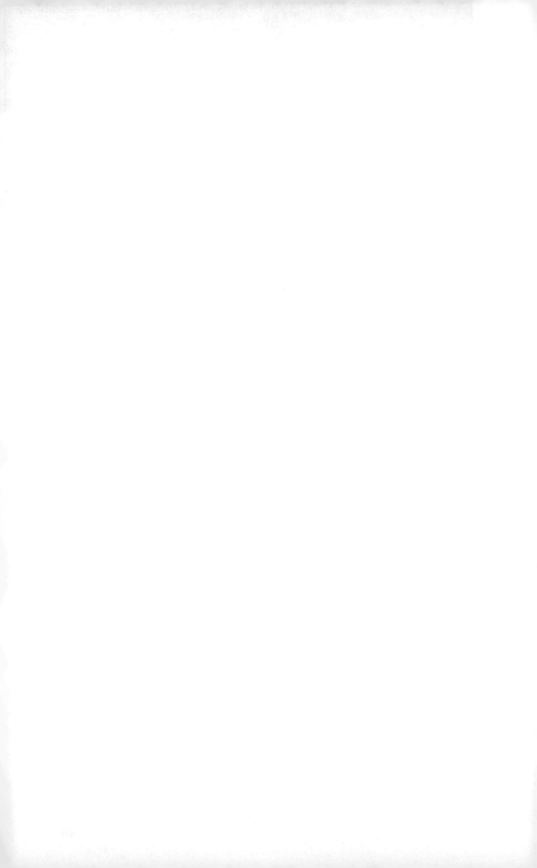

CONTRIBUTORS

BASEM ABDELMALAK, MD, Staff Anesthesiologist and Director, Departments of General Anesthesiology and Outcomes Research, The Cleveland Clinic, Cleveland, Ohio

MATTHEW S. ABRAHAMS, MD, Assistant Professor and Regional Anesthesia Fellowship Director, Department of Anesthesiology and Perioperative Medicine, Oregon Health and Sciences University, Portland, Oregon

DAVID B. AUYONG, MD, Staff Anesthesiologist, Department of Anesthesiology, Virginia Mason Medical Center, Seattle, Washington

CHRISTOPHER BERNARDS, MD, Department of Anesthesiology, Virginia Mason Medical Center, Seattle, Washington

JUAN P. CATA, MD, Staff Anesthesiologist, Departments of General Anesthesiology and Outcomes Research, The Cleveland Clinic, Cleveland, Ohio

RALF E. GEBHARD, MD, Associate Professor, Departments of Anesthesiology and Orthopedics and Rehabilitation, Miller School of Medicine, University of Miami, Miami, Florida

RALPH GERTLER, MD, DESA, Consultant Anesthesiologist, Department of Anesthesiology and Intensive Care Medicine, German Heart Center of the State of Bavaria, Technical University Munich, Munich, Germany

LAURA HAMMEL, MD, Assistant Professor, Department of Anesthesiology and Critical Care, University of Wisconsin Hospital and Clinics, Madison, Wisconsin

BRIAN E. HARRINGTON, MD, Staff Anesthesiologist, Billings Clinic Hospital, Billings, Montana

ZOLTAN HEVESI, MD, Professor, Department of Anesthesiology, University of Wisconsin Hospital and Clinics, Madison, Wisconsin

JEAN-LOUIS HORN, MD, Professor and Director of Regional Anesthesia, Department of Anesthesiology and Perioperative Medicine, Oregon Health and Sciences University, Portland, Oregon

ROBERT L. HSIUNG, MD, Staff Anesthesiologist, Department of Anesthesiology, Virginia Mason Medical Center, Seattle, Washington

GIRISH P. JOSHI, MBBS, MD, FFARCSI, Professor of Anesthesiology and Pain Management; Director of Perioperative Medicine and Ambulatory Anesthesia, University of Texas Southwestern Medical Center, Dallas, Texas

KINNARI P. KHATRI, MD, Fellow, Regional Anesthesia, Department of Anesthesiology, UIC Medical Center, University of Illinois at Chicago, Chicago, Illinois

GREGORY N. KOZLOV, DO, Resident, Department of Anesthesiology, Advocate Illinois Masonic Medical Center, Chicago, Illinois

ROBERT S. LAGASSE, MD, Associate Professor, Department of Anesthesiology, Yale School of Medicine, New Haven, Connecticut

JACQUELINE M. LEUNG, MD, MPH, Professor, Department of Anesthesia and Perioperative Care, University of California, San Francisco, California

DETLEF OBAL, MD, DESA, Assistant Professor, Department of Anesthesiology and Perioperative Medicine, University of Louisville Hospital, Louisville, Kentucky

SARAH OSWALD, MD, Assistant Professor, Department of Anesthesiology, UIC Medical Center, University of Illinois at Chicago, Chicago, Illinois

EDWARD POLLAK, MD, Quality Assurance Director and Vice Chief, Department of Anesthesiology and Perioperative Medicine, William Beaumont Hospital, Royal Oak, Michigan

MAUNAK V. RANA, MD, Director, Pain Management, Advocate Illinois Masonic Medical Center; Clinical Assistant Professor of Anesthesiology, University of Illinois-Chicago Medical Center, Chicago, Illinois

KAREN J. ROETMAN, MD, Department of Anesthesiology, Virginia Mason Medical Center, Seattle, Washington

LEELACH ROTHSCHILD, MD, Assistant Professor, Department of Anesthesiology, UIC Medical Center, University of Illinois at Chicago, Chicago, Illinois

LAURA P. SANDS, PhD, Professor, School of Nursing, Purdue University, West Lafayette, Indiana

JOSHUA SEBRANEK, MD, Assistant Professor, Department of Anesthesiology, University of Wisconsin Hospital and Clinics, Madison, Wisconsin

TIFFANY L. TSAI, BA, Research Associate, Department of Anesthesia and Perioperative Care, University of California, San Francisco, California

ANUPAMA WADHWA, MBBS, Associate Professor, Department of Anesthesiology and Perioperative Medicine, University of Louisville Hospital, Louisville, Kentucky

GUY WEINBERG, MD, Professor, Department of Anesthesiology, UIC Medical Center, University of Illinois at Chicago; Staff Physician, Jesse Brown VA Medical Center, Chicago, Illinois

ADVANCES IN
Anesthesia

CONTENTS

Measuring the Clinical Competence of Anesthesiologists
By Robert S. Lagasse and Edward Pollak

Ultrasound in Central Venous Cannulation
By David B. Auyong and Robert L. Hsiung

Peripheral Blocks of the Chest and Abdomen
By Matthew S. Abrahams and Jean-Louis Horn

Postdural Puncture Headache
By Brian E. Harrington

Current Concepts in the Management of Systemic Local Anesthetic Toxicity
By Kinnari P. Khatri, Leelach Rothschild, Sarah Oswald, and Guy Weinberg

Biomarkers: Understanding, Progress, and Implications in the Perioperative Period

By Basem Abdelmalak and Juan P. Cata

Single or Multiple Guidance Methods for Peripheral Nerve Blockade in Modern-Day Practice of Regional Anesthesia

By Anupama Wadhwa, Ralf E. Gebhard, and Detlef Obal

CONTENTS continued

The Anesthetic Management of Adult Patients with Organ Transplants Undergoing Nontransplant Surgery
By Laura Hammel, Joshua Sebranek, and Zoltan Hevesi

Perioperative Implications of Obstructive Sleep Apnea
By Karen J. Roetman and Christopher Bernards

An Update on Postoperative Cognitive Dysfunction

By Tiffany L. Tsai, Laura P. Sands, and Jacqueline M. Leung

Advances in Anesthesia 28 (2010) 1–14

ADVANCES IN ANESTHESIA

Herbal Supplements and Nutraceuticals: Perioperative Considerations

Maunak V. Rana, MD[a,b,*], Gregory N. Kozlov, DO[c]

[a]Pain Management, Advocate Illinois Masonic Medical Center, 836 West Wellington Avenue #4815, Chicago, IL 60657, USA
[b]University of Illinois - Chicago Medical Center, Chicago, IL, USA
[c]Department of Anesthesiology, Advocate Illinois Masonic Medical Center, 836 West Wellington Avenue, #4815, Chicago, IL 60657, USA

HERBAL SUPPLEMENTS AND ANESTHESIA

Herbal medicines have become enormously popular in recent years: nearly 20 million Americans are using herbal supplements for their purported health benefits including promotion of cardiac health, mental health, genitourinary health, and preventive health. These nutraceutical supplements are used in hopes of slowing the aging process, preventing the onset of dementia, lowering cholesterol, maintaining vision, enhancing immunity, and improving cardiovascular health. Society may be ingesting these supplements as an alternative to more expensive prescription drugs and as natural treatments with the goal of minimizing side effects that may accompany prescription medications. In 2007, Americans spent $34 billion on herbals and vitamins [1]. A recent survey revealed that the average person using supplements is older than 50 years, Caucasian, female, married, college-educated, and in a higher socioeconomic class [2].

Despite the common use of these agents, 70% of patients using these supplements neglect to tell their physician that they are taking them unless they are specifically asked. As a result, physicians may not be aware of potentially problematic substances and drug interactions of herbal medications with prescription drugs. Although these agents are often marketed as innocuous, the intake of these herbal medicines may pose health risks to patients.

The Dietary Health and Supplement Act of 1994 [3] defines herbal preparations as dietary supplements; therefore, they are not subject to the same rigorous safety and efficacy standards that prescription and over-the-counter medications must meet. For these supplements to be withdrawn from the market, the Food and Drug Administration (FDA) must prove a lack of safety [4].

*Corresponding author. Pain Management, Advocate Illinois Masonic Medical Center, 836 West Wellington Avenue #4815, Chicago, IL 60657. E-mail address: maunakr@gmail.com.

0737-6146/10/$ – see front matter
doi:10.1016/j.aan.2010.07.001

Despite various salubrious effects of herbals, the possibility of detrimental side effects exists, especially when multiple supplements are used in combination. From 1985 to 1997, nearly 200 deaths were directly attributed to the use of herbal supplements [5]. Because the use of these dietary supplements is prevalent and increasing, an understanding of their possible interactions with commonly used anesthetic drugs as well as potential untoward effects is crucial for anesthesiologists and perioperative physicians.

Popular herbals that merit discussion include:

1. St John's wort
2. Echinacea
3. *Ginkgo biloba*
4. Saw palmetto
5. Garlic
6. Ginger
7. Ginseng
8. Valerian
9. Ma Huang/Ephedra
10. Kava kava
11. Omega-3 fatty acids.

St John's Wort

St John's wort, derived from the flowering tops of the perennial plant *Hypericum perforatum* native to Europe and Asia, was brought to North America by European settlers. According to legend, the eponymous St John's wort arose from the head of John the Baptist after his beheading. Patients may use this herb for its anxiolytic, sedative, bronchodilatory, and antidepressant effects, and as an analgesic for peptic ulcer disease and hemorrhoids [6]. Hyperforin and hypericin are believed to be 2 of the principal active constituents of St John's wort responsible for its beneficial effects [7]. St John's wort is available in a variety of preparations to treat various ailments. The suggested dose to treat depression is 300 mg, standardized to 0.3% hypericin, taken orally 3 times daily for 4 to 6 weeks; alternatively, a tea can be brewed from 2 to 4 g of the herb in 1 to 2 cups of water [7].

The mechanism of action of St John's wort remains unknown, as in vitro and in vivo studies have reached different conclusions: in vitro studies demonstrate inhibition of monoamine oxidase isoforms, whereas in vivo studies demonstrate inhibition of γ-aminobutyric acid (GABA) receptors [8]. The antidepressant effects of the herbal may be a result of GABA inhibition. The potential for undesired side effects with concomitant administration of monoamine oxidase inhibitors (MAOIs), amphetamines, selective serotonin reuptake inhibitors (SSRIs), trazodone, tricyclic antidepressants, narcotics, and cold and flu medications exists [9]. Furthermore, St John's wort has been implicated in one case of hypertensive crisis in a 41-year-old psychiatric patient [10].

Interactions with β-sympathomimetic agents such as Ma Huang or pseudoephedrine may instigate a hypertensive crisis. St John's wort, when taken in combination with other SSRIs such as fluoxetine or paroxetine, may cause serotonergic syndrome, which is manifested by tremors, hyperthermia, autonomic dysfunction, hallucinations, myoclonus, and possibly death [11–13]. Photosensitivity is another common side effect of St John's wort, therefore caution is advised when administering other drugs, such as tetracycline and piroxicam, which have similar adverse effects. In addition, caution is advised with patients concurrently using MAOIs. Further research is needed to elucidate the exact interactions and effects, but caution and awareness should be the rule in the perioperative period.

Echinacea

Echinacea is produced from the dried roots and rhizomes of the *Echinacea angustifolia* or *Echinacea pallida* plants. Fresh juice, made from the nonroot portions of the *Echinacea purpurea* plant, is also available [6]. Patients commonly take this herbal supplement to treat the following ailments: abscesses, eczema, burns, liver cancer [13], colorectal cancer [14], upper respiratory tract infections, urinary tract infections, varicose leg ulcers, and skin wounds [6].

The recommended dosage of echinacea is 6 to 9 mL of juice daily, or 900 to 1000 mg of powder orally 3 times daily, or 0.75 to 1.5 mL of tincture orally 2 to 5 times daily. In addition, echinacea can be brewed as a tea using 4 g of herb brewed in boiling water for 10 minutes. Using echinacea for 10 to 14 days is thought to provide maximal benefit; experts recommend taking this herb for no longer than 8 weeks, as the immune enhancing effects may be decreased by this time [6].

Certain patient populations may not benefit from echinacea therapy: individuals infected with human immunodeficiency virus, patients with AIDS, patients with collagen vascular disease, and patients suffering from multiple sclerosis (echinacea stimulates the immune system [14], therefore autoimmune diseases that are treated with immunosuppressant drugs may have a negative interaction with echinacea).

Echinacea is an inhibitor of the cytochrome P-450 3A4 hepatic microsomal system, one of the key metabolic enzyme pathways involved in drug metabolism. This effect can become a concern in patients concomitantly taking drugs that are metabolized by this system, including phenytoin, rifampin, rocuronium, and local anesthetics; caution is advised because there may be prolonged clinical effects of these agents [15]. Awareness of this interaction is important for anesthesia providers.

Ginkgo Biloba

Prized by Chinese herbalists for centuries, Western interest in ginkgo as a nonpharmacologic treatment of Alzheimer disease has intensified lately as more and more people have become interested in alternative medicines and therapies [16]. Ginkgo extract is derived from the leaves of the kew tree, also known as the maidenhair tree or *Ginkgo biloba* tree. Patients use Ginkgo to treat such ailments as asthma, dementia, hearing loss, SSRI-induced erectile dysfunction, memory loss, and senile macular degeneration, and to enhance alertness [6]. In

France and Germany, ginkgo is among the leading prescriptions for poor circulation and dementia, whereas in the United States ginkgo is available only as an over-the-counter dietary supplement [6]. Ginkgo is among the most popular herbal supplements in the United States, with sales exceeding $150 million [17].

Commonly recommended dosages of ginkgo are, for dementia, 120 to 240 mg orally twice to thrice daily and for poor leg circulation, vertigo, or tinnitus, 120 to 160 mg orally twice to thrice daily [6].

Awareness of possible adverse effects of ginkgo is imperative for the anesthesiologist, as ginkgo is the third best-selling herbal product in the United States [15]. Although relatively safe, possible untoward effects of the herb include nausea, vomiting [18], headache, seizures, and increased risk of bleeding (the maximum recommended dose is 240 mg thrice a day). Furthermore, several case reports detailing morbidities of ginkgo exist: subarachnoid hemorrhage, subdural hematoma, and hyphema [19–22]. The additive effects of ginkgo with aspirin, warfarin, enoxaparin, heparin, abciximab, and other anticoagulant and antiplatelet agents may contraindicate neuraxial anesthetic techniques, as clotting ability may be unpredictable. The terpene lactone components of ginkgo (ginkgolides) inhibit blood clotting via inhibition of platelet aggregation [21–23]. Perioperative physicians may better assess the degree to which a patient is anticoagulated using platelet function analysis and/or coagulation studies. Common drug interactions include a decreased efficacy of anticonvulsants when administered with ginkgo [23]. Also, the seizure threshold is lowered in patients taking tricyclic antidepressants with ginkgo [23]. It is recommended that gingko be discontinued 36 hours before surgery to decrease the risk of side effects [24].

Saw Palmetto

Saw palmetto is harvested from the brown-black berries of the American dwarf palm, *Serenoa repens/Sabal serrulata*. Historically, saw palmetto was listed as a treatment for genitourinary tract ailments in the *National Formulary* from 1906 to 1950 [6]. At present, patients use saw palmetto to treat benign prostate hypertrophy (BPH), to decrease gynecomastia [6], to improve libido, to increase sperm production, and to reduce fluid retention.

The recommended dose of the available preparations for BPH is 320 mg orally in 2 equal doses, continued for 3 months [6].

Possible concerns for the anesthesiologist and perioperative physician include an elevation in blood pressure and a theoretical potentiation of blood-thinning agents [6].

Garlic

Garlic, botanically known as *Allium sativum*, is one of the most studied medicinal herbs. The use of garlic to treat various maladies has been traced back not only to the ancient China but also to western Europe [25]. Supplements of garlic are prepared from either dried cloves that have been crushed into powder or are made from garlic oil. Of note, products that claim to be "odor-free" may lack medicinal value, because it appears that the beneficial effects of garlic come from the sulfur-containing allicin, the chemical that imparts garlic with its distinctive aroma [6]. Garlic has been used to treat asthma, tinea pedis, constipation, diabetes, fungal infection, heavy-metal poisoning, hypertension, and hypercholesterolemia [6].

The commonly recommended dose of garlic for treating elevated cholesterol is 600 to 900 mg orally once daily [6]. Alternatively, 4 g of fresh garlic or 8 mg of garlic oil can be taken. The World Health Organization (WHO) 1999 monograph recommends these doses: 2 to 5 g fresh garlic, 0.4 to 1.2 g dried powder, 2 to 5 mg oil, 300 to 1000 mg extract, or any other formulation containing 2 to 5 mg allicin [6]. The formulation of garlic most often used in clinical trials is Kwai (Lichtwer Pharma, Köln, Germany); it is available as a nonenteric-coated dehydrated garlic powder formulation standardized for 1.3% allicin.

Garlic impairs platelet aggregation and has been associated with reports of bleeding. Based on this fact it should be used cautiously, if at all, in patients with peptic ulcer disease or intracranial bleeding, and in patients receiving concurrent antiplatelet or anticoagulation therapy or nonsteroidal anti-inflammatories, or with other drug-related hemostatic issues [26]. There is a case report of a spontaneous spinal/epidural hematoma in a patient using excessive amounts of garlic [27]. Other important adverse effects of garlic include dizziness, nausea, asthma exacerbations, hypothyroidism, and exacerbation of gastroesophageal reflux disease [6].

Garlic's effect on platelet aggregation is complex and is caused by several mechanisms: garlic reduces thromboxane formation from arachidonic acid, inhibits phospholipase activity, and inhibits the incorporation of arachidonate into platelet phospholipids [28,29].

The anesthesiologist caring for patients being treated with garlic therapy should be especially cognizant for surgical hemostasis. Physicians should be vigilant perioperatively for the possibility of excessive bleeding both intra- and postoperatively [28]. Furthermore, garlic has been reported to interact with the P450 enzyme system [30], which also may affect concomitant drug metabolism.

Ginger

Although ginger, *Zingiber officinale*, has attractive purple-green flowers, herbalists value its root more than any other part of the plant. Ginger may be used to treat common ailments such as arthritis, motion sickness, nausea, muscle pain and swelling, and bacterial infections, due to its property as an antioxidant [6]. In addition, ginger has been demonstrated to be an effective cure for hyperemesis gravidarum in the obstetric population [31].

The dose of ginger depends on indication: the dose for nausea is powdered ginger 500 to 1000 mg orally, or fresh ginger root 1000 mg orally [6].

Despite the possible benefits of ginger therapy, certain concerns exist with the excessive intake of this agent. Ginger is a potent inhibitor of thromboxane-synthetase. and may also interfere with platelet aggregation [32,33]; therefore, intake of ginger may increase bleeding time [34] and other tests that evaluate platelet function. In a patient with a history of bleeding or bruising, anesthesiologists should consider evaluating alteration in platelet function status before proceeding with a neuraxial or regional anesthetic technique. Ginger has been implicated as a source of arrhythmia, drowsiness, and excessive sedation, side effects of which perioperative physicians should be aware [6].

Ginseng

For over 2000 years, ginseng has been used in traditional Asian medicine to treat such ailments as depression, diabetes, hypertension, fluid retention, overactive thymus, and insomnia. Ginseng has also been used as an aphrodisiac, as a sedative, and to enhance the body's stress response [6]. Commercially prepared American ginseng is extracted from the *Panax quinquefolius* plant, and Asian (Korean and Japanese) varieties are derived from the *Panax ginseng* plant. The Asian variety undergoes more post-harvest processing to isolate the extract and, because of this, it is more sought after for its medicinal properties. The recommended dose of ginseng is 0.5 to 2 g of dry ginseng root daily, or 200 to 600 mg of ginseng extract daily in 2 divided doses [6].

Ginseng has adaptogenic properties, augmenting adrenal steroid production via a central mechanism [35]. Hypoglycemic properties of ginseng are believed to be due to ginsenoside Rb2 and panaxans I, J, K, and L [36–40]. Ginseng has been known to cause the following adverse effects: impotence, hypertension, chest pain, headache, blurred vision, epistaxis [41], insomnia, nausea, vomiting, nervousness, tachycardia, and vaginal bleeding.

Ginseng abuse syndrome is caused by the combination of ginseng with other stimulants, resulting in diarrhea, hypertension, restlessness, insomnia, depression, poor appetite, swelling, and unusual sense of well-being [6]. Ginseng, oral hypoglycemics, and insulin may interact synergistically [6]; blood glucose levels should be assessed perioperatively. The possibility of an acute manic episode exists when patients undergoing MAOI treatment use ginseng because of the additive effects of ginseng and the MAOIs [42–44]. For the anesthesiologist, it is important to be aware of the hypertensive effects of ginseng as well as its antiplatelet properties. Because many anesthetic agents themselves cause hemodynamic instability, the added variable of ginseng may make hemodynamic management challenging. It has been recommended that ginseng should be discontinued at least 1 week before surgery [45].

Siberian ginseng, *Eleutherococcus senticosus*, belonging to the same family as panax or Asian ginseng, is used as a treatment for inflammation and insomnia due to anxiety, and to improve exercise tolerance, regulate blood pressure, and stimulate the circulatory and immune systems. The recommended dose is 500 to 2000 mg orally, daily for no more than 3 weeks [6].

Possible adverse effects of Siberian ginseng include diarrhea, difficulty in concentrating, dizziness, hypertension, nervousness, and an unusual sense of well-being. Siberian ginseng has an adverse interaction with digoxin, barbiturates, and vitamins B1, B2, and C. Siberian ginseng, just as American and

Asian ginseng, has a potent hypoglycemic effect [6]. Blood glucose levels should be ascertained before any procedure.

Ephedra (Ma Huang)

Ephedra is a herbal supplement that has been used in Chinese medicine to promote weight loss and to increase energy, and as a treatment for asthma and bronchitis [45]. Ephedra contains a combination of adrenergic alkaloids including ephedrine, pseudoephedrine, norephedrine, methylephedrine, and norpseudoephedrine [46]. Ephedrine is a noncatecholamine sympathomimetic agent with α-1, β-1, and β-2 activity acting at adrenergic receptors and releasing endogenous norepinephrine [45]. Patients chronically taking ephedra may be catecholamine depleted. Although ephedrine is safely administered by trained anesthesiologists intraoperatively as perioperative therapy for hypotension, unsupervised use by untrained laypersons is potentially dangerous because of the possibility of vasospasm of coronary and cerebral arteries and other sympathomimetic effects, including myocardial infarction and thrombotic stroke [47]. In addition, ephedra has been implicated in hypersensitivity myocarditis characterized by cardiomyopathy with lymphocytic and eosinophilic infiltrates [48]. The elimination half-life of ephedra is 5.2 hours, with 70% to 80% of the herb excreted unchanged in the urine; therefore, it should be discontinued at least 24 hours before surgery [49,50].

Although now of historical significance due to the sporadic use of halothane anesthesia, special consideration should be paid to patients undergoing halothane general anesthesia, because halothane sensitizes the myocardium to exogenous catecholamines, and ventricular arrhythmias may develop [51]. Theoretically, a similar concern exists in patients taking ephedra who receive high doses of desflurane and experience an increase in circulating catecholamines. Furthermore, long-term ephedra use results in tachyphylaxis of its sympathomimetic effects secondary to depletion of endogenous catecholamine stores, which may contribute to perioperative hemodynamic instability. Therefore, direct-acting sympathomimetics are the preferred agents to treat hypotension and bradycardia in these circumstances [45].

Despite the FDA ban on the sale of supplements containing ephedra, this supplement is reported as being readily available from various international Web sites [52].

Hoodia Gordonii

Tribesmen have traditionally used *Hoodia gordonii*, a cactus native to Southeastern Africa, during times of starvation to ease their hunger [53]. For the same reason, currently it is a popular weight loss supplement in the United States. Its pharmacologically active constituents include steroidal glycosides (P57AS3 or P57), and steroidal derivates: gordonosides, and calogenin glycosides [53]. MacLean and Luo [54] studied P57 isolated from hoodia, and determined in a rat model that cerebroventricular administration of P57 resulted in an increase in the adenosine triphosphate concentrations of hypothalamic neurons; this in turn was the hypothesized mechanism of appetite reduction.

Table 1	
Herbals that may interfere with hemostasis	
Garlic	Decreases platelet aggregation
Ginkgo biloba	Synergistic relationship with anticoagulants
Saw palmetto	Potentiation of blood thinning agents. Some formulations of saw palmetto have been contaminated with coumadin [70]
Ginger	Inhibits thromboxane synthetase and decreases platelet aggregation
Green tea	Effects likely due to the caffeine content, raises prothrombin time and activated partial thromboplastin time
Fish oil	Decreases platelet aggregation
Ginseng	Decreases platelet aggregation

Human research is lacking, and there are few data concerning its efficacy or safety profile. P57 has also been shown to inhibit CYP3A4 activity, which may affect drug metabolism within the liver [55].

Green Tea

Green tea, *Camellia sinensis*, has been enjoyed in Asia for centuries and recently, green tea and its purified extract has been used in Western medicine as adjuvant treatment of obesity, hyperlipidemia, hypertension, and atherosclerosis [6]. Epigallocatechin-3-gallate (EGCG) is the principal active agent in green tea and is credited for providing an anticancer effect; it accounts for 40% of its total polyphenol content [56]. Other constituents of green tea that may affect the anesthetic management of patients include caffeine, theophylline, and proanthocyanidins (tannins) [57].

Specific doses of green tea to obtain maximal benefits have not been established, because most investigations have studied brewed green tea rather than an extract tablet (tablets vary from 100 to 750 mg of green tea extract) [58]. One cup of tea contains approximately 80 to 100 mg of polyphenols and approximately 50 mg of caffeine [58].

Most of the adverse effects of green tea are attributed to its caffeine content, therefore some experts recommend drinking decaffeinated green tea rather than green tea in its natural form. However, it is unknown whether decaffeinated tea has the same health benefits as natural green tea [59,60]. Caffeine is a central nervous system stimulant and a diuretic, increasing urine volume as well as urine sodium and potassium concentrations, thus potentially decreasing sodium and potassium concentrations in the blood. Furthermore, caffeine may worsen incontinence, may increase the production of stomach acid, and may exacerbate peptic ulcer symptoms [58]. Therefore, persons with concurrent advanced liver disease should use caffeine and green tea

Table 2	
Herbals causing excessive sedation	
Kava kava	Potentiates benzodiazepines and barbiturates
Ginger	Used as a single agent may cause drowsiness
Valerian	Potentiates sedatives and central nervous system depressants

Table 3	
Herbals that may cause hemodynamic instability	
St John's wort	Possibility of hypertensive crisis exists
Saw palmetto	May elevate blood pressure
Ginger	May cause arrhythmia
Ginseng	May cause tachycardia. May cause falsely high or falsely low digoxin levels depending the assay used [67]. Discontinue 7 days before surgery
Siberian ginseng	May elevate blood pressure. May cause falsely high or falsely low digoxin levels depending the assay used [71]
Ephedra	Patients may be catecholamine depleted; direct-acting sympathomimetics are the preferred agents to treat hypotension and bradycardia
Green tea	Tannin content renders atropine less effective [59]; adenosine less effective as well [43]
Fish oil	May lower blood pressure
Valerian	Possibility of arrhythmia exists

cautiously, as blood caffeine concentrations may accumulate [57]. In laboratory and animal studies, caffeine has been found to hinder blood clotting because it raises prothrombin time and partial thromboplastin time [58,59]. Furthermore, the tannins in green tea may reduce absorption and bioavailability of codeine, atropine, and iron supplements [44]. Use of green tea in infants has been associated with impaired iron metabolism and microcytic anemia [58]. Furthermore, the tannin content of green tea may inhibit the hemodynamic effects of adenosine [59].

Omega-3 Fatty Acids

Derived from either plant or fish sources, omega-3 polyunsaturated fatty acids are used primarily to treat elevated cholesterol levels. Typical dietary sources of these fatty acids include salmon, mackerel, sardines, albacore tuna, herring, soy, tofu, flax seed, walnuts, and canola oil. Because Alaskan and Greenland Inuits had favorable lipid profiles and a lower incidence of coronary artery disease as compared with non-Inuit cohorts, it was postulated that their diet, which is high in omega-3 fatty acids, was responsible for this difference. Subsequent studies addressing this fact demonstrated that people who ate fish weekly did in fact have lower mortality from coronary artery disease [61,62].

In the United States, 2 servings of fish per week is the current recommendation for people to reap the benefits of omega-3 fatty acids. It has been postulated

Table 4	
Herbals interfering with the efficacy of other drugs	
Echinacea	Inhibitor of cytochrome P-450 3A4
Hoodia gordonii	P57, the active constituent, is a potent inhibitor of cytochrome P-450 3A4
Ginkgo biloba	May decrease the efficacy of anticonvulsants
Green tea	The caffeine component decreases the efficacy of codeine

that fish oils have several mechanisms of cardiac protection including antiarrhythmic effects, a reduction in serum triglyceride levels, decreased platelet aggregation, an anti-inflammatory effect via enhanced production of nitric oxide (endothelium-derived relaxing factor), and a modest decrease in blood pressure [63,64].

Although further study is necessary to validate these positive effects, many patients take fish oils for these perceived benefits, therefore knowledge of the effects of omega-3 oils is important for the anesthesiologist. Hemostasis can be an issue during surgery as well as planning for regional or neuraxial techniques. Coagulation studies should be obtained before any neuraxial or regional procedure in a patient who has a history of bleeding and bruising and concomitant use of omega-3 oils.

Kava Kava

Kava kava has been a popular beverage in the South Pacific for its ability to induce a tranquil, euphoric state and for its sociable effects [65]. Historically, women chewed the leaves, mixing the chewed leaves with coconut milk or other fruit juices [6]. For children diagnosed with attention-deficit/hyperactivity disorder a liquid extract is given orally (1:1 weight/volume fresh plant or 1:4 weight/volume dry plant) in a recommended dose of 5 to 15 drops diluted in their favorite beverage 2 to 3 times daily. The adult dose for anxiety is 100 to 250 mg 1 to 3 times per day as needed, standardized to contain 30% kavalactones per dose. When used solely as a sleep aid, 250 to 500 mg at bedtime is the recommended dose [6].

Kava kava may cause hallucinations, dermopathy, and visual changes [66–68]. Kava kava can also produce antinociceptive effects mediated through nonopioid-dependent pathways [69,70]. In addition, anesthesiologists should be aware that the use of kava kava may potentiate barbiturates and benzodiazepines, leading to excessive sedation [71].

Valerian

Valerian comes from the perennial plant *Valeriana officinalis*, which is native to Eurasia and cultivated worldwide. Valerian is used as a sleep aid, as treatment of muscle spasms (particularly in Europe), and to treat restlessness [6].

For sleep disorders, the recommended dosage is 400 to 900 mg of standardized valerian extract 30 to 60 minutes before bedtime. Doses greater than 2.5 g may result in liver injury [6].

Adverse effects of valerian include blurry vision, excitability, headache, insomnia, arrhythmia, and nausea. Producing dose-dependent sedation and

Table 5	
Herbals affecting blood glucose levels	
Ginseng	Lowers glucose levels; evaluate glucose levels before surgery
Siberian ginseng	Lowers glucose levels; evaluate glucose levels before surgery

hypnosis via GABA receptors, valerian may potentiate the effects of central nervous system depressants and sedative hypnotics [72].

SUMMARY

Herbal medications are being used by the general population for various purported health benefits, including the treatment of cardiovascular, endocrine, psychiatric, and neurologic disorders [73] along with, and in addition to, prescription therapies. Patients may ingest these agents to treat maladies and health conditions "naturally." Nutraceuticals, despite being derived from natural compounds, do have significant side effects and risks that have shown themselves in research studies [29], and may present some risk to patients. These possible side effects, coupled with a decreased regulation versus traditional prescription medicines, can lead to previously unanticipated consequences, including most commonly an increased risk of perioperative bleeding [74]. These side effects may occur with increased doses of the herbal medication and also with combination therapy with other nutraceuticals or prescription medicines. Because of the widespread use of these agents by patients, anesthesiologists as perioperative physicians must be aware of these agents and the risks they pose to their patients in the perioperative period (Tables 1–5).

References

[1] Marchione M, Stobbe M. Americans spend $34B for alternative medicine. Newsday (NY): The Associated press; July 31, 2009.

[2] Harrison RA, Holt D, Pattison DJ. Who and how many people are taking herbal supplements? A survey of 21,923 adults. Int J Vitam Nutr Res 2004;74:183–6.

[3] Dietary Supplement Health and Education Act, 1994, PL 103-417 (180 Stat 2126).

[4] Marwick C. Growing use of medicinal botanicals forces assessment by drug regulators. JAMA 1995;273:607.

[5] Tan PH, Chou AK, Peng JS. Accidental shock during epidural anesthesia in a patient with NSAID-induced hyporeninemic hypoalderosteronism. J Clin Anesth 1997;9:424–7.

[6] Fetrow Charles W, Avila Juan. The complete guide to herbal medicines. New York: Simon and Schuster; 2000.

[7] Susan Budavari, editor. Merck index. 11th edition. Rahway (NJ): Merck and Co; 1989. p. 4799.

[8] Kaye A, Sabar R, Vig S, et al. Nutraceuticals—current concepts and the role of the anesthesiologist. Am J Anesthesiol 2000;27(8):467–71.

[9] Gordon JB. SSRI and St. John's wort: possible toxicity? Am Fam Physician 1998;57:950–3.

[10] Patel S, Robinson R, Burk M. Hypertensive crisis associated with St. John's wort. Am J Med 2002;112(6):507–8.

[11] Ness J, ShermanFT, Pan CX. Alternative medicine: what the data say about the common herbal therapies. Geriatrics 1999;54(10):33–43.

[12] Czekalla J, Gastpar M, Hübner WD, et al. The effect of hypericum extract on cardiac conduction as seen in the electrocardiogram compared to that of imipramine. Pharmacopsychiatry 1997;30(Suppl 2):86–8.

[13] Lersch C, Zeuner M, Bauer A. Stimulation of the immune response in outpatients with hepatocellular carcinomas by low doses of cyclophosphamide (LDCY), echinacea purpurea extracts (echinacein), and thymostimulin. Arch Geschwulstforsch 1990;60:379–83.

[14] Lersch C, Zeuner M, Bauer A. Nonspecific immunostimulation with low doses of cyclophosphamide (LDCY), thymostimulin, and echinacea purpurea extract (echinacein) in

patients with far advanced colorectal cancers. preliminary results. Cancer Invest 1992;10:343–8.

[15] Kaye A, Sabar R, Vig S, et al. Nutraceuticals—current concepts and the role of the anesthesiologist. Am J Anesthesiol 2000;27(7):405–7.

[16] LeBars PL, Katz MM, Berman N. A placebo controlled, double-blind randomized trial of an extract of gingko biloba for dementia. JAMA 1997;278:1327–32.

[17] Blumenthal M. Herb sales down 3% in mass market retail stores. HerbalGram 2000;49:68.

[18] Pittler MH, Ernst E. Ginkgo biloba extract for the treatment of intermittent claudication: a meta-analysis of randomized trials. Am J Med 2000;108(4):276–81.

[19] Rosenblatt M, Mindel J. Spontaneous hyphema associated with ingestion of Ginkgo biloba extract. N Engl J Med 1997;336:1108.

[20] Rowin J, Lewis SL. Spontaneous bilateral subdural hematomas associated with chronic Ginkgo biloba ingestion have also occurred. Neurology 1996;46:1775–6.

[21] Gilbert GJ. Ginkgo biloba. Neurology 1997;48:1137.

[22] Vale S. Subarachnoid hemorrhage associated with Ginkgo biloba. Lancet 1998;352:36.

[23] Miller LG. Herbal medicinals. Arch Intern Med 1998;158:2200–11.

[24] Memorial Sloan Kettering Cancer Center. About herbs, botanicals, and other products. Available at: http://www.mskcc.org/mskcc/html/69235.cfm. Accessed January 12, 2010.

[25] Brace LD. Cardiovascular benefits of garlic (Allium sativum L). J Cardiovasc Nurs 2002; 16(4):33–49.

[26] Kiesewetter H, Jung F, Jung EM, et al. Effects of garlic coated tablets in peripheral arterial occlusive disease. Clin Investig 1993;71(5):383–6.

[27] Rose KD, Croissant PD, Parliament CF, et al. Spontaneous epidural hematoma with associated platelet dysfunction from excessive garlic ingestion: a case report. Neurosurgery 1990;26(5):880–1.

[28] Bordia A. Effect of garlic on human platelet aggregation in vitro. Atherosclerosis 1978;30: 355–60.

[29] LePoncin Lafitte M, Rapin J, Rapin JR, et al. Effects of Ginkgo biloba on changes induced by quantitative cerebral microembolization in rats. Arch Int Pharmacodyn Ther 1980;243: 236–44.

[30] Krucoff MW, Costello R, Mark D, et al. Complementary and alternative medical therapy in cardiovascular care. In: Fuster V, O'Rourke RA, Walsh RA, et al, editors. Hurst's the heart. 12th edition. NewYork: McGrawHill; 2007. Available at: http://www.accessmedicine.com.lp.hscl.ufl.edu/content.aspx?aID=3077596. Accessed January 12, 2010.

[31] Fischer-Rasmussen W, Kjaer SK, Dahl C. Ginger treatment of hyperemesis gravidarum. Eur J Obstet Gynecol Reprod Biol 1991;38(1):19–24.

[32] Guh JH, Ko FN, Jong TT, et al. Antiplatelet effect of gingerol isolated from Zingiber officinale. J Pharm Pharmacol 1995;47(4):329–32.

[33] Wendel HP, Heller W, Gallimore MJ, et al. The prolonged activated clotting time (ACT) with aprotinin depends on the type of activator used for measurement. Blood Coagul Fibrinolysis 1993;4(1):41–5.

[34] Backon J. Ginger: inhibition of thromboxane synthetase and stimulation of prostacyclin: relevance for medicine and psychiatry. Med Hypotheses 1986;20:271–8.

[35] Ng TB, Li WW, Yeung HW. Effects of ginsenosides, lectins and Momordica charantia insulin like peptide on corticosterone production by isolated rat adrenal cells. J Ethnopharmacol 1987;21:21–9.

[36] Yokozawa T, Kobayashi T, Oura H, et al. Studies on the mechanism of hypoglycemic activity of ginsenoside-Rb2 in streptozotocin-diabetic rats. Chem Pharm Bull 1895;33:869–72.

[37] Oshima Y, Konno C, Hikono H. Isolation and hypoglycemic activity of panaxans I, J, K, and L, glycans of panax ginseng roots. J Ethnopharmacol 1985;14:255–9.

[38] Konno C, Murakami M, Yoshiteru O, et al. Isolation and hypoglycemic activity of panaxans Q, R, S, R, and U: glycans of panax ginseng roots. J Ethnopharmacol 1985;14:69–74.

[39] Konno C, Murakami M, Yoshiteru O, et al. Isolation and hypoglycemic activity of panaxans A, B, C, D, and E, glycans of panax ginseng roots. Planta Med 1984;50:436–8.

[40] Tokmoda M, Shimada K, Konno M, et al. Partial structure of Panax A: a hypoglycemic glycan of panax ginseng roots. Planta Med 1984;50:436–8.

[41] Hammond TG, Whitworth JA. Adverse reactions to ginseng. Med J Aust 1981;1:492.

[42] Shader RI, Greenblatt DJ. Phenelzine and the dream machine ramblings and reflections. J Clin Psychopharmacol 1985;5:65.

[43] Jones BD, Runikis AM. Interactions of ginseng with phenylzine. J Clin Psychopharmacol 1987;7:201–2.

[44] Brinker F. Herb contraindications and drug interactions. 3rd edition. Sandy (OR): Eclectic Medical Publications; 2001.

[45] Ang-Lee MK, Moss J, Yuan CS. Herbal medicines and perioperative care. JAMA 2001;286: 208–16.

[46] Gurley BJ, Gardner SF, Hubbard MA. Content versus label claims in ephedra-containing dietary supplements. Am J Health Syst Pharm 2000;57:963–9.

[47] Haller CA, Benowitz NL. Adverse cardiovascular and central nervous system events associated with dietary supplements containing ephedra alkaloids. N Engl J Med 2000;343: 1833–8.

[48] Zaacks SM, Klein L, Tan CD, et al. Hypersensitivity myocarditis associated with ephedra use. J Toxicol Clin Toxicol 1999;37:485–9.

[49] White LM, Gardner SF, Gurley BJ, et al. Pharmacokinetics and cardiovascular effects of ma-huang (Ephedra sinica) in normotensive adults. J Clin Pharmacol 1997;37:116–22.

[50] Gurley BJ, Gardner SF, White LM, et al. Ephedrine pharmacokinetics after the ingestion of nutritional supplements containing Ephedra sinica (ma huang). Ther Drug Monit 1998;20: 439–45.

[51] Rozien MF. Anesthetic implications of concurrent diseases. In: Miller RD, editor. Anesthesia. 4th edition. New York: Churchill Livingstone Inc; 1994. p. 903–1014.

[52] Ephedra for sale. Available at: http://www.supplementlifestyle.com/. Accessed February 23, 2010.

[53] Memorial Sloan Kettering Cancer Center. About herbs, botanicals, and other products. Available at: http://www.mskcc.org/mskcc/html/69255.cfm. Accessed July 10, 2009.

[54] MacLean DB, Luo LG. Increased ATP content/production in the hypothalamus may be a signal for energy-sensing of satiety: studies of the anorectic mechanism of a plant steroidal glycoside. Brain Res 2004;1020(1–2):1–11.

[55] Madgula VL, Avula B, Pawar RS, et al. In vitro metabolic stability and intestinal transport of P57AS3 (P57) from Hoodia gordonii and its interaction with drug metabolizing enzymes. Planta Med 2008;74(10):1269–75.

[56] Tosetti F, Ferrari N, De Flora S. Angioprevention: angiogenesis is a common and key target for cancer chemopreventive agents. FASEB J 2002;16:2–14.

[57] Memorial Sloan Kettering Cancer Center. About herbs, botanicals, and other products. Available at: http://www.mskcc.org/mskcc/html/69247.cfm. Accessed July 27, 2009.

[58] Green tea (Camelia sinensis). Available at: http://www.mayoclinic.com/health/green-tea/NS_patient-green_tea. Accessed July 27, 2009.

[59] Huang MT, Lee CY, Ho CT. Effects of tea, decaffeinated tea, and caffeine on UVB light-induced complete carcinogenesis in SKH-1 mice: demonstration of caffeine as a biologically important constituent of tea. Cancer Res 1997;57:2623–9.

[60] Memorial Sloan Kettering Cancer Center. About herbs, botanicals, and other products. Available at: http://www.mskcc.org/mskcc/html/69247.cfm. Accessed March 22, 2010.

[61] Burr ML, Fehily AM, Gilbert JF, et al. Effects of changes in fat, fish, and fibre intakes on death and myocardial reinfarction: diet and reinfarction trial (DART). Lancet 1989;2:757–61.

[62] Kromhout D, Bosschieter EB, de Lezenne CC. The inverse relation between fish consumption and 20-year mortality from coronary heart disease. N Engl J Med 1985;312:1205–9.

[63] Marckmann P, Gronbaek M. Fish consumption and coronary heart disease mortality. A systematic review of prospective cohort studies. Eur J Clin Nutr 1999;53:585–90.

[64] Von Schacky C, Angerer P, Kothny W. The effect of dietary omega-3 fatty acids on coronary atherosclerosis. A randomized, double-blind, placebo-controlled trial. Ann Intern Med 1999;130:554–62.

[65] Leak JA. Herbal medicine: Is it an alternative or an unknown? A brief review of popular herbals used by patients in a pain and symptom management practice setting. Curr Rev Pain 1999;3:226–36.

[66] Garner LF, Klinger JD. Some visual effects caused by the beverage kava. J Ethnopharmacol 1985;13(3):307–11.

[67] Winslow LC, Kroll DJ. Herbs as medicines. Arch Intern Med 1998;158:2192–9.

[68] Dasgupta A, Reyes MA. Effect of Brazilian, Indian, Siberian, Asian, and North American ginseng on serum digoxin measurement by immunoassays and binding of digoxin-like immunoreactive components of ginseng with Fab fragment. Am J Clin Pathol 2005; 124(2):229–36.

[69] Jamleson DD, Duffield PH. The antinociceptive actions of kava components in mice. Clin Exp Pharmacol Physiol 1990;17(7):495–507.

[70] Singh YN. Effects of kava on neuromuscular transmission and muscular contractility. J Ethnopharmacol 1983;7(3):267–76.

[71] Gruenwald J, Brendler T, Jaenicke C, et al. PDR for herbal medicines. 1st edition. Montvale (NJ): Medical Economics Company; 1998. p.1043–5.

[72] Carrasco MC, Vallejo JR, Pardo-de-Santayana M, et al. Interactions of Valeriana officinalis L. and Passiflora incarnata L. in a patient treated with lorazepam. Phytother Res 2009; 23(12):1795–6.

[73] Smith PF, Maclennan K, Darlington CL. The neuroprotective properties of the Ginkgo biloba leaf: a review of the possible relationship to platelet-activating factor (PAF). J Ethnopharmacol 1996;50:131–9.

[74] Srivastava KC. Evidence for the mechanism by which garlic inhibits platelet aggregation. Prostaglandins Leukot Med 1986;22(3):313–21.

Advances in Anesthesia 28 (2010) 15–33

ADVANCES IN ANESTHESIA

Modern Understanding of Intraoperative Mechanical Ventilation in Normal and Diseased Lungs

Ralph Gertler, MD, DESA[a], Girish P. Joshi, MBBS, MD, FFARCSI[b],*

[a]Department of Anesthesiology and Intensive Care Medicine, German Heart Center of the State of Bavaria, Technical University Munich, Lazarettstr. 36, 80636 Munich, Germany
[b]Department of Anesthesiology and Pain Management, University of Texas Southwestern Medical Center, 5323 Harry Hines Boulevard, Dallas, TX 75390-9068, USA

Acute lung injury (ALI) and acute respiratory distress syndrome (ARDS) are devastating occurrences in medical and surgical patients. Their prevalence in ventilated patients is around 40% [1] with mortalities approaching 40% to 50% [2]. Mechanical ventilation strategies introduced in the last 2 decades have led to a significant reduction in the associated mortality [3,4]. Applying these strategies during general anesthesia would represent a substantial shift in commonly applied ventilatory management of the intraoperative period. This article provides guidance for mechanical ventilation in the perioperative setting for the healthy patient as well as the patient with diseased lungs.

BASIC GOALS OF MECHANICAL VENTILATION

The primary goal of mechanical ventilation is to supply oxygen (O_2) and to remove carbon dioxide (CO_2). Thus, 2 interrelated processes must occur: ventilation, the movement of air between the environment and the alveoli; and gas exchange, the transfer of O_2 and CO_2 between the alveolar gas and the mixed venous blood entering the lungs. Another goal includes prevention of anesthesia-related adverse effects, mainly atelectasis, as well as prevention of ventilator-induced lung injury (VILI).

PULMONARY MECHANICS AND GAS EXCHANGE DURING ANESTHESIA

General anesthesia induces significant changes to the basic lung function. The change from the upright position to the supine position reduces functional residual capacity (FRC) by 15% to 20%. Loss of muscle tone induces a change

*Corresponding author. E-mail address: girish.joshi@utsouthwestern.edu.

0737-6146/10/$ – see front matter
doi:10.1016/j.aan.2010.07.002

in the balance of elastic recoil and chest compliance leading to reduced lung volumes [5], increased shunting across the lung, and a further reduction in FRC [6]. The change in lung compliance and the reduction in FRC promote airway closure and induce compression atelectasis. Microatelectasis can be detected in up to 90% of patients undergoing general anesthesia and can involve up to 5% to 20% of the total gas exchange area [5]. Also, absorption atelectasis is common when high inspired O_2 concentrations (FiO_2) are applied [7]. It occurs when less gas enters the alveolus than is removed by uptake into the blood. In the perioperative period, compression and absorption atelectasis are the 2 major mechanisms for the occurrence of atelectasis.

General anesthesia is also associated with an increased alveolar dead space. The reduction in FRC moves all lung areas down on their pressure-volume curve. Therefore, in conditions of general anesthesia and mechanical ventilation, apical alveoli located on the linear part of this curve are best ventilated but less perfused for gravitational reasons. Increased alveolar pressure and reduced pulmonary artery pressure may further decrease apical perfusion. These changes in alveolar dead space reduce the efficacy of alveolar ventilation in eliminating CO_2 and increase the arterial-to-end-tidal CO_2 gradient.

Mechanical ventilation leads to ventilation-perfusion (V/Q) mismatch, more pronounced in the posterodorsal areas, and causes changes in the function of surfactant [8]. In addition, volatile anesthetics reduce hypoxic pulmonary vasoconstriction (HPV), also known as the Euler-Liljestrand reflex. Venous admixture increases and the alveolar-arterial O_2 pressure gradient increases. Under 2 minimum alveolar concentrations of isoflurane, HPV is reduced by almost 50% [5].

In summary, the right-to-left shunting increases from 1% to 5% observed in the healthy, upright, spontaneously ventilating adult to 15% to 20% in the patient who is supine, anesthetized, and ventilated. Therefore, oxygenation is moderately compromised during general anesthesia, despite increase in FiO_2 [5]. Also, atelectasis occurring during general anesthesia may promote injury to alveoli resulting from recurrent shear stress caused by opening and closing of the atelectatic areas (ie, atelectrauma).

TRADITIONAL INTRAOPERATIVE VENTILATION STRATEGIES

In the intraoperative period, the traditional mode of ventilation has been a volume-control mode with moderately high tidal volumes (10–12 mL/kg), low respiratory rates (8–10 breaths/min), I/E ratio (1:2), slightly increased FiO_2 (30%–50%), and zero end-expiratory pressure. The reasons for using twice the physiologic tidal volumes stem from the concern that small tidal volumes can lead to loss of lung volume and hypoxemia caused by right-to-left shunting [9,10]. Volume-control ventilation (VCV) modes are preferred, because they provide fixed tidal volume, even during changes in compliance of chest wall and lungs that can occur during surgery (eg, caused by changes in patient's position, external pressure on the thorax, and changing degrees of muscle relaxation).

The traditional goal of ventilation is to maintain mild hypocapnia (ie, end-tidal CO_2 [$ETCO_2$] around 30 to 35 mm Hg). This goal is probably intended to achieve an apneic threshold, defined as the highest arterial CO_2 tension at which a subject remains apneic, which is approximately 4 or 5 mm Hg less than resting arterial CO_2 tension achieved during spontaneous ventilation. However, the benefits of maintaining mild intraoperative hypocapnia remain controversial. Recent evidence suggests that mild hypercapnia (ie, $ETCO_2$ values around 40–50 mm Hg) can improve tissue oxygenation through improved tissue perfusion and oxygenation resulting from increased cardiac output and vasodilatation as well as increased O_2 off-loading from the shift of the oxyhemoglobin dissociation curve to the right [11–13]. In addition, mild hypercapnia and mild respiratory acidosis attenuate or dampen the inflammation caused by ischemia-reperfusion, established bacterial pneumonia [14], and endotoxin-induced lung injury. However, hypercapnia and acidosis may increase intracranial pressure as well as increase pulmonary vascular resistance, and thereby increase right ventricular workload [15]. Therefore, it should be avoided in select patient populations.

CONCERNS WITH TRADITIONAL VENTILATION STRATEGIES

One of the major concerns of mechanical ventilation is development of VILI, which is caused by volutrauma and barotrauma resulting in an enhanced systemic inflammatory response with worsening oxygenation. One hour of mechanical ventilation alone without surgery in healthy patients did not lead to an increase in measured inflammatory parameters [16]. Choi and colleagues [17] compared the use of tidal volumes of 12 mL/kg without positive end-expiratory pressure (PEEP) with tidal volumes of 6 mL/kg with PEEP of 10 cm H_2O in patients undergoing major abdominal surgery. Bronchiolar lavage was performed before and after 5 h of mechanical ventilation. Lavage fluid from the high tidal volume group showed a pattern of leakage of plasma into the alveoli consistent with alveolar lung injury. This study suggests that, even in patients with no lung disease, the use of large tidal volumes without PEEP causes systemic inflammation and lung injury. The severity of this injury seems to be directly related to the duration of mechanical ventilation and usually remains subclinical.

An observational study found a 25% incidence of ALI/ARDS within 5 days of mechanical ventilation [18]. The development of lung injury was associated with the initial ventilator settings and correlated with an odds ratio of 1.6 for peak airway pressures greater than 30 cm H_2O and an odds ratio of 1.3 for each milliliter of tidal volume exceeding 6 mL/kg predicted body weight. Perioperative ALI becomes clinically important when injurious ventilation patterns are used in patients who have other concomitant lung injuries, such as pulmonary resection, cardiopulmonary bypass, or transfusion related lung injury (see later discussion).

Edema, secretions, and infiltrations all contribute to worsening pulmonary dynamics measured as a decreased static and dynamic compliance, which increase peak airway pressure, regardless of the mode of ventilation. However, peak inspiratory pressure (PIP) reflects the proximal airway pressure and not the alveolar pressure. Therefore, in the setting of reduced compliance or reduced thoracic expansion, high pressures may not induce lung injury [19]. A better approximation of end-tidal alveolar pressure is obtained by using the plateau pressure in a VCV mode. A plateau pressure of greater than 35 cm H_2O has also been implicated in the development of VILI [20].

Overall, volume rather than pressure seems to be the culprit, coining the term volutrauma instead of the traditional expression of barotrauma. Taken together, all studies in healthy patients, as well as in patients at risk, show that ventilation with large tidal volumes for a longer time period may represent a primary hit or an additional hit in cases of extrapulmonary injury [17,21–25]. In patients with pulmonary injury, even shorter periods of harmful ventilation can cause exaggerated injuries to the lung, possibly triggering a systemic inflammatory response.

VILI encompasses 3 different entities: overinflation of alveoli, high-permeability type pulmonary edema (presents as a protein-rich expression of lung fluid), and lung inflammation, also called biotrauma. During ALI, regional compliance heterogeneity creates a functional baby lung. Normal or large tidal volumes delivered to a reduced number of ventilated alveoli can lead to further distention of lung areas that are already overdistended. The alveolar endothelial membrane is altered by mechanical distortion, increased transmural pressure, surfactant inactivation, and the immigration of inflammatory cells. Secondary changes include emphysemalike lesions, lung cysts, and bronchiectasis in nondependant and caudal lung regions [26].

DETERMINATION OF OPTIMAL TIDAL VOLUME

In the intensive care unit (ICU) setting, ventilation with lung volumes of 6 to 8 mL/kg ideal body weight (IBW), as well as peak inspiratory plateau pressures of less than 30 cm H_2O, is now considered the standard of care [27,28]. The ARDSnet study has demonstrated a reduction in mortality from 40% to 31% when a population of patients with ARDS/ALI was ventilated with half the tidal volume (6 vs 12 mL/kg, IBW) [29]. This approach reduces volutrauma caused by high tidal volumes and barotrauma secondary to shear stress related to high airway pressures. Furthermore, biotrauma, a combination of lung and distant organ injury caused by systemic inflammatory response, is reduced [30]. Lower intraoperative tidal volumes of 6.7 mL/kg versus 8.3 mL/kg IBW and avoidance of excessive fluid infusion resulted in reduced respiratory failure after pneumonectomy [31]. Similarly, protective ventilation strategies reduce lung injury and time on the ventilator after esophageal cancer surgery [32].

Intraoperative mechanical ventilation should be similar to that in the ICU setting because of the difficulty in diagnosing ALI/ARDS and the potential for multiple hits caused by intraoperative volutrauma [33]. Therefore, lung protective patterns of intraoperative mechanical ventilation using physiologic tidal volumes and appropriate PEEP should be considered.

ROLE OF PEEP AND RECRUITMENT MANEUVERS

Concerns of atelectasis from general anesthesia as well as the use of low tidal volumes have generated a considerable interest in maneuvers designed to prevent and recruit atelectatic lung regions. PEEP prevents alveolar collapse and maintains end-expiratory lung volumes recruited during inspiration. However, the appropriate level of PEEP is controversial [34]. Attempts to optimize alveolar recruitment by increasing PEEP may be either poorly effective [35] or deleterious because of overinflation of more compliant lung regions [36]. This overinflation counteracts the beneficial effects from low tidal volumes and limited airway pressure ventilation [37].

A recent meta-analysis concluded that, in patients with ALI/ARDS, lower tidal volumes reduced hospital mortality regardless of low or high levels of PEEP. However, higher PEEP levels required 50% fewer interventions for rescue therapy in patients with severe hypoxemia, and reduced mortality in this population [38–40]. The appropriate PEEP values in patients with noncompliant thoraces or increased abdominal pressure are not known, because this patient population was excluded in most of the studies.

Overall, selection of PEEP level should take into consideration lung morphology and regional distribution [41]. Higher levels of PEEP may be appropriate when the loss of aeration is diffuse and involves all lung regions, commonly referred to as white lung [41]. In addition, higher PEEP levels can be beneficial without adding harm from overdistention, provided plateau pressures were kept to less than 30 cm H_2O [34]. Moderate PEEP levels of around 10 cm H_2O should maintain a balance between aeration and overinflation when the loss of aeration is localized and focally distributed (in which the lung behaves as several compartments).

Application of PEEP alone may not always reverse atelectasis and improve arterial oxygenation [42]. The application of 5 cm H_2O of PEEP without prior recruitment was similar to application of no PEEP [43]. In contrast, PEEP of 10 cm H_2O without recruitment consistently reopened some collapsed lung tissue [44]. In 1963, Bendixen and colleagues [45] suggested that periodic deep breaths prevent progressive atelectasis and intrapulmonary shunting. To reexpand the atelectatic lung, it may be necessary to use a vital capacity maneuver with higher inflation pressures, referred to as a recruitment or Lachmann maneuver [46]. Inspiratory pressures of 30 cm H_2O are required to reexpand half of the anesthesia-induced atelectatic lung, but PIPs of up to 40 cm H_2O may be needed to fully reverse anesthesia-induced collapse of healthy lungs, and even higher pressures may be required if the patient is grossly obese [47]. The duration of recruitment maneuver should generally be at least 7 to 8 seconds [48]. Most of the reexpanded lung tissue should remain inflated for about 40 minutes [49]. During a recruitment maneuver, arterial blood pressure should be closely monitored because of its potential to reduce preload and induce hypotension. In a pig model, recruitment maneuvers, applied every 6 hours, had no negative effect on alveolocapillary membrane integrity as measured by extravascular lung water, pulmonary clearance, and light microscopy [50].

Recruitment maneuvers should not be used routinely, and should be restricted for the rapid reversal of loss of aeration from disconnections from the ventilator, for example, to perform tracheal suctioning [51]. The primary aim of lung recruitment should be to achieve arterial saturation greater than or equal to 90% at FiO_2 less than or equal to 0.6. In cases of severe hypoxemia, adjunctive interventions (eg, prone positioning, inhaled nitric oxide, or extracorporeal oxygenation) may be considered.

Ideally, lung recruitability should be assessed by dynamic lung imaging techniques, which would allow the determination of the best physiologic PEEP. In addition, the use of transpulmonary pressure would allow the assessment of the detrimental effects of low tidal volumes. Until this becomes widely available, optimal ventilator settings would include tidal volumes of 6 mL/kg IBW and the maximum PEEP based on the upper limit of airway pressure. In the perioperative setting, maintaining a PEEP of 5 cm H_2O from preoxygenation to the tracheal extubation should reduce atelectasis [52]. Intermittent recruitment maneuvers may be necessary, which should be followed by sufficient PEEP to maintain alveolar unit expansion [49]. Vital capacity maneuvers without subsequently applied PEEP proved to be ineffective for increasing lung volumes and increasing gas exchange [53].

In summary, both PEEP and recruitment maneuvers complement each other and are considered components of the open lung concept. However, recruitment maneuvers during general anesthesia cannot at this time be generally recommended for routine use, and may be best applied in certain circumstances such as ventilation with high FiO_2 and after cardiopulmonary bypass.

DETERMINATION OF OPTIMAL RESPIRATORY RATE

Optimal respiratory rate implies selecting the best compromise between 2 opposing goals: CO_2 elimination and avoidance of the development of intrinsic (auto) PEEP. With the use of lower tidal volumes, higher respiratory rates may be necessary to maintain adequate CO_2 levels. Higher respiratory rates shorten expiratory times, which may result in intrinsic PEEP. In general, respiratory rates can be increased to 20 to 30 breaths/min without generating significant intrinsic PEEP in healthy patients. However, if higher respiratory rates are used, it may be necessary to monitor inspiratory and expiratory flows. If the end-expiratory flow remains zero, respiratory rates can be increased without the risk of intrinsic PEEP formation [54].

SETTING INSPIRED O_2 CONCENTRATIONS

Intraoperative FiO_2 is frequently increased to compensate for the gas exchange impairment related to anesthesia. However, use of excessive O_2 concentrations is potentially deleterious for the lungs and other organs. Application of 100% O_2 for 24 hours has been reported to cause tracheobronchial irritation and pulmonary toxicity leading to irreversible fibrosis [55]. In the intraoperative period, even short-term high FiO_2 may result in absorption atelectasis, which can exaggerate the effects of other stressors to the lung such as stretch injury secondary to inappropriately high tidal volumes or airway pressures [56,57]. High FiO_2 has been linked to poor regulation of blood glucose levels [58] and increased systemic vascular tone [59].

FiO_2 of 0.8 during surgery and until 2 hours after major colorectal surgery correlated with reduced surgical site infection (SSI) rate and postoperative complications [60]. The incidence of postoperative nausea and vomiting (PONV) may also be reduced by higher FiO_2 [61]. However, these early results have not been confirmed in subsequent studies involving other surgeries [62,63]. A recent meta-analysis did not support a beneficial effect of higher FiO_2 on PONV [64]. Another meta-analysis found that the use of higher FiO_2 resulted in an absolute SSI risk reduction of 3% and relative risk reduction of 25% [65]. However, other measures for improving tissue oxygenation, such as temperature control [66], fluid and sympathetic tone management [67], and avoidance of hypocapnia, may prove to be equally important in reducing infections and improving wound healing [68]. When using high FiO_2, lung protective ventilation strategies should be implemented to avoid complications of mechanical ventilation and O_2 toxicity [57,69]. Therefore, a low-O_2 strategy may preserve lung function and improve arterial oxygenation better than high-O_2 therapy during elective surgery [70]. The clinical relevance of these observations currently awaits further confirmation.

MODES OF VENTILATION

The VCV mode is most commonly used in the operating room. In recent years, anesthesia ventilators have improved and increasingly approach ICU ventilator features including synchronized intermittent mandatory ventilation (SIMV), pressure-controlled ventilation (PCV), and pressure support ventilation (PSV), as well as improved monitoring of respiratory mechanics (ie, pressure-volume loops). These newer ventilator features offer flexibility to anesthesiologists, particularly in the management of challenging patients such as those with morbid obesity and pulmonary disease (eg, asthma and chronic obstructive pulmonary disease [COPD]) as well as in challenging situations (eg, severe hypoxemia and hypercarbia).

PCV

In PCV mode, the airway pressure is fixed and the tidal volume changes with resistance and compliance of chest wall and lungs as well as duration of inspiration. During PCV, the peak pressure is achieved rapidly and maintained for the duration of inspiration, which allows delivery of tidal volumes that are similar to VCV, but at lower PIP, assuming similar compliance. In addition, the decelerating gas flow during PCV improves the distribution of gas flow to the lungs [71]. Furthermore, PCV allows delivery of a more homogeneous tidal volume to all areas of the lung, and quicker delivery of tidal volume with greater time for gas exchange, which improves lung compliance and oxygenation.

Unlike VCV, in which the tidal volume is predetermined, inspiratory pressures must be individualized for each patient to ensure adequate ventilation while using PCV. Also, use of PCV requires increased vigilance because the intraoperative lung compliance/resistance can be highly variable (eg, changes in degree of neuromuscular blockade, abdominal packing, surgeons hand on the patient's chest), which can decrease tidal volumes and contribute to the development of hypercarbia and atelectasis [72]. Volume-guaranteed PCV, as a new ventilatory mode, may prove useful in addressing these limitations in the future.

PSV

Although commonly used in the ICU setting, PSV is a new intraoperative mode of mechanical ventilation. PSV augments the patient's spontaneous breaths and reduces the work of breathing. PSV improves gas exchange and prevents perioperative atelectasis in patients breathing spontaneously through supralaryngeal devices (eg, laryngeal mask airway) or tracheal tubes [73–75]. In addition, PSV with or without SIMV may reduce the need for neuromuscular blockers and deep levels of anesthesia. Furthermore, PSV may be used at the end of surgery while the patient is recovering from residual anesthesia and muscle relaxants.

However, as in PCV, the ability of PSV to deliver an adequate tidal volume is dependent on patients' respiratory mechanics, and therefore vigilance is paramount. Volume-guaranteed PSV is designed to address these concerns by adjusting the pressure support to deliver a preset tidal volume [76,77]. Although promising, the literature is mixed regarding clinical validation of intraoperative PSV [78].

MONITORING OF PULMONARY MECHANICS

Monitoring during mechanical ventilation typically includes PIP, mean airway pressure, and plateau pressure. The PIP is measured at the end of the insufflation time, whereas the plateau pressure is measured at the end of the inspiratory pause. The PIP is a function of the inspiratory flow as well as respiratory system compliance and resistance. Inspiratory flow depends on the tidal volume and the inspiratory time, which is a function of respiratory rate and the inspiratory/expiratory ratio. The plateau pressure depends on the tidal volume and the compliance of the respiratory system as a whole. With constant tidal volume and inspiratory time, peak and plateau airway pressures provide information on the resistance and compliance of the respiratory system. Increases in resistance result in an increase in the PIP but not the plateau pressure. In contrast, a reduction in compliance increases the peak and plateau pressures to the same extent. Therefore, pressure curve monitoring is helpful in diagnosing tracheal tube obstruction or kinking, bronchospasm, or reduced respiratory system compliance caused by retractors, pneumoperitoneum, respiratory muscles activation, or changes in patient positioning.

Real-time monitoring of pulmonary mechanics can allow for the individualization of ventilator settings [79]. Modern ICU ventilators display in real time, breath by breath, flow, volume, and pressure at the mouth curves, both as a function of time and as a loop. Data from curve analysis help understand the interaction between patient and ventilator. The pressure-volume loops can be used to characterize pulmonary mechanics and the changes induced by various pulmonary pathologies [80] as well as to identify the onset of alveolar overdistention; presence of large areas of collapsed, but recruitable, lung units; and best PEEP [81]. The flow-volume loops assess resistance and allow identification of pulmonary obstruction, monitoring of the efficacy of therapeutic interventions, [82] as well as detection of leaks and intrinsic PEEP.

Although monitoring of pulmonary mechanics offers the potential to tailor ventilatory strategies based on individual patient needs, there is no consensus on how such information should be interpreted or applied to clinical decision making [80].

SPECIAL PATIENT POPULATION AND SITUATIONS
Postoperative Ventilation after Tracheal Extubation (Noninvasive Ventilation)

One of the most common postoperative pulmonary complications is atelectasis with the consequent risks of pneumonia and acute respiratory failure. Postoperative respiratory compromise can occur in patients with morbid obesity and/or obstructive sleep apnea, as well as those with pulmonary disease, particularly those patients undergoing cardiac, thoracic, or major abdominal surgery. This postoperative respiratory compromise may persist for weeks.

Noninvasive ventilation (NIV) can reduce the need for tracheal intubation and mechanical ventilation in patients with respiratory compromise. NIV compensates for the loss of respiratory function, reduces the work of breathing, and improves gas exchange by improving alveolar recruitment. Most studies evaluating NIV have reported reduced postoperative atelectasis and pneumonia rate [83]. With the use of NIV, the indications for tracheal intubation and mechanical ventilation have become stringent, including severe respiratory failure as indicated by minute ventilation greater than 15 L/min, PaO_2/FiO_2 ratios less than 120 mm Hg, and diffuse or patchy densities on chest radiograph representing more diffuse and severe lung injury. Additional indications include the presence of marked metabolic derangements, shock states, and impaired ability to protect the airway [84,85].

Before initiating NIV, it is necessary to prepare the patient by adequate positioning and explanation of the procedure. After an initial setting of PEEP at 7 to 10 cm H_2O, the inspiratory pressure setting is slowly increased by 2 cm H_2O until patient comfort improves, respiratory rate decreases, and tidal volumes of 6 to 8 mL/kg are achieved [86]. Peak pressures of greater than 20 cm H_2O should be avoided in an effort to avoid gastric insufflation and abdominal distention. NIV can be used intermittently (eg, for 60–90 minutes) every couple of hours until the respiratory status is improved. Concerns about anastomotic dehiscence after thoracic or abdominal surgery have been expressed, but do not seem to be validated as long as the limitations on PIP are observed [86,87].

PATIENTS WITH COPD

COPD describes at least 3 disease entities: emphysema, peripheral airway disease, and chronic bronchitis. Patients with COPD are at increased risk for lung injury in the perioperative period. Emphysema is almost exclusively an expiratory disease, whereas asthma and chronic bronchitis have both inspiratory and expiratory components. Emphysema is associated with gas trapping, which leads to development of intrinsic PEEP, often referred to as dynamic hyperinflation. COPD can lead to the development of cystic air spaces in the lung parenchyma known as bullae, which are often asymptomatic until they occupy more than 50% of the hemithorax. Severe hyperinflation can cause secondary impairment of cardiac venous return and result in hemodynamic instability with acute right heart failure.

Mechanical ventilation may expand existing bullae, promoting the risk of rupture, tension pneumothorax, and bronchopleural fistula. An important goal of intraoperative ventilation is to optimize expiration while preventing air trapping and intrinsic PEEP formation. This goal can be achieved by using prolonged expiratory times and/or reducing the respiratory rate. In addition, the PIPs should be less than 35 cm H_2O to reduce the risk of bullae rupture. Overall, this might necessitate the acceptance of hypercapnia.

Direct measurement of intrinsic PEEP is not possible with current anesthesia ventilators. Therefore, indirect indicators, such as the slope of the expiratory phase of the capnogram, may be used. In patients with hemodynamic instability in whom high intrinsic PEEP is suspected, disconnecting the patient from the ventilator might improve venous return and thus improve hemodynamic status. In modern anesthesia ventilators, the expiratory duration may be set according to an observed expiratory flow limitation on a flow-time loop.

Small airway collapse may be prevented by the application of external PEEP to stent the airway open [88]. In spontaneously breathing patients, external PEEP can reduce the work of breathing required to trigger the ventilator [89]. The use of inhalation anesthetics, as well as prophylactic postoperative NIV, may prevent postextubation respiratory failure [90]. In addition, broncholytic therapy should be continued throughout the perioperative period.

Patients Who are Obese

Obesity is associated with a reduction in FRC, increased PIP during positive pressure ventilation, and a decrease in lung compliance [91]. The expiratory flow limitation and development of intrinsic PEEP may further increase the work of breathing at rest. These changes increase the risk for perioperative pulmonary complications [92].

Lung protective ventilation strategies in the obese would include the use of PCV [93] with tidal volumes around 8 mL/kg IBW and a PEEP of 10 cm H_2O [94]. In addition, acceptance of mild hypercapnia may limit the need for increased PIP. It is important to avoid hyperventilation (and hypocapnia), because this may result in metabolic alkalosis and lead to postoperative hypoventilation.

Preoxygenation with FiO_2 of 1.0 and PEEP of 10 cm H_2O has been shown to prevent atelectasis while improving oxygenation during induction of anesthesia in patients who are obese [95]. In one study, a PEEP of 10 cm H_2O in patients with mean BMI of 51 kg/m^2 improved intraoperative compliance and oxygenation [96]. Another study concluded that a PEEP of 15 cm H_2O provided the greatest benefit in terms of FRC improvement and gas exchange without hemodynamic compromise [97]. Optimal PEEP level should reduce intrinsic PEEP as detected by flow measurements. Recruitment maneuvers are beneficial in patients who are obese and should be applied in particular during laparoscopic surgery [98]. However, the effects of recruitment maneuvers are short lasting and often limited by hemodynamic instability.

In the postoperative period, supplemental O_2 is beneficial for most patients; however, it should be administered with caution as it may reduce hypoxic respiratory drive and increase the incidence and duration of apneic episodes. Because patients who are obese often have unrecognized sleep apnea, recurrent hypoxemia may be treated better with continuous positive airway pressure (CPAP) or bilevel positive airway pressure along with O_2 rather than O_2 alone.

Patients with Pneumoperitoneum

The insufflation of CO_2 into the abdomen creates a hypercapnic physiology pattern, with up to 20% more CO_2 elimination and a restrictive respiratory pattern similar to the patient who is obese, which is usually limited to the duration of the pneumoperitoneum. In the obese, lung compliance is reduced, resistance is increased, and oxygenation is worsened even before the creation of pneumoperitoneum [99], and the reversal of atelectasis is slower [100]. Also, creation of pneumoperitoneum can lead to mainstem intubation with a brisk reduction in pulmonary function immediately after insufflation.

The increase in alveolar ventilation during CO_2 insufflation can be achieved either by increasing tidal volume or increasing respiratory rate. Because VCV increases peak and plateau pressures and puts the patient at risk for VILI, PCV may be beneficial [93,101,102]. Recruitment maneuvers before [103] and after pneumoperitoneum improve lung function in normal patients [104] as well as in patients who are moderately obese [98,105]. The application of PEEP of 10 to 15 cm H_2O improves V/Q mismatch and improves oxygenation as well as ventilation [106].

In summary, optimal ventilator settings in patients undergoing procedures requiring a pneumoperitoneum include a tidal volume of 6 to 8 mL/kg along with moderate PEEP levels of around 10 cm H_2O, and the application of multiple recruitment maneuvers before and after insufflation.

Patients at Risk for Intraoperative Pulmonary Complications (eg, Cardiopulmonary Bypass Exposure)

Cardiopulmonary bypass may cause lung injury that can be aggravated by injurious ventilation patterns. Zupancich and colleagues [25] compared the use of high tidal volumes (10–12 mL/kg) plus low PEEP (2–3 cm H_2O) with a lung protective strategy with low tidal volumes (8 mL/kg) plus high PEEP

(10 cm H_2O) in patients ventilated for 6 hours after coronary artery bypass surgery. Serum and bronchiolar lavage levels of the inflammatory cytokines were significantly increased at 6 hours only in the high tidal volume group. However, another similar study failed to observe any benefits of a lung protective strategy [23]. Nevertheless, there is the suggestion of benefit for lung protective ventilation during cardiac surgery.

Similar evidence is available for thoracic procedures as well as in patients with sepsis and lung contusion, but their coverage is beyond the scope of this article.

Patients in Prone Position

Overall, FRC and oxygenation is improved on assuming a prone position in normal people [107] and patients who are obese [108]. Although ventilation is not affected by posture, perfusion is always dorsally distributed [109], so ventilation-perfusion matching improves along the vertical axis in the prone position [110]. These findings are more pronounced in patients with ALI [111]. The abdomen must be able to move freely and not impede respiratory mechanics and venous return.

Pediatric Patients

Smaller elastic retraction forces and a lower relaxation volume predispose children less than 7 years of age to more airway collapse than adults [112], particularly with the use of high FiO_2. As with adults, atelectasis is more pronounced

Table 1
Summary of recommendations for perioperative mechanical ventilation and degree of evidence

CPAP 6–10 cm H_2O during preoxygenation before induction of anesthesia	Reduces atelectasis	A
	Improves arterial oxygenation	B
	Prolongs nonhypoxic apnea time	B
Pressure-controlled ventilation	Reduces peak airway pressure	B
	Does not improve gas exchange	B
Tidal volumes 6–8 mL/kg	Reduces alveolar inflammation	A
	Reduces postoperative pulmonary dysfunction in patients at high risk	A
PEEP 5–10 cm H_2O	Reduces alveolar inflammation in association with low tidal volume ventilation	A
	Improves arterial oxygenation in the morbidly obese	A
	Improves arterial oxygenation during 1-lung ventilation	A
	Prevents derecruitment after vital capacity maneuver	B
FiO_2 0.8 intraoperatively	May reduce wound infection after abdominal surgery	A
	May protect cardiovascular system	A
	No effect on incidence of PONV	B
	May increase absorption atelectasis	B

in the caudal and dependent lung regions [43]. The levels of PIPs that are adequate to reopen small airways and alveoli have not been studied in children, but may be lower in healthy children undergoing surgery [113–115].

In a small study (n = 46 children), it was shown that a PEEP of 6 cm H_2O prevented changes caused by higher Fio_2. Therefore, PEEP levels in children of 5 to 6 cm H_2O may be advocated [43,116]. In contrast with adults, no pediatric studies have been conducted to confirm that a lung protective strategy of low tidal volume and pressure limitation is optimal. Nevertheless, based on adult and animal studies, it can be extrapolated that lung protective ventilation might also be beneficial in children [117].

SUMMARY

In recent years there has been significant attention directed toward the detrimental pulmonary, cardiovascular, and inflammatory consequences of mechanical ventilation that may adversely influence perioperative outcome. An evidence-based approach to mechanical ventilation should reduce perioperative lung injury and improve surgical outcome (Table 1). Use of a lung protective strategy including low tidal volumes of 6 to 8 mL/kg with an initial PEEP of 5 to 10 cm H_2O and plateau pressures limited to 30 cm H_2O seems to be protective against VILI. Optimal strategies vary by clinical situation (ie, healthy vs diseased or injured lung).

The recent advances in intraoperative ventilation modalities and the ability to better monitor respiratory mechanics offer the perioperative anesthesiologist many opportunities to customize the ventilation strategy to the needs of individual patients. However, with this advanced technology comes the need for better understanding of pulmonary physiology and mechanics to assess which ventilation strategy would improve patient outcomes. There is a need for more studies evaluating the benefits of pulmonary monitoring and improved ventilators, which might allow better perioperative strategies as well as the evaluation of the use of advanced ventilation modes such as closed-loop (automated) artificial ventilation, automatic tube compensation, and proportional assist ventilation.

References

[1] Roupie E, Lepage E, Wysocki M, et al. Prevalence, etiologies and outcome of the acute respiratory distress syndrome among hypoxemic ventilated patients. SRLF Collaborative Group on Mechanical Ventilation. Societe de Reanimation de Langue Francaise. Intensive Care Med 1999;25:920.

[2] Lewandowski K. Epidemiological data challenge ARDS/ALI definition. Intensive Care Med 1999;25:884.

[3] Hickling KG, Henderson SJ, Jackson R. Low mortality associated with low volume pressure limited ventilation with permissive hypercapnia in severe adult respiratory distress syndrome. Intensive Care Med 1990;16:372.

[4] Hickling KG, Walsh J, Henderson S, et al. Low mortality rate in adult respiratory distress syndrome using low-volume, pressure-limited ventilation with permissive hypercapnia: a prospective study. Crit Care Med 1994;22:1568.

[5] Hedenstierna G, Edmark L. The effects of anesthesia and muscle paralysis on the respiratory system. Intensive Care Med 2005;31:1327.

[6] Wahba RW. Perioperative functional residual capacity. Can J Anaesth 1991;38:384.

[7] Magnusson L, Spahn DR. New concepts of atelectasis during general anaesthesia. Br J Anaesth 2003;91:61.

[8] Woo SW, Berlin D, Hedley-Whyte J. Surfactant function and anesthetic agents. J Appl Physiol 1969;26:571.

[9] Bendixen HH. Atelectasis and shunting. Anesthesiology 1964;25:595.

[10] Suter PM, Fairley B, Isenberg MD. Optimum end-expiratory airway pressure in patients with acute pulmonary failure. N Engl J Med 1975;292:284.

[11] Akca O, Doufas AG, Morioka N, et al. Hypercapnia improves tissue oxygenation. Anesthesiology 2002;97:801.

[12] Fleischmann E, Herbst F, Kugener A, et al. Mild hypercapnia increases subcutaneous and colonic oxygen tension in patients given 80% inspired oxygen during abdominal surgery. Anesthesiology 2006;104:944.

[13] Hager H, Reddy D, Mandadi G, et al. Hypercapnia improves tissue oxygenation in morbidly obese surgical patients. Anesth Analg 2006;103:677.

[14] Chonghaile MN, Higgins BD, Costello J, et al. Hypercapnic acidosis attenuates lung injury induced by established bacterial pneumonia. Anesthesiology 2008;109:837.

[15] Feihl F, Perret C. Permissive hypercapnia. How permissive should we be? Am J Respir Crit Care Med 1994;150:1722.

[16] Wrigge H, Zinserling J, Stüber F, et al. Effects of mechanical ventilation on release of cytokines into systemic circulation in patients with normal pulmonary function. Anesthesiology 2000;93:1413.

[17] Choi G, Wolthuis EK, Bresser P, et al. Mechanical ventilation with lower tidal volumes and positive end-expiratory pressure prevents alveolar coagulation in patients without lung injury. Anesthesiology 2006;105:689.

[18] Gajic O, Dara SI, Mendez JL, et al. Ventilator-associated lung injury in patients without acute lung injury at the onset of mechanical ventilation. Crit Care Med 2004;32:1817.

[19] Dreyfuss D, Soler P, Basset G, et al. High inflation pressure pulmonary edema. Respective effects of high airway pressure, high tidal volume, and positive end-expiratory pressure. Am Rev Respir Dis 1988;137:1159.

[20] Esteban A, Anzueto A, Frutos F, et al. Characteristics and outcomes in adult patients receiving mechanical ventilation: a 28-day international study. JAMA 2002;287:345.

[21] Miranda DR, Gommers D, Papadakos PJ, et al. Mechanical ventilation affects pulmonary inflammation in cardiac surgery patients: the role of the open-lung concept. J Cardiothorac Vasc Anesth 2007;21:279.

[22] Wolthuis EK, Choi G, Dessing MC, et al. Mechanical ventilation with lower tidal volumes and positive end-expiratory pressure prevents pulmonary inflammation in patients without preexisting lung injury. Anesthesiology 2008;108:46.

[23] Wrigge H, Uhlig U, Baumgarten G, et al. Mechanical ventilation strategies and inflammatory responses to cardiac surgery: a prospective randomized clinical trial. Intensive Care Med 2005;31:1379.

[24] Wrigge H, Uhlig U, Zinserling J, et al. The effects of different ventilatory settings on pulmonary and systemic inflammatory responses during major surgery. Anesth Analg 2004;98:775.

[25] Zupancich E, Paparella D, Turani F, et al. Mechanical ventilation affects inflammatory mediators in patients undergoing cardiopulmonary bypass for cardiac surgery: a randomized clinical trial. J Thorac Cardiovasc Surg 2005;130:378.

[26] Treggiari MM, Romand JA, Martin JB, et al. Air cysts and bronchiectasis prevail in nondependent areas in severe acute respiratory distress syndrome: a computed tomographic study of ventilator-associated changes. Crit Care Med 2002;30:1747.

[27] Ventilation with lower tidal volumes as compared with traditional tidal volumes for acute lung injury and the acute respiratory distress syndrome. The Acute Respiratory Distress Syndrome Network. N Engl J Med 2000;342:1301.

[28] Petrucci N, Iacovelli W. Lung protective ventilation strategy for the acute respiratory distress syndrome. Cochrane Database Syst Rev 2007;3:CD003844.

[29] Slutsky AS. Lung injury caused by mechanical ventilation. Chest 1999;116:9S.

[30] Ranieri VM, Giunta F, Suter PM, et al. Mechanical ventilation as a mediator of multisystem organ failure in acute respiratory distress syndrome. JAMA 2000;284:43.

[31] Fernandez-Perez ER, Keegan MT, Brown DR, et al. Intraoperative tidal volume as a risk factor for respiratory failure after pneumonectomy. Anesthesiology 2006;105:14.

[32] Michelet P, D'Journo XB, Roch A, et al. Protective ventilation influences systemic inflammation after esophagectomy: a randomized controlled study. Anesthesiology 2006;105:911.

[33] Schultz MJ, Haitsma JJ, Slutsky AS, et al. What tidal volumes should be used in patients without acute lung injury? Anesthesiology 2007;106:1226.

[34] Gattinoni L, Caironi P. Refining ventilatory treatment for acute lung injury and acute respiratory distress syndrome. JAMA 2008;299:691.

[35] Cakar N, der Kloot TV, Youngblood M, et al. Oxygenation response to a recruitment maneuver during supine and prone positions in an oleic acid-induced lung injury model. Am J Respir Crit Care Med 2000;161:1949.

[36] Rouby JJ. Lung overinflation. The hidden face of alveolar recruitment. Anesthesiology 2003;99:2.

[37] Pinhu L, Whitehead T, Evans T, et al. Ventilator-associated lung injury. Lancet 2003;361:332.

[38] Meade MO, Cook DJ, Guyatt GH, et al. Ventilation strategy using low tidal volumes, recruitment maneuvers, and high positive end-expiratory pressure for acute lung injury and acute respiratory distress syndrome: a randomized controlled trial. JAMA 2008;299:637.

[39] Mercat A, Richard JC, Vielle B, et al. Positive end-expiratory pressure setting in adults with acute lung injury and acute respiratory distress syndrome: a randomized controlled trial. JAMA 2008;299:646.

[40] Putensen C, Theuerkauf N, Zinserling J, et al. Meta-analysis: ventilation strategies and outcomes of the acute respiratory distress syndrome and acute lung injury. Ann Intern Med 2009;151:566.

[41] Rouby JJ, Lu Q, Goldstein I. Selecting the right level of positive end-expiratory pressure in patients with acute respiratory distress syndrome. Am J Respir Crit Care Med 2002;165:1182.

[42] Bindslev L, Hedenstierna G, Santesson J, et al. Airway closure during anaesthesia, and its prevention by positive end expiratory pressure. Acta Anaesthesiol Scand 1980;24:199.

[43] Tusman G, Bohm SH, Tempra A, et al. Effects of recruitment maneuver on atelectasis in anesthetized children. Anesthesiology 2003;98:14.

[44] Tokics L, Hedenstierna G, Strandberg A, et al. Lung collapse and gas exchange during general anesthesia: effects of spontaneous breathing, muscle paralysis, and positive end-expiratory pressure. Anesthesiology 1987;66:157.

[45] Bendixen HH, Hedley-Whyte J, Laver MB. Impaired oxygenation in surgical patients during general anesthesia with controlled ventilation. A concept of atelectasis. N Engl J Med 1963;269:991.

[46] Lachmann B. Open up the lung and keep the lung open. Intensive Care Med 1992;18:319.

[47] Rothen HU, Sporre B, Engberg G, et al. Re-expansion of atelectasis during general anaesthesia: a computed tomography study. Br J Anaesth 1993;71:788.

[48] Rothen HU, Neumann P, Berglund JE, et al. Dynamics of re-expansion of atelectasis during general anaesthesia. Br J Anaesth 1999;82:551.

[49] Rothen HU, Sporre B, Engberg G, et al. Reexpansion of atelectasis during general anaesthesia may have a prolonged effect. Acta Anaesthesiol Scand 1995;39:118.

[50] Magnusson L, Tenling A, Lemoine R, et al. The safety of one, or repeated, vital capacity maneuvers during general anesthesia. Anesth Analg 2000;91:702.

[51] Lu Q, Capderou A, Cluzel P, et al. A computed tomographic scan assessment of endotracheal suctioning-induced bronchoconstriction in ventilated sheep. Am J Respir Crit Care Med 2000;162:1898.

[52] Rusca M, Proietti S, Schnyder P, et al. Prevention of atelectasis formation during induction of general anesthesia. Anesth Analg 2003;97:1835.

[53] Dyhr T, Laursen N, Larsson A. Effects of lung recruitment maneuver and positive end-expiratory pressure on lung volume, respiratory mechanics and alveolar gas mixing in patients ventilated after cardiac surgery. Acta Anaesthesiol Scand 2002;46:717.

[54] Richecoeur J, Lu Q, Vieira SR, et al. Expiratory washout versus optimization of mechanical ventilation during permissive hypercapnia in patients with severe acute respiratory distress syndrome. Am J Respir Crit Care Med 1999;160:77.

[55] Bonikos DS, Bensch KG, Ludwin SK, et al. Oxygen toxicity in the newborn. The effect of prolonged 100 per cent O_2 exposure on the lungs of newborn mice. Lab Invest 1975;32:619.

[56] Grocott HP. Oxygen toxicity during one-lung ventilation: is it time to re-evaluate our practice? Anesthesiol Clin 2008;26:273.

[57] Sinclair SE, Altemeier WA, Matute-Bello G, et al. Augmented lung injury due to interaction between hyperoxia and mechanical ventilation. Crit Care Med 2004;32:2496.

[58] Bandali KS, Belanger MP, Wittnich C. Does hyperoxia affect glucose regulation and transport in the newborn? J Thorac Cardiovasc Surg 2003;126:1730.

[59] Harten JM, Anderson KJ, Angerson WJ, et al. The effect of normobaric hyperoxia on cardiac index in healthy awake volunteers. Anaesthesia 2003;58:885.

[60] Greif R, Akca O, Horn EP, et al. Supplemental perioperative oxygen to reduce the incidence of surgical-wound infection. Outcomes Research Group. N Engl J Med 2000;342:161.

[61] Greif R, Laciny S, Rapf B, et al. Supplemental oxygen reduces the incidence of postoperative nausea and vomiting. Anesthesiology 1999;91:1246.

[62] Meyhoff CS, Wetterslev J, Jorgensen LN, et al. Effect of high perioperative oxygen fraction on surgical site infection and pulmonary complications after abdominal surgery: the PROXI randomized clinical trial. JAMA 2009;302:1543.

[63] Pryor KO, Fahey TJ 3rd, Lien CA, et al. Surgical site infection and the routine use of perioperative hyperoxia in a general surgical population: a randomized controlled trial. JAMA 2004;291:79.

[64] Orhan-Sungur M, Kranke P, Sessler D, et al. Does supplemental oxygen reduce postoperative nausea and vomiting? A meta-analysis of randomized controlled trials. Anesth Analg 2008;106:1733.

[65] Qadan M, Akca O, Mahid SS, et al. Perioperative supplemental oxygen therapy and surgical site infection: a meta-analysis of randomized controlled trials. Arch Surg 2009;144:359.

[66] Kurz A, Sessler DI, Lenhardt R. Perioperative normothermia to reduce the incidence of surgical-wound infection and shorten hospitalization. Study of Wound Infection and Temperature Group. N Engl J Med 1996;334:1209.

[67] Gottrup F, Firmin R, Rabkin J, et al. Directly measured tissue oxygen tension and arterial oxygen tension assess tissue perfusion. Crit Care Med 1987;15:1030.

[68] Hunt TK, Pai MP. The effect of varying ambient oxygen tensions on wound metabolism and collagen synthesis. Surg Gynecol Obstet 1972;135:561.

[69] Kabon B, Kurz A. Optimal perioperative oxygen administration. Curr Opin Anaesthesiol 2006;19:11.

[70] Zoremba M, Dette F, Hunecke T, et al. The influence of perioperative oxygen concentration on postoperative lung function in moderately obese adults. Eur J Anaesthesiol 2010;27(6):501-7.

[71] Davis K Jr, Branson RD, Campbell RS, et al. Comparison of volume control and pressure control ventilation: is flow waveform the difference? J Trauma 1996;41:808.

[72] Duggan M, Kavanagh BP. Pulmonary atelectasis: a pathogenic perioperative entity. Anesthesiology 2005;102:838.

[73] Bosek V, Roy L, Smith RA. Pressure support improves efficiency of spontaneous breathing during inhalation anesthesia. J Clin Anesth 1996;8:9.

[74] Zoremba M, Aust H, Eberhart L, et al. Comparison between intubation and the laryngeal mask airway in moderately obese adults. Acta Anaesthesiol Scand 2009;53:436.

[75] Zoremba M, Kalmus G, Dette F, et al. Effect of intra-operative pressure support vs pressure controlled ventilation on oxygenation and lung function in moderately obese adults. Anaesthesia 2010;65:124.

[76] MacIntyre NR. New modes of mechanical ventilation. Clin Chest Med 1996;17:411.

[77] Ranieri VM. Optimization of patient-ventilator interactions: closed-loop technology to turn the century. Intensive Care Med 1997;23:936.

[78] Jaber S, Delay JM, Matecki S, et al. Volume-guaranteed pressure-support ventilation facing acute changes in ventilatory demand. Intensive Care Med 2005;31:1181.

[79] Lucangelo U, Bernabe F, Blanch L. Lung mechanics at the bedside: make it simple. Curr Opin Crit Care 2007;13:64.

[80] de Chazal I, Hubmayr RD. Novel aspects of pulmonary mechanics in intensive care. Br J Anaesth 2003;91:81.

[81] Roupie E, Dambrosio M, Servillo G, et al. Titration of tidal volume and induced hypercapnia in acute respiratory distress syndrome. Am J Respir Crit Care Med 1995;152:121.

[82] Dolovich MB, Ahrens RC, Hess DR, et al. Device selection and outcomes of aerosol therapy: evidence-based guidelines: American College of Chest Physicians/American College of Asthma, Allergy, and Immunology. Chest 2005;127:335.

[83] Pelosi P, Jaber S. Noninvasive respiratory support in the perioperative period. Curr Opin Anaesthesiol 2010;23:233.

[84] Antonelli M, Conti G, Moro ML, et al. Predictors of failure of noninvasive positive pressure ventilation in patients with acute hypoxemic respiratory failure: a multi-center study. Intensive Care Med 2001;27:1718.

[85] Rana S, Jenad H, Gay PC, et al. Failure of non-invasive ventilation in patients with acute lung injury: observational cohort study. Crit Care 2006;10:R79.

[86] Jaber S, Delay JM, Chanques G, et al. Outcomes of patients with acute respiratory failure after abdominal surgery treated with noninvasive positive pressure ventilation. Chest 2005;128:2688.

[87] Michelet P, D'Journo XB, Seinaye F, et al. Non-invasive ventilation for treatment of postoperative respiratory failure after oesophagectomy. Br J Surg 2009;96:54.

[88] Marini JJ. Positive end-expiratory pressure in severe airflow obstruction: more than a "one-trick pony"? Crit Care Med 2005;33:1652.

[89] Blanch L, Bernabe F, Lucangelo U. Measurement of air trapping, intrinsic positive end-expiratory pressure, and dynamic hyperinflation in mechanically ventilated patients. Respir Care 2005;50:110.

[90] Hill NS, Brennan J, Garpestad E, et al. Noninvasive ventilation in acute respiratory failure. Crit Care Med 2007;35:2402.

[91] Pelosi P, Croci M, Ravagnan I, et al. The effects of body mass on lung volumes, respiratory mechanics, and gas exchange during general anesthesia. Anesth Analg 1998;87:654.

[92] Rose DK, Cohen MM, Wigglesworth DF, et al. Critical respiratory events in the postanesthesia care unit. Patient, surgical, and anesthetic factors. Anesthesiology 1994;81:410.

[93] Cadi P, Guenoun T, Journois D, et al. Pressure-controlled ventilation improves oxygenation during laparoscopic obesity surgery compared with volume-controlled ventilation. Br J Anaesth 2008;100:709.

[94] Soni N, Williams P. Positive pressure ventilation: what is the real cost? Br J Anaesth 2008;101:446.

[95] Neumann P, Rothen HU, Berglund JE, et al. Positive end-expiratory pressure prevents atelectasis during general anaesthesia even in the presence of a high inspired oxygen concentration. Acta Anaesthesiol Scand 1999;43:295.

[96] Pelosi P, Ravagnan I, Giurati G, et al. Positive end-expiratory pressure improves respiratory function in obese but not in normal subjects during anesthesia and paralysis. Anesthesiology 1999;91:1221.

[97] Erlandsson K, Odenstedt H, Lundin S, et al. Positive end-expiratory pressure optimization using electric impedance tomography in morbidly obese patients during laparoscopic gastric bypass surgery. Acta Anaesthesiol Scand 2006;50:833.

[98] Whalen FX, Gajic O, Thompson GB, et al. The effects of the alveolar recruitment maneuver and positive end-expiratory pressure on arterial oxygenation during laparoscopic bariatric surgery. Anesth Analg 2006;102:298.

[99] Sprung J, Whalley DG, Falcone T, et al. The effects of tidal volume and respiratory rate on oxygenation and respiratory mechanics during laparoscopy in morbidly obese patients. Anesth Analg 2003;97:268.

[100] Eichenberger A, Proietti S, Wicky S, et al. Morbid obesity and postoperative pulmonary atelectasis: an underestimated problem. Anesth Analg 2002;95:1788.

[101] Balick-Weber CC, Nicolas P, Hedreville-Montout M, et al. Respiratory and haemodynamic effects of volume-controlled vs pressure-controlled ventilation during laparoscopy: a cross-over study with echocardiographic assessment. Br J Anaesth 2007;99:429.

[102] De Baerdemaeker LE, Van der Herten C, Gillardin JM, et al. Comparison of volume-controlled and pressure-controlled ventilation during laparoscopic gastric banding in morbidly obese patients. Obes Surg 2008;18:680.

[103] Park HP, Hwang JW, Kim YB, et al. Effect of pre-emptive alveolar recruitment strategy before pneumoperitoneum on arterial oxygenation during laparoscopic hysterectomy. Anaesth Intensive Care 2009;37:593.

[104] Cakmakkaya OS, Kaya G, Altintas F, et al. Restoration of pulmonary compliance after laparoscopic surgery using a simple alveolar recruitment maneuver. J Clin Anesth 2009;21:422.

[105] Almarakbi WA, Fawzi HM, Alhashemi JA. Effects of four intraoperative ventilatory strategies on respiratory compliance and gas exchange during laparoscopic gastric banding in obese patients. Br J Anaesth 2009;102:862.

[106] Loeckinger A, Kleinsasser A, Hoermann C, et al. Inert gas exchange during pneumoperitoneum at incremental values of positive end-expiratory pressure. Anesth Analg 2000;90:466.

[107] Pelosi P, Croci M, Calappi E, et al. The prone positioning during general anesthesia minimally affects respiratory mechanics while improving functional residual capacity and increasing oxygen tension. Anesth Analg 1995;80:955.

[108] Pelosi P, Croci M, Calappi E, et al. Prone positioning improves pulmonary function in obese patients during general anesthesia. Anesth Analg 1996;83:578.

[109] Glenny RW, Lamm WJ, Albert RK, et al. Gravity is a minor determinant of pulmonary blood flow distribution. J Appl Physiol 1991;71:620.

[110] Nyren S, Radell P, Lindahl SG, et al. Lung ventilation and perfusion in prone and supine postures with reference to anesthetized and mechanically ventilated healthy volunteers. Anesthesiology 2010;112:682.

[111] Douglas WW, Rehder K, Beynen FM, et al. Improved oxygenation in patients with acute respiratory failure: the prone position. Am Rev Respir Dis 1977;115:559.

[112] Mansell A, Bryan C, Levison H. Airway closure in children. J Appl Physiol 1972;33:711.

[113] Gaver DP 3rd, Samsel RW, Solway J. Effects of surface tension and viscosity on airway reopening. J Appl Physiol 1990;69:74.

[114] Naureckas ET, Dawson CA, Gerber BS, et al. Airway reopening pressure in isolated rat lungs. J Appl Physiol 1994;76:1372.
[115] Polgar G, Weng TR. The functional development of the respiratory system from the period of gestation to adulthood. Am Rev Respir Dis 1979;120:625.
[116] Tusman G, Bohm SH, Vazquez de Anda GF, et al. 'Alveolar recruitment strategy' improves arterial oxygenation during general anaesthesia. Br J Anaesth 1999;82:8.
[117] Marraro GA. Protective lung strategies during artificial ventilation in children. Paediatr Anaesth 2005;15:630.

Advances in Anesthesia 28 (2010) 35–57

ADVANCES IN ANESTHESIA

Measuring the Clinical Competence of Anesthesiologists

Robert S. Lagasse, MD[a],*, Edward Pollak, MD[b]

[a]Department of Anesthesiology, Yale School of Medicine, 333 Cedar Street, TMP 3, New Haven, CT 06520-8051, USA
[b]Department of Anesthesiology and Perioperative Medicine, William Beaumont Hospital, 3601 West Thirteen Mile Road, Royal Oak, MI 48073, USA

THE PROBLEM IN PERSPECTIVE

Why is so much attention directed at judging physician competence in the United States? Much of this attention has been thrust on health care practitioners by the Institute of Medicine (IOM). The IOM was chartered in the United States in 1970 by the National Academy of Sciences. According to the Academy's 1863 charter, its charge is to enlist distinguished members of the appropriate professions in the examination of policy matters pertaining to public health and to act as an adviser to the federal government on issues of medical care, research, and education. In 1998, the Quality of Health Care in America Project was initiated by the IOM with the goal of developing strategies that would result in a threshold improvement in quality in the subsequent 10 years [1].

Toward that goal, the Quality of Health Care in America Project published a series of reports on health care quality in the United States. The first in the series was entitled *To Err Is Human: Building a Safer Health System.* This report on patient safety addressed a serious issue affecting the quality of our health care, specifically human error. This first report began by quoting 2 large US studies, one conducted in Colorado and Utah and the other in New York, which found that adverse events occurred in 2.9% and 3.7% of hospitalizations, respectively. In the Colorado and Utah hospitals, 8.8% of adverse events led to death, compared with 13.6% in New York hospitals. In both of these studies, more than half of these adverse events resulted from medical errors and, according to the IOM, could have been prevented [1].

When extrapolated to the more than 33.6 million hospital admissions in the United States during 1997, the results of these studies implied that 44,000 to 98,000 Americans avoidably die each year as a result of medical errors. Even when using the lower estimate, death caused by medical errors becomes the eighth leading cause of death in the United States. More people die in a given

*Corresponding author. E-mail address: BobLagasse@yahoo.com.

0737-6146/10/$ – see front matter
doi:10.1016/j.aan.2010.07.003

year as a result of medical errors than from motor vehicle accidents (43,458), breast cancer (42,297), or AIDS (16,516). The IOM estimated the costs of preventable adverse events, including lost income, lost household production, disability, and health care costs, to be between 17 and 29 billion dollars annually; health care expenditures constitute more than half of these costs [1].

The IOM did attempt to do more than point out the problems. As mentioned earlier, the goal of the Quality of Health Care in America Project was to develop strategies to substantially improve health care quality in a 10-year period. The strategies recommended by the IOM fell into a 4-tiered framework as follows:

1) Establish a national focus to create leadership, research, tools, and protocols to enhance the nation's knowledge base about safety
2) Identify and learn from errors through immediate mandatory reporting efforts, as well as encouragement of voluntary efforts, both with the aim of making sure the system continues to be made safer for patients
3) Raise standards and expectations for improvements in safety through the actions of oversight organizations, group purchasers, and professional groups
4) Create safety systems within health care organizations through the implementation of safe practices at the delivery level [1].

The IOM believed that the delivery level would be the ultimate target of all their recommendations. By way of example, anesthesiology was cited as an area in which impressive improvements in safety had been made at the delivery level. The initial report of the Quality of Health Care in America Project stated, "As more and more attention has been focused on understanding the factors that contribute to error and on the design of safer systems, preventable mishaps have declined. Studies, some conducted in Australia, the United Kingdom and other countries, indicate that anesthesia mortality is about 1 death per 200,000 to 300,000 anesthetics administered, compared with 2 deaths per 10,000 anesthetics in the early 1980s [1]." The reference cited for this marked improvement in anesthesia-related mortality does not describe the study that resulted in the lower rate quoted by the IOM and does not have an author listed [2]. Some believe that the IOM's claim of improved anesthesia mortality resulted from a study by John Eichhorn, who examined 11 cases of major intraoperative accidents that had been reported to a malpractice insurance carrier between 1976 and 1988 [3]. In an effort to remove disease and postoperative care as contributing factors, Eichhorn's study considered only patients with an American Society of Anesthesiologists (ASA) Physical Status of I or II who died intraoperatively. Therefore, 5 intraoperative anesthesia-related deaths out of an insured population of 1,001,000 ASA Physical Status I or II patients resulted in a mortality of 1 per 200,200 in which anesthesia was considered the sole contributor [4]. In a 2002 review of the published literature, anesthesia-related mortality in less exclusive general patient populations ranged from 1 in 1388 anesthetics to 1 in 85,708 anesthetics, and preventable anesthetic mortality ranged from 1 in 1707 anesthetics to 1 in 48,748 anesthetics.

When anesthesia-related death is defined as a perioperative death to which human error on the part of the anesthesia provider has contributed, as determined by peer review, then anesthesia-related mortality is estimated to be approximately 1 death per 13,000 anesthetics [3].

As noted in the corrective strategies listed earlier, error reporting and peer review were among the recommendations of the IOM report. It was believed that a nationwide, mandatory public-reporting system should be established for the collection of standardized information about adverse events that result in death or serious patient harm. Despite this aggressive approach, the Quality of Health Care in America Project also saw a role for voluntary, confidential reporting systems. Their initial report recommended that voluntary reporting systems be encouraged to examine the less severe adverse events and that these reports be protected from legal discoverability. In this model, information about the most serious adverse events that result in harm to patients, and which are subsequently found by peer review to result from human errors, would not be protected from public disclosure. For less severe events, public disclosure was not recommended by the IOM because of concerns that fear about legal discoverability of information might undermine efforts to analyze errors to improve safety [1].

In the second report from the Quality of Health Care in America Project, the IOM described the gap between our current health care system and an optimal health care system as a "quality chasm." They went on to say that efforts to close this gap should include analysis and synthesis of the medical evidence, establishment of goals for improvement in care processes and outcomes, and development of measures for assessing quality of care. This second report also emphasized the importance of aligning payment policies with quality improvement, and changing the ways in which health professionals are regulated and accredited [5].

This article examines the quality chasm as it applies to anesthesiologists, and current efforts to close the gap. The current methods of judging clinical competence, such as licensure and certification, in contrast to the evolving Accreditation Council for Graduate Medical Education (ACGME) outcomes project and the American Board of Anesthesiology (ABA) Maintenance of Certification in Anesthesiology (MOCA), are investigated. The traditional role of peer review in judging clinical competence and its importance in affecting changes in physician behavior are delineated. The article also takes a critical look at the ability of existing national database registries, such as the National Practitioner Data Bank (NPDB), to judge clinical competence, and compares this with the mission and vision of the emerging Anesthesia Quality Institute (AQI). The taboo areas of judging clinical competence for the aging anesthesiologist and those returning to the work force after recovery from substance abuse disorders are also examined.

LICENSURE AND CERTIFICATION
The 10th Amendment of the United States Constitution authorizes states, and other licensing jurisdictions, such as United States territories and the District of

Columbia, to establish laws and regulations to protect the health, safety, and welfare of their citizens. Medicine is a regulated profession because of the potential harm to the public if an incompetent or impaired physician is allowed to practice. To protect the public from incompetent or impaired physicians, state medical boards license physicians, investigate complaints, discipline those who violate the law, conduct physician evaluations, and facilitate rehabilitation of physicians where appropriate. There are currently 70 state medical boards authorized to regulate allopathic and osteopathic physicians.

Obtaining an initial license to practice medicine in the United States is a rigorous process. State medical boards universally ensure that physicians seeking licensure have met predetermined qualifications that include graduation from an approved medical school, postgraduate training of 1 to 3 years, background checks of professional behavior with verification by personal references, and passage of a national medical licensing examination. All states currently require applicants to pass the United States Medical Licensing Examination (USMLE), or past equivalent. Passing the USMLE is a 3-step process. Step 1 assesses whether the applicant understands and can apply the basic sciences to the practice of medicine, including scientific principles required for maintenance of competence through lifelong learning. This assessment is in the form of an examination made up of multiple-choice questions with one best answer. Step 2 assesses the clinical knowledge and skills essential for the provision of safe and competent patient care under supervision. The clinical knowledge assessment is also in the form of an examination made up of multiple-choice questions, but the clinical skills assessment uses standardized patient models to test an applicant's ability to gather information from patients, perform physical examinations, and communicate their findings to patients and colleagues. Step 3 assesses whether an applicant can apply medical knowledge and understanding of biomedical and clinical science in the unsupervised practice of medicine, with emphasis on patient management in ambulatory settings. This part of the USMLE also takes the form of an examination made up of multiple-choice questions. Although initial medical licensure relies heavily on examinations composed of multiple-choice questions, most agree that it is a moderately rigorous process with sufficient state oversight to assure initial physician competence and to provide a measure of valuable public protection [6].

Although the achievement of licensure to practice medicine is generally accepted as adequate assurance of initial competence, the processes in place for assessment of continuing competence have raised increasing concern among medical professionals, licensing authorities, and other interested parties, including the general public. After physicians are initially licensed, they must renew their license to practice medicine every 2 to 3 years to continue their active status. During this renewal process, physicians must show that they have maintained acceptable standards of professional conduct and medical practice as shown by a review of the NPDB, the Federation Physician Data Center, and other sources of public information held by the states. In most states, physicians must also show they have participated in a program of continuing medical education and are in good health. These criteria are often satisfied by a declaration by the physician that he or she has completed approximately 40 hours of continuing medical education over the past 2 years, and has continued in the active practice of medicine with no known physical or mental impediments to that practice. The renewal process does not involve an examination of knowledge, practical demonstration of competence, or peer review of practice [7].

PEER REVIEW

In 1986, Governor Mario Cuomo of New York State announced his plan to have physician credentials periodically recertified as part of the renewal process for medical licensure. He convened the New York State Advisory Committee on Physician Recredentialing, which subsequently recommended physicians be given 3 options for satisfying the requirements of relicensure. These options included: (1) specialty board certification and recertification, (2) examination of knowledge and problem-solving ability, and (3) peer review in accord with standardized protocols. In 1989, the New York State Society of Anesthesiologists (NYSSA) began developing a model program of quality assurance and peer review to meet the evolving requirements for the recredentialing and relicensure of anesthesiologists in New York State. In that same year, the ASA endorsed a peer review model, developed by Vitez [8,9], which created error profiles for comparison of practitioners. The NYSSA modified this model for the purpose of recredentialing and relicensure of anesthesiologists with the belief that standardized peer review was the only appropriate method for identifying patterns of human error in anesthesiologists [10]. The NYSSA hoped that a standardized peer review model would permit development of a statewide clinical profile containing the performance of all anesthesiologists practicing in the state. Conventional statistical methods would then be used to compare the clinical profiles of individual anesthesiologists with the statewide profile to identify outliers who may need remediation.

The NYSSA model program was never instituted in New York State because the recommendations of the New York State Advisory Committee on Physician Recredentialing were never enacted into New York public health law. Many statewide professional review boards, and the NPDB, track deviations from accepted standards of care, but lack individual denominator data to determine error rates. Therefore, the concept of identifying clinical outliers among anesthesiologists by error profiles has never been tested and may not be feasible. Individual denominator data are available to departments of anesthesiology in the form of administrative billing data and, when combined with a structured peer review model, can produce individual rates of human error. However, it is unlikely that the number of patients treated by an anesthesiologist offers enough statistical power to use rate of human error as a feasible means of judging clinical competence.

In a recent study of 323,879 anesthetics administered at a university practice using a structured peer review of adverse events, 104 of these adverse events were attributed to human error for a rate of 3.2 per 10,000 anesthetics. With this knowledge, faculty of this university practice were asked what rate of human error by an anesthesiologist would indicate the need for remedial training, and suggest incompetence. The median human error rates believed to indicate the need for remedial training and suggest incompetence were 10 and 12.5 per 10,000 anesthetics, respectively. Power analysis tells us that, if we were willing to be wrong about 1 out of 100 anesthesiologists judged to be incompetent (alpha error of 0.01) and 1 out 20 anesthesiologists judged to be competent (beta error of 0.05), then sample sizes of 21,600 anesthetics per anesthesiologist would be required [11]. Even at these unacceptably high levels of alpha and beta error, an appropriate sample size could require more than 2 decades to collect. Therefore, the concept of using human error rates to judge clinical competence is not feasible and this has implications for all database registries designed for this purpose.

CLOSED CLAIMS AND THE NPDB

The *Health Care Quality Improvement Act of 1986* led to the establishment of the NPDB, an information clearinghouse designed to collect and release certain information related to the professional competence and conduct of physicians. The establishment of the NPDB was believed to be an important step by the US Government to enhance professional review efforts by making certain information concerning medical malpractice payments and adverse actions publicly available. As noted earlier, the NPDB lacks the denominator data necessary to determine individual provider error rates to judge clinical competence. Even if individual denominator data were available, malpractice closed claims data are also likely to lack the statistical power necessary to be a feasible measure of clinical competence. For example, in a study of 37,924 anesthetics performed at a university health care network between 1992 and 1994, 18 cases involved legal action directed at an anesthesia provider. An anesthesiologist was the sole defendant named in 2 malpractice claims, only one of which resulted in a $60,000 award. A single letter of intent also named an anesthesiologist as the sole defendant. In the 15 additional legal actions, an anesthesia provider was named as codefendant in 3 claims and implicated in 12 letters of intent. The incidence of all legal actions against the anesthesia practitioners in this sample was 4.7 per 10,000 anesthetics, and the single judgment against a practitioner in this sample represents a closed claims incidence of 0.26 per 10,000 anesthetics [12].

More importantly, there may be no relationship between malpractice litigation and human errors by anesthesiologists. In the sample that yielded 18 cases involving legal action, there were a total of 229 adverse events that resulted in disabling patient injuries. Of these 229 disabling patient injuries, 13 were considered by peer review to have resulted from human error, or deviations from the standard of care, on the part of the anesthesia provider. The rate of anesthetist error leading to disabling patient injuries, therefore, was 3.4 per 10,000 anesthetics. Comparison of legal action and deviations from the standard of care showed the 2 groups to be statistically unrelated. None of the 13 cases in which a disabling injury was caused by deviations from the standard of care, as determined by peer review, resulted in legal action; and none of the 18 cases involving legal action was believed to be due to human error on the part of the anesthesia provider. Therefore, closed malpractice claims lack both statistical power and face validity as a measure of competence [12].

INDICATORS OF CLINICAL COMPETENCE AND FACE VALIDITY

Malpractice claims are not the only indicator of clinical competence that may lack validity. The first anesthesia clinical indicators developed in the United States came from the Joint Commission (TJC), formerly known as the Joint Commission on Accreditation of Healthcare Organizations. These original 13 anesthesia clinical indicators (Box 1) were adverse perioperative events that were intended to trigger a peer review process to assess the contribution of anesthesia care. Before the release of these indicators in 1992, TJC conducted alpha testing for face validity and ease of data collection in a limited number of health care facilities. After their initial release, these indicators were subjected to beta testing, in which similar characteristics were evaluated in a broader range of health care organizations. Following the completion of the beta phase in 1993, the original 13 anesthesia clinical indicators were

---

Box 1: Anesthesia clinical indicators drafted in 1992 by TJC[a]

Central nervous system complication during or within 2 postprocedure days*

Peripheral neurologic deficit during or within 2 postprocedure days*

Acute myocardial infarction during or within 2 postprocedure days*

Cardiac arrest during or within 1 postprocedure day*

Unplanned respiratory arrest during or within 1 postprocedure day

Death of patients during or within 2 postprocedure days*

Unplanned admission of patients to the hospital within 1 postprocedure day

Unplanned admission of patients to the intensive care unit within 1 postprocedure day

Fulminant pulmonary edema developed during or within 1 postprocedure day

Aspiration pneumonitis occurring during or within 2 postprocedure days

Postural headache within 4 postprocedure days after spinal or epidural anesthesia

Dental injury during procedure involving anesthesia care

Ocular injury during procedure involving anesthesia care

[a] The original 13 anesthesia clinical indicators developed in the United States by TJC were reduced to 5 perioperative performance indicators* after testing for face validity and feasibility of data collection.

reduced by TJC to 5 perioperative performance indicators in an effort to make them applicable to a broader range of institutions and to emphasize that these adverse outcomes are not specific to errors in anesthesia care.

Similarly, a recent systematic review by Haller and colleagues [13] identified 108 clinical indicators related to anesthesia care, and nearly half of these measures were affected by some surgical or postoperative ward care. Using the definitions of Donabedian [14], 42% of these indicators were process measures, 57% were outcome measures, and 1% related to structure. All were felt to have some face validity, but validity assessment relied solely on expert opinion 60% of the time. Perhaps more disconcerting, the investigators found that only 38% of proscriptive process measures were based on large randomized control trials or systematic reviews [13].

METRIC ATTRIBUTES

Although showing the validity of performance measures should be necessary for judging clinical competence, it may not be sufficient when these performance measures are intended to influence physician reimbursement for patient care. In 2005, a group of 250 physicians and medical managers from across the United States convened a conference to produce a consensus statement on how "outcomes-based compensation arrangements should be developed to align health care toward evidence-based medicine, affordability and public accountability for how resources are used." This consensus statement recommended several important attributes for measures included in pay-for-performance (P4P), or value-based compensation, programs. These attributes included high volume, high gravity, strong evidence basis, a gap between current and ideal practice, and good prospects for quality improvement, in addition to the already discussed reliability, validity, and feasibility [15]. A high-volume measure examines frequently experienced processes and outcomes of care, or common structural attributes, whereas high gravity implies that there is a large potential effect on health associated with the metric. Although most agree that there should be evidence of linkage between a change in a measure and its related outcomes, it must be accepted that this linkage can be dynamic. Take, for example, the changing evidence linkage between the use of perioperative β-blockers and its effect on perioperative cardiac events in certain patient populations. Therefore, performance measure must be maintained in a manner similar to practice guidelines with periodic assessments of the evidence and gap. As the gap between current and ideal practice closes, P4P measures are likely to be retired by payers [15].

GUIDING PRINCIPLES FOR THE MANAGEMENT OF PERFORMANCE MEASURES

In 1997, the ASA established the Ad Hoc Committee on Performance Based Credentialing, which created Guidelines for Delineation of Clinical Privileges. These guidelines suggest that performance measures, compared with benchmarks, should be considered in the delineation of clinical privileges in anesthesiology. Because national benchmarks did not exist, the Ad Hoc Committee on Performance Based Credentialing became the standing Committee on Performance and Outcome Measures (CPOM), in 2001. The first order of business for CPOM was to develop Guidelines for (Performance & Outcomes) Database Management by the American Society of Anesthesiologists that has evolved into Guiding Principles for the Management of Performance Measures by the American Society of Anesthesiologists. This document, last modified in 2005, describes the development and maintenance of clinical indicators (clinical outcomes, processes of care, and perceptions of care) and administrative indicators (resource use and personnel management) by the ASA. These indicators, or performance measures, could then be collected and stored in a relational database along with demographic data about providers. The ASA did not believe that participation should be required for any aspect of their database registry, but did recognize that, with time, there may be increasing external pressures to participate. In 2005, CPOM believed these pressures were likely to come from national, regional, or local organizations that demand evidence of participation in an outcomes database system, or require the comparison of the outcomes of groups or individual providers with national benchmarks [16]. Carolyn Clancy, Director of the Agency for Healthcare Research and Quality (AHRQ), confirmed this sentiment in July 2009, when she stated that physicians who want to obtain government funds should prepare themselves by using registries to collect data [17].

CLINICAL OUTCOME REGISTRIES AND THE AQI

In October 2008, the ASA House of Delegates approved funding for the AQI that was chartered in December of the same year. Although established by the ASA, the AQI is a separate organization that intends to become the primary source of information for performance measurement, and subsequent quality improvement, in the clinical practice of anesthesiology. This information is managed in the National Anesthesia Clinical Outcomes Registry (NACOR). The AQI expects to have 20 anesthesia groups participating in NACOR by the end of 2010. Currently, the bulk of the data being collected are electronic claims data, but the plan for the future is to collect data from automated anesthesia records [18].

Although an administrative data source answers questions about case type and case length, it is not suited for judging physician performance. The validity of administrative data to measure clinical performance, or lend applicability to risk adjustment, has been challenged. Lee and colleagues [19] showed that administrative data could fail to detect up to 55% of cases of preexisting renal disease, nearly 65% of previous myocardial infarctions, and 75% of preexisting cerebrovascular disease. In a more recent study, Romano and colleagues [20] compared National Surgical Quality Improvement Project (NSQIP) data, which were manually abstracted from medical records, with AHRQ Patient Safety Indicators, which were collected via the administrative system based on International Classification of Diseases, Ninth Revision (Clinically

Modified) (ICD-9-CM), and found that the latter missed 44% of cases of pulmonary embolus or deep venous thrombosis, 68% of postoperative sepsis, 71% of wound dehiscence, and 80% of the occurrences of postoperative respiratory failure. This lack of validity of administrative data, and the perception that the federal government lacks sufficient concern over assuring validity in hospital comparison data that are made public, have led some anesthesiologists to suggest that the best course of action for AQI would be to combine forces with the American College of Surgeons (ACS) in the development of NSQIP in the public sector [21].

The NSQIP was developed by the Veterans Health Administration (VHA) in response to a 1986 congressional mandate to report risk-adjusted surgical outcomes annually, and to compare their outcomes with national averages. Perioperative performance measurement had not advanced to the point at which risk-adjusted national averages existed. In response, NSQIP developed risk-adjustment models for 30-day morbidity and mortality after major surgery in 8 surgical subspecialties and for all operations combined.

Measuring only performance and making the data public seems to have had a profound effect. In NSQIP's first 10 years, the 30-day postoperative mortality decreased by 27%. Beginning with a 30-day mortality of 3.1% for major surgery in 1991, it decreased to 2.2% in 2002. An even more dramatic decline has been seen in postoperative morbidity. The number of patients undergoing major surgery in the NSQIP who experienced one or more of 20 predefined postoperative complications decreased from 17.8% to 9.8% in 10 years. The median length of stay declined by 5 days. Although data are unpublished, NSQIP administrators believed that these initial results justified the cost [22].

The cost of NSQIP data collection and analysis has been quoted at approximately $38 per case. The VHA database is expanding by approximately 100,000 cases annually and currently has more than 1 million cases. Thus, the cost to date has been more than $38 million dollars, yet private sector hospitals are still lining up to participate as they expand this project beyond the VHA hospitals under the auspices of the ACS. In ACS NSQIP, each hospital is expected to pay $35,000 annually, plus the cost of a trained nurse data collector, which should be about $50,000 per year, depending on regional wages. The VHA made this investment because of a 1986 Congressional mandate to compare their outcomes with national benchmarks after accusations of substandard care for veterans. When compared with 14 academic centers in the private sector, the VHA showed comparable morbidity and mortality, but that was after the VHA had maximized their initial improvement. Maybe continued improvement is no longer possible, leaving the continued high cost of database management unjustified [22].

Physician Consortium for Performance Improvement

External pressures to improve accountability for the practice of anesthesiology have come from several sources. In 1997, the American Medical Association (AMA) introduced the American Medical Accreditation Program (AMAP), in partnership with state and county medical associations and national medical specialty societies, as a method for physicians to submit their credentials to multiple health care organizations in a single approved format. Physicians who were associated with multiple health plans and hospitals underwent fragmented and duplicative processes for credentialing, and were often evaluated against multiple, and sometimes conflicting, criteria [23]. Before AMAP, no nationally recognized program existed for individual physician accreditation. To satisfy the increasing demand for physician accountability, this standardized credentialing system was to include AMAP-approved physician level performance measures. Although AMAP failed from a business standpoint [24], it spawned the Physician Consortium for Performance Improvement (PCPI), an amalgam of committees that previously advised AMAP. This physician-led consortium included representatives of the 24 national medical specialty societies comprising the American Board of Medical Specialties (ABMS) and was charged with developing evidence-based clinical performance measures that would enhance quality of patient care and foster accountability. Today, PCPI comprises more than 170 national medical specialty societies, state medical societies, the ABMS member boards, Council of Medical Specialty Societies, health care professional organizations, federal agencies, individual members and others interested in improving the quality of patient care and accountability of physicians.

Performance Measures Relevant to Anesthesiology

As of October 2007, the PCPI, in conjunction with the ASA, had produced 5 measures relevant to anesthesiology and critical care [25]. These measures are geared toward:

1. Reducing surgical site infection through appropriate timing of prophylactic antibiotics
2. Preventing catheter-related bloodstream infections through adherence to a catheter insertion protocol
3. Improving perioperative temperature management by using active warming devices
4. Reducing stress ulcer disease through prophylaxis of ventilated patients
5. Preventing ventilator-associated pneumonia through head elevation.

Other measures relevant to anesthesiologists are shown in Box 2.

Although these measures were designed for individual quality improvement, PCPI believes that these measures are appropriate for accountability if methodological, statistical, and implementation rules are achieved. Because these are process measures, risk adjustment is not required as long as appropriate exclusions are applied to the denominator when measuring compliance rates. For process measures, PCPI provides 3 categories of reasons for which a patient may be excluded from the denominator of an individual measure: medical reasons (eg, not indicated or contraindicated); patient reasons (eg, patient declines for economic, social or religious reasons); or system reasons (eg, resources not available, or payor-related limitations) [26].

> **Box 2: Performance measures relevant to the practice of anesthesiology**
>
> *Measures copyrighted by the AMA PCPI*
>
> Timing of Prophylactic Antibiotics – Administering Physician©
>
> Prevention of Ventilator-Associated Pneumonia – Head Elevation©
>
> Prevention of Catheter-Related Bloodstream Infections (CRBSI) – Catheter Insertion Protocol©
>
> Stress Ulcer Disease (SUD) Prophylaxis Considered in Ventilated Patients©
>
> Perioperative Temperature Management© for Surgical Procedures
>
> *Measures under development/consideration by the AMA PCPI*
>
> Perioperative Cardiac Risk Assessment (History and Current Symptoms)
>
> Avoidance of Electrocardiogram Overuse (for patients undergoing low-risk surgical procedures)
>
> Perioperative Continuation of β-Blockers
>
> *Measures proposed by the ASA Committee on Performance and Outcomes Measurement in 2007[a]*
>
> Pencil-Point Spinal Needles – Reduction of Postdural Puncture Headache
>
> Management of Postoperative Hypothermia
>
> Patient Education – Postoperative Analgesia
>
> Preoperative Fasting Status (Clear Liquids)
>
> Treatment of Postoperative Shivering with Meperidine
>
> [a] These proposed measures are committee work products and not necessarily endorsed by the ASA.

Physician Quality Reporting Initiative

The first 3 PCPI measures listed earlier have already been incorporated into the Center for Medicare and Medicaid Services (CMS) Physician Quality Reporting Initiative (PQRI). In this pay-for-reporting initiative, successfully reporting on 80% of the patients included in all 3 measures can earn up to 2% of the total Medicare Part B allowed charges for covered professional services [27]. Reporting is carried out via the Medicare claims form as CPT II codes/modifiers. Although PQRI is currently a pay-for-reporting initiative with positive financial incentives, it is likely to evolve into a pay-for-performance system with negative financial incentives for poor performers.

Judging Clinical Competence Under Special Circumstances

Although judging clinical competence is difficult for all physicians, certain situations make this a particularly daunting task for anesthesiologists. These situations include physicians in training, physicians approaching the end of their careers, and physicians returning to work after recovering from a substance abuse disorder. Common to these situations is the dynamic nature of clinical competence and the potential for rapid change. Rapid changes in clinical competence can be associated with patient harm, if the warning signs are not recognized and appropriate steps are not taken.

Anesthesiologists in Training

The most straightforward time to evaluate a physician's competence is when they are in training, because evaluation during medical education is the most developed. At this stage the obstacles to certification are significant. Accredited medical schools and residencies are overseen by the Accreditation Council of Graduate Medical Education (ACGME), which has established guidelines for the competency-based educational component of graduate medical education. There are formal requirements for continuous performance evaluation with feedback to students and residents. In addition, residents are required to evaluate their programs to ensure that their educational needs are being met. The ABMS has established certification as a rigorous process, in which success requires passing written and oral board examinations. Thus, initial certification is, in many ways, the gold standard against which future physician evaluation should be measured.

The ACGME is a private, nonprofit council that evaluates and accredits medical residency programs in the United States. ACGME's Outcome Project requires residency programs to teach 6 core competencies, create tools to assess learning of the competencies, and to use the assessment data for program and resident improvement. The ACGME summarizes the change from a minimal threshold model to one that looks at the success of programs in teaching the 6 core competencies.

In the competency-based model, toward which the Outcome Project is directed, programs are asked to show how residents have achieved competency-based educational objectives and, in turn, how programs use information drawn from evaluation of those objectives to improve the educational experience of the residents. The minimal threshold model identifies whether a program has the potential to educate residents; the competency-based model examines whether the program is educating them.

The 6 core competencies are:

- patient care
- medical knowledge
- practice-based learning and improvement
- interpersonal and communication skills
- professionalism
- systems-based practice.

Traditionally, anesthesia residents have been evaluated directly by their supervising faculty members, and in many cases they are judged by their performance on the In-Training Examination. The Outcome Project asks for more rigorous and detailed evaluation of residents. It seeks reliable tools to assess each of the competencies listed earlier. Global resident evaluations and In-Training Examinations should remain, but training programs need to have more refined performance evaluation tools [28]. The University of Florida, for example, has attempted to connect resident evaluation to evidence-based clinical outcomes. Clinical process measures are identified with high levels of existing data supporting their use (eg, aspirin for acute myocardial infarction). Next, the residents are evaluated in terms of success in applying these measures. Then, the feedback is used to improve resident performance and patient care. Clinical deficiencies can be used to help improve the program, and therefore to identify gaps in didactics [29].

Anesthesiology programs are likely to have a more difficult time implementing high-quality evidence-based outcomes measures to evaluate resident performance than other specialty training programs, such as internal medicine. As noted earlier, the lack of valid, risk-adjusted, outcome measures in anesthesiology makes comparative performance assessment difficult. The limited number of evidenced-based performance measures makes it impossible to use such data to evaluate overall resident performance. A concrete example of this is the resident who times the administration of prophylactic antibiotics perfectly, but thinks that every episode of tachycardia in the operating room should immediately be treated with β-blockers.

The mission of the ABMS is:

> To provide assurance to the public that a physician specialist certified by a Member Board of the ABMS has successfully completed an approved educational program and evaluation process, which includes an examination designed to assess the knowledge, skills, and experience required to provide quality patient care in that specialty [30].

On further examination, one might challenge the underlying significance of performance measurement during medical school and residency training. One might even challenge the belief that certified practitioners are better than noncertified practitioners. However, starting with medical school, lack of professional behavior is predictive of poor career performance. In a 2005 publication in the *New England Journal of Medicine*, a group from the University of California at San Francisco reported that disciplinary action among practicing physicians by medical boards is strongly associated with unprofessional behavior in medical school. They concluded "professionalism should have a central role in medical academics and throughout one's medical career" [31]. The same group found that examination performance and professionalism ratings during internal medicine residency were associated with a lower risk of subsequent disciplinary action [32]. Within anesthesiology, there has been validation of the faculty evaluation of residents' clinical skills as a predictor of their subsequent success on the certification examination. Furthermore, there is a strong association between failure of the certification examination and deficiency in personality traits associated with successful practice of anesthesiology [33]. A more recent study showed the expected connection between success on the ABA In-Training Examination (taken during residency) and shortest time to ABA certification [34].

Certification and quality are also linked once resident training is completed. In both cardiology and surgery, several studies have found an association between certification and compliance with guidelines and, in some cases, lower mortality [35].

In addition, a study of midcareer anesthesiologists links poor outcomes to nonboard-certified physicians [36]. Thirty-day mortality and failure-to-rescue rates were higher for noncertified anesthesiologists than for their certified counterparts in midcareer. The investigators looked at midcareer anesthesiologists to allow ample time to have attempted certification, and to exclude older physicians who trained when there was less emphasis on board certification. Although this retrospective review of Medicare claims data suggests an association between lack of ABA certification and poor outcomes, it cannot prove causation. The hospitals with more noncertified anesthesiologists had poorer outcomes, but the patients who go to such hospitals may also be different (less healthy in both measured and unmeasured dimensions) than those who go to hospitals with certified anesthesiologists.

The Aging Anesthesiologist

A combination of demographic and economic factors has led to forecasts predicting continued demand for older anesthesiologists. An older population has increased need for surgery, and this, combined with the shortage of anesthesiologists trained in the 1990s, leads to a future shortfall in anesthesiologists to care for these patients [37]. In addition, the recent downturn in retirement accounts may lead to physicians opting to work later in life. Aging anesthesiologists present particular challenges for at least 2 reasons. First, the scope of the problem is enormous: all anesthesiologists are aging. Second, there is no discreet moment at which one's practice goes from experienced to obsolete. Losing skills parallels physical aging: it happens gradually, but eventually it happens to all of us.

Katz [38] highlighted the myriad of complex issues facing the aging anesthesiologist in a review article. Although potentially we gain wisdom and experience as we age, we are also subject to physical and mental changes that may impede our ability to continue to practice safely in the dynamic operating room environment. Normal age-associated physical and cognitive decline makes the practice of anesthesiology particularly challenging as we age. Contrary to the widely held assumption that age-related cognitive decline typically occurs in our 70s, recent evidence suggests it begins in our 20s. Timothy Salthouse and his laboratory at the University of Virginia have examined decline across 4 cognitive dimensions: vocabulary, pattern recognition speed, memory, and reasoning. Vocabulary increases into our 50s, but all other components of cognitive function show substantial decline beginning in our 20s (Fig. 1). The magnitude of the age-related cognitive decline in speed, pattern recognition, and memory are more substantial

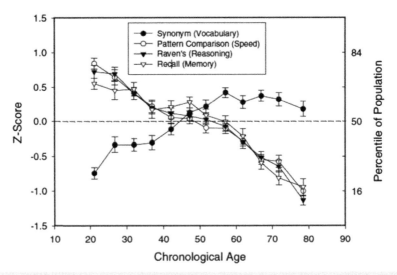

Fig. 1. Cognitive function declines linearly with age starting in our 20s. Means (and standard errors) of performance in four cognitive tests as a function of age. Each data point is based on between 52 and 150 adults. (*Data from* Salthouse TA. What and when of cognitive aging. Curr Dir Psychol Sci 2004;13:140–4.)

than most of us realize: "Performance for adults in their early 20s was near the 75th percentile in the population, whereas the average for adults in their early 70s was near the 20th percentile" [39].

In light of such significant cognitive decline, how can anesthesiologists continue to function well into their 50s and 60s? First, cognitive ability is only one element of successful performance of a task. We draw on motivation and persistence, as well as patience, which may not decline with age. Second, we can adapt our environment to avoid negative consequences of our cognitive decline. Anesthesia is often practiced in a care team model. In that setting, a physician may hide diminished skills by allowing others to do the more challenging tasks. Even in a personally administered care setting, those organizing the schedule may often assign less complicated cases to those with limited skills. Familiarity of environment (practice setting/case mix) may minimize cognitive challenges as we age. In addition, safe care demands that we ask for help when we have trouble with a given task; thus, it is good practice to seek help. Salthouse and his colleagues found that increases in knowledge and experience may offset cognitive decline; for example, older adults perform remarkably well on crossword puzzles compared with their younger counterparts.

Because anesthesiology is a form of shift work, it is important to remark on the interaction between aging and shift work. The effect is not at all straightforward. Age is associated with well-recognized patterns of sleep disturbance, but vigilance under conditions of extreme sleep deprivation is diminished more in younger than in older workers [40]. Conversely, need for recovery (an index of fatigue) after shift work is increased in older workers [41]. Older workers perform well, remaining vigilant during long shifts, but have more trouble with recovery from those shifts. Aging anesthesiologists would be expected, then, still to perform well at night but to have more trouble with the postcall recovery.

Clinical competence, as judged by ABA certification, is not based on a recertification examination for anyone who has been certified since 1999. Therefore, those anesthesiologists whose training is most out of date are exempt from the MOCA recertification process. Residencies have only recently incorporated lifelong learning as a competency required of their graduates, and previous anesthesiology professional training may not have adequately prepared the aging anesthesiologist for the challenges they face. Those anesthesiologists participating in MOCA are required to maintain professional standing acceptable to the ABA and to show cognitive expertise through written examination every 10 years. In addition, MOCA requires practice performance assessment and improvement that includes simulation-based education during the 10-year cycle. If MOCA evolves from simulation-based education to simulation-based assessment at more frequent intervals, it may offer another means of competency assessment for the aging anesthesiologist.

Acting on age-related decline in competency does have legal implications. These legal issues can be complex, but some background information is useful. The Age Discrimination in Employment Act of 1967 (ADEA) protects individuals who are 40 years of age or older from employment discrimination based on age. There are some notable exceptions and the 2 most important are:

1. The employer is terminating an individual's employment for good cause.

ADEA is not meant to prohibit termination with cause. If there are reasonable grounds for termination with cause, ADEA does not prevent that.

2. Age is a Bona Fide Occupational Qualification (BFOQ).

This is the basis on which pilots and police officers are often age limited: age is an essential proxy to protect public safety.

The burden of proof for BFOQ lies with the employer and can be severe. For example, the Supreme Court found that just because airlines can limit pilot duties, this does not mean that pilots cannot continue to work as flight engineers [42,43]. According to a 2005 study by Altman Weil, a law firm consultancy, 57% of law firms with 100 or more attorneys enforce a mandatory retirement age, which typically ranges from ages 65 to 75 years [44]. Most law firms are arranged as partnerships among owners and, therefore, may be exempt from the age discrimination claims that would arise if an employer were to have a mandatory retirement for employees. Employers using the BFOQ defense against charges of age discrimination must show either: (1) that it is reasonable to believe that all or most employees of a certain age cannot perform the job safely, or (2) that it is impossible or highly impractical to test employees' abilities to tackle all tasks associated with the job on an individualized basis. For example, an employer who refuses to hire anyone more than 60 years old as a pilot has a potential BFOQ defense if there is a reasonable basis for concluding that pilots aged 60 years or older pose significant safety risks, or that it is not feasible to test older pilots individually. In light of the substantial legal burden on employers wishing to enact age-based retirement rules, mandatory retirement policies are likely to continue to face legal hurdles preventing them from becoming widespread within anesthesiology. Therefore, a more feasible goal is to develop practical performance measures, and to enhance CME requirements; replacing educational vacations with simulation-based training.

Recovery from Substance Abuse Disorders

It is widely known that anesthesiologists are at risk for substance abuse. According to one study, there is a 34% increased rate of death from accidental overdose [45]. Another study showed a 7-fold increase in risk of substance abuse among anesthesia residents compared with other fields [46]. Although the impaired physician would likely be one whose performance is poor, there are no clear data to support this hypothesis. Many believe that impairment itself implies a substantial performance deficiency in a field whose motto is "Vigilance." We lack the technology and infrastructure to perform rigorous simulation assessments required to show retained competence of older anesthesiologists. In time, computer-based simulation exercises may reassure us that an aging physician is still fit for the task (analogous to Federal Aviation Administration pilot requirements). By contrast, there is no examination, peer review, or simulation training for a physician recovering from a substance abuse disorder that could establish conclusively if or when it is safe to return to work.

Most providers with a history of substance abuse are allowed to return to work with mandatory surveillance. Despite this, there is a tremendous relapse rate. High rates of recidivism likely stem from easy access to drugs, stressful work conditions, and poorly understood physiologic predisposition to addiction [47]. Coexisting psychiatric illness and family history have been found to be predictive of relapse [48]. In a study of drug- and alcohol-abusing patients who underwent liver transplantation, an additional predictor of relapse included being less than 1 year beyond a time of previous alcohol abuse [49]. A recent editorial from the Mayo Clinic, published in *Anesthesiology*, called for a sea change in our approach to the impaired anesthesiologist. They called for a "one strike and you're out" policy that would bar the substance-abusing physician from future anesthesia practice. Substance abusers could retrain in another field of medicine that has fewer environmental triggers for relapse [50].

Assessing the fitness of a recovering addict to return to work has some features in common with assessing the competency of a resident or an aging physician. However, an important distinction is that in one case we are assessing quality of medical care and in the other we are looking for signs that a poorly understood clandestine behavior or disease is recurring or remains in remission. For the recovering addict there is little evidence to show that they are at low risk for relapse. The ethical questions raised here are common to many of these issues. How should we balance the rights of the individual against the rights of the community? Is it really just to maintain that there is no course of treatment an impaired physician could undergo, and no amount of time without relapse, that would allow the likelihood of safe practice? And, although we may believe that we are standing on principle, are we really? If the principle is to absolutely protect our patients from physicians who are potentially impaired, then should we not strictly apply an age limit in the field (if it were legal) because practitioners in their 70s and 80s are more likely to suffer from dementia? Substance abuse presents many of the same issues as aging; in both cases, it is a challenge to evaluate competence in an environment with the potential for rapid change and the potential for patient harm.

Policing Our Own in Anesthesiology

Many physicians ask, "If we had an independent measure of a licensed, certified practitioner's competence, would we really need to use it?" Should not physicians themselves determine whether or not they are competent? The answer is, definitely not. Human beings are poor at assessing their own expertise. According to the British philosopher Bertrand Russell, "the trouble with the world is that the stupid are cocksure, and the intelligent are full of doubt" [51]. The problem has come to be known as the Kruger-Dunning effect [52]. These 2 psychologists studied competence in many areas and found that in virtually every area:

1. Incompetent individuals overestimate their own level of skill
2. Incompetent individuals fail to recognize genuine skill in others
3. Incompetent individuals fail to recognize the extremity of their inadequacy.

It is difficult, unwise, and ultimately dangerous, to depend on self-assessment as a way of safeguarding patients from unskilled practitioners. Most professions suffer from this same problem, as discussed in the recent book, *Why We Make Mistakes* [53].

In a recent article in the *New England Journal of Medicine*, 2 leaders of the modern patient safety movement addressed the lack of individual accountability within hospitals [54]. Wachter and Pronovost provide a scathing assessment of the failure of hospitals and physicians to police their colleagues on such basic measures as hand hygiene. Virtually all of the focus of modern patient safety literature has focused on system failures, which are important, but there has been little attention to the consequences of the failing physician. In many cases, one's colleagues know that a practitioner is a low performance outlier and yet fail to intervene. This situation happens in many cases because there is little institutional, or departmental, support for genuinely holding physicians accountable. Generally speaking, only when there is a negative financial consequence, such as incomplete charts or malpractice litigation, do hospitals hold practitioners truly accountable. In situations as obvious as failure to wash one's hands, hospitals and departments usually look the other way.

Wachter and Pronovost summarize the problem as follows. In the first decade of the patient safety movement, the focus was on systems issues and engineering solutions (eg, computerized order entry and checklists). However, identification of system-wide safety problems is hindered when employees fail to report near misses or mistakes. Creating a culture for hospital workers to speak up when they see signs of an unsafe environment within their organization has been conflated with a false imperative to create a no-blame culture. No-blame must not become no-consequences-for-any-action, no matter how dangerous, or how clear the rules. The concept that we constantly hold physicians accountable to a high set of standards is the justification for many of our own professional societies' assertions that government should leave physician regulation to physicians. Wachter and Pronovost conclude that without self-regulation we will face more public regulation:

> Part of the reason we must do this is that if we do not, other stakeholders, such as regulators and state legislatures, are likely to judge the reflexive invocation of the "no blame" approach as an example of guild behavior — of the medical profession circling its wagons to avoid confronting harsh realities, rather than as a thoughtful strategy for attacking the root causes of most errors. With that as their conclusion, they will be predisposed to further intrude on the practice of medicine, using the blunt and often politicized sticks of the legal, regulatory, and payment systems [54].

SUMMARY

Physicians are granted a great deal of autonomy and self-governance as a profession uniquely entrusted to protect their patients. Every major professional medical body attempts to conform to the Hippocratic Oath to "do no harm." This practice contrasts with a norm of allowing physicians to completely self-determine whether they are competent to care for patients, when they should retire, and when it is safe to return to work after recovering from a substance abuse disorder. Anesthesiologists are not required to wait for a death or major disability before limiting a colleague from practicing anesthesia. There must be a point at which loss of skills and obsolescence of knowledge compel us to prevent an anesthesiologist from continuing to treat patients. In an idealized society, that point should come before patient safety is jeopardized. This goal does not begin with a culture of blame and shame, but neither does it stem from a relativistic attitude that any licensed practitioner is equally good as any other. It is a myth that physicians are somehow different from pilots or athletes. Given enough time, through the process of normal aging, all of us lose the requisite skills to practice safely. Defining a specific age at which that happens is likely to be impossible, but the reality is no different for anesthesiologists than it is for pilots. As is often noted, the consequences for the pilot working with outdated skills are more dire for the pilot than they are for a physician. Despite this, independent regulatory bodies still require commercial pilots to undergo rigorous simulator-based assessments twice a year and prohibit them from working beyond age 65 years. In anesthesiology we need to demand independent assessment of competence even for senior members. "Grandfathering in" makes no sense when patient safety and competence are at issue. Anesthesiology, as a profession, must embrace the science of performance measurement and overcome the barriers to judging clinical competence. If anesthesiology is going to remain at the forefront of the patient safety movement, judging clinical competence is going to require better quality metrics with improved statistical power and appropriate risk adjustment, genuine peer assessment of valid indicators, and frequent written examination and assessments in simulated clinical environments.

References

[1] Committee on Quality of Health Care in America, Institute of Medicine. To err is human: building a safer health care system. In: Kohn L, Corrigan JM, Donaldson MS, editors. Washington, DC: National Academy Press; 1999. p. 241.

[2] Sentinel events: approaches to error reduction and prevention. Jt Comm J Qual Improv 1998;24:175–86.

[3] Lagasse RS. Anesthesia safety: model or myth? A review of the published literature and analysis of current original data. Anesthesiology 2002;97:1609–17.

[4] Eichhorn JH. Prevention of intraoperative anesthesia accidents and related severe injury through safety monitoring. Anesthesiology 1989;70:572–7.

[5] Committee on Quality of Health Care in America, Institute of Medicine. Crossing the quality chasm: a new health system for the 21st century. Washington, DC: National Academy Press; 2001. p. 364.

[6] Federation of State Medical Boards. Available at: http://www.fsmb.org/. Accessed August 27, 2010.

[7] Physician Accountability for Physician Competence. Available at: http://innovationlabs.com/ summit. Accessed August 27, 2010.

[8] Vitez TS. A model for quality assurance in anesthesiology. J Clin Anesth 1990;2:280–7.

[9] Vitez T. Judging clinical competence. Park Ridge (IL): American Society of Anesthesiologists; 1989.

[10] Gabel RA. Quality assurance/peer review for recredentialing/relicensure in New York State. Int Anesthesiol Clin 1992;30:93–101.

[11] Lagasse R, Akerman M. The power of peer review: human error rates as a measure of anesthesiologists' clinical competence [abstract]. American Society of Anesthesiologists Annual Meeting. San Diego (CA); 2010. p. A386.

[12] Edbril SD, Lagasse RS. Relationship between malpractice litigation and human errors. Anesthesiology 1999;91:848–55.

[13] Haller G, Stoelwinder J, Myles PS, et al. Quality and safety indicators in anesthesia: a systematic review. Anesthesiology 2009;110:1158–75.

[14] Donabedian A. Explorations in quality assessment and monitoring: the criteria and standards of quality. Ann Arbor (MI): Health Administration Press; 1982.

[15] Fourth Annual Disease Management Outcome Summit. Outcomes-based compensation: pay-for-performance design principles. Nashville (TN): American Healthways, Inc; 2004.

[16] Committee on Performance and Outcome Measures. Annual Report to the ASA House of Delegates. Park Ridge (IL): American Society of Anesthesiologists; 2005.

[17] Johnstone R. Convergence of large group studies and individual performance measures. ASA Newsl 2010;74(5):10–1.

[18] Dutton R. Counterpoint: out with the old, in with the new. ASA Newsl 2010;74(5):18–9.

[19] Lee DS, Donovan L, Austin PC, et al. Comparison of coding of heart failure and comorbidities in administrative and clinical data for use in outcomes research. Med Care 2005;43: 182–8.

[20] Romano PS, Mull HJ, Rivard PE, et al. Validity of selected AHRQ Patient Safety Indicators based on VA National Surgical Quality Improvement Program data. Health Serv Res 2009;44:182–204.

[21] Glance L. A roadmap for the AQI – one anesthesiologist's opinion. ASA Newsl 2010;74(5): 16–7.

[22] Lagasse RS. The right stuff: Veterans Affairs National Surgical Quality Improvement Project. Anesth Analg 2008;107:1772–4.

[23] Kmetik K. Physician performance measurement and improvement in the American Medical Accreditation Program (AMAPSM), Clinical practice applications. Hanover: Medical Outcomes Trust; 1998.

[24] Frieden J. AMAP is dead (American Medical Accreditation Program). Ob Gyn News, March 15. Farmington Hills (MI): Gale Group; 2000.

[25] Committee on Performance and Outcome Measures. Annual Report to the ASA House of Delegates. Park Ridge (IL): American Society of Anesthesiologists; 2007.

[26] American Society of Anesthesiologists and Physician Consortium for Performance Improvement® Anesthesiology and Critical Care Physician Performance Measurement Set. Chicago (IL): American Medical Association; 2007.

[27] Centers for Medicare & Medicaid Services - PQRI Overview. Available at: https://www.cms.gov/pqri/. Accessed August 27, 2010.

[28] Tetzlaff JE. Assessment of competency in anesthesiology. Anesthesiology 2007;106: 812–25.

[29] Haan C, Edwards F, Poole B, et al. A model to begin to use clinical outcomes in medical education. Acad Med 2008;83:574–80.

[30] Jones JW, McCullough LB, Richman BW. Who should protect the public against bad doctors? J Vasc Surg 2005;41:907–10.

[31] Papadakis MA, Teherani A, Banach MA, et al. Disciplinary action by medical boards and prior behavior in medical school. N Engl J Med 2005;353:2673–82.

[32] Papadakis MA, Arnold GK, Blank LL, et al. Performance during internal medicine residency training and subsequent disciplinary action by state licensing boards. Ann Intern Med 2008;148:869–76.

[33] Slogoff S, Hughes FP, Hug CC Jr, et al. A demonstration of validity for certification by the American Board of Anesthesiology. Acad Med 1994;69:740–6.

[34] McClintock JC, Gravlee GP. Predicting success on the certification examinations of the American Board of Anesthesiology. Anesthesiology 2010;112:212–9.

[35] Sutherland K, Leatherman S. Does certification improve medical standards? BMJ 2006;333:439–41.

[36] Silber JH, Kennedy SK, Even-Shoshan O, et al. Anesthesiologist board certification and patient outcomes. Anesthesiology 2002;96:1044–52.

[37] Tremper KK, Shanks A, Morris M. Five-year follow-up on the work force and finances of United States anesthesiology training programs: 2000 to 2005. Anesth Analg 2007;104:863–8.

[38] Katz JD. Issues of concern for the aging anesthesiologist. Anesth Analg 2001;92:1487–92.

[39] Salthouse TA. What and when of cognitive aging. Curr Dir Psychol Sci 2004;13:140–4.

[40] Adam M, Retey JV, Khatami R, et al. Age-related changes in the time course of vigilant attention during 40 hours without sleep in men. Sleep 2006;29:55–7.

[41] Kiss P, De Meester M, Braeckman L. Differences between younger and older workers in the need for recovery after work. Int Arch Occup Environ Health 2008;81:311–20.

[42] Western Airlines v Criswell 472, US 400.

[43] Ford K, Notestine K, Hill R. Fundamentals of employment law: tort and insurance practice section. 2nd edition. Chicago (IL): American Bar Association; 2000.

[44] Jones L. ABA takes stand against mandatory retirement. Natl Law J; 2007. Available at: http://www.law.com/jsp/nlj/PubArticleNLJ.jsp?id=900005488594&slreturn=1&hbxlogin=1. Accessed August 28, 2010.
[45] Alexander BH, Checkoway H, Nagahama SI, et al. Cause-specific mortality risks of anesthesiologists. Anesthesiology 2000;93:922–30.
[46] Talbott GD, Gallegos KV, Wilson PO, et al. The Medical Association of Georgia's Impaired Physicians Program. Review of the first 1000 physicians: analysis of specialty. JAMA 1987;257:2927–30.
[47] Bryson EO, Silverstein JH. Addiction and substance abuse in anesthesiology. Anesthesiology 2008;109:905–17.
[48] Domino KB, Hornbein TF, Polissar NL, et al. Risk factors for relapse in health care professionals with substance use disorders. JAMA 2005;293:1453–60.
[49] Gedaly R, McHugh PP, Johnston TD, et al. Predictors of relapse to alcohol and illicit drugs after liver transplantation for alcoholic liver disease. Transplantation 2008;86:1090–5.
[50] Berge KH, Seppala MD, Lanier WL. The anesthesiology community's approach to opioid- and anesthetic-abusing personnel: time to change course. Anesthesiology 2008;109: 762–4.
[51] Russell B. Marriage and morals. New York: Liveright; 1957.
[52] Kruger J, Dunning D. Unskilled and unaware of it: how difficulties in recognizing one's own incompetence lead to inflated self-assessments. J Pers Soc Psychol 1999;77:1121–34.
[53] Hallinan JT. Why we make mistakes: how we look without seeing, forget things in seconds, and are all pretty sure we are way above average. 1st edition. New York: Broadway Books; 2009.
[54] Wachter RM, Pronovost PJ. Balancing "no blame" with accountability in patient safety. N Engl J Med 2009;361:1401–6.

Advances in Anesthesia 28 (2010) 59–79

ADVANCES IN ANESTHESIA

Ultrasound in Central Venous Cannulation

David B. Auyong, MD, Robert L. Hsiung, MD*

Department of Anesthesiology, Virginia Mason Medical Center, 1100 Ninth Avenue, MS: B2-AN, Seattle, WA 98101, USA

Ore than 5 million central venous catheters (CVCs) are placed yearly [1] for a multitude of indications, and this number is expected to increase due to an aging population. With demands to prevent medical errors coupled with the improvement of portable ultrasound technology, the role of ultrasound guidance in central vein catheterization grows increasingly important. This article is not another meta-analysis, but looks at the significant history behind ultrasound's prominence in guiding central venous access and provides the rationale as to why ultrasound should be adopted in current anesthesia practice. The second part of this article reviews the technical skills with which to achieve success with ultrasound in central venous access.

By the 1980s, ultrasound in central venous catheterization had already been well described [2,3]. Many of the initial studies comparing ultrasound to surface landmarks had differing methodologies that made generalization difficult. For example, the ultrasound-guided dynamic technique is likely superior to the static technique, that is, real-time guidance (visualization and identification of the relevant anatomic structures, tracking the progression of the needle, and confirmation of the guidewire within the target central vein) as compared with ultrasound being used for the sole purpose of anatomic identification and subsequent surface marking before needle insertion [4,5], yet each is considered ultrasound-assisted. In addition, there are differences in what constitutes a failure (number of attempts, an absolute time in procedure, or carotid puncture). Another confounding variation is which surface landmark approach ultrasound is to be judged against, as there are numerous landmark-based approaches. Even in this decade there are still studies [6,7] comparing the "superiority" of one landmark-based approach over another, yet it is uncertain how much operator experience and frequency of CVC placements contributes to success and complication.

Two meta-analyses are worth reviewing, as they are the most frequently cited, and often the basis for recommendations for the use of ultrasound

*Corresponding author. E-mail address: Robert.Hsiung@vmmc.org.

0737-6146/10/$ – see front matter
doi:10.1016/j.aan.2010.07.004

guidance in central venous cannulation. Randolph and colleagues [8] identified 8 randomized controlled trials comparing ultrasound guidance versus traditional surface landmark-based techniques. There was a decrease in the number of placement failures in both internal jugular (relative risk [RR] 0.26; 95% confidence interval [CI] 0.11–0.58) and subclavian veins (RR 0.11; 95% CI 0.02–0.56) when ultrasound was used. The number of attempts before success also decreased with the use of ultrasound (RR 0.60; 95% CI 0.45–0.79). Of note, operator experience was not reported in many of the studies, and it was uncertain if there was any prior formal training or exposure to ultrasound concepts and equipment. In addition, the use of color flow Doppler and 2-dimensional (2D) ultrasound were mixed and considered to be equivalent.

In 2003, Hind and colleagues [9] performed a larger meta-analysis consisting of 18 trials (1646 patients) comparing 2D ultrasound with landmark-based techniques, specifically looking at failed catheter placement, catheter placement complications, number of attempts, and time to cannulation. Their results were more conclusive, as ultrasound decreased failed catheter placements both for internal jugular (RR 0.36; 95% CI 0.11–1.19) and for subclavian vein approaches (RR 0.09; 95% CI 0.02–0.38). As most of the data were based on the internal jugular approach, the time to catheterization with ultrasound was faster, 180 seconds, versus the landmark-based technique of 192 seconds ($P<.0001$). Though statistically significant, 12 seconds may not confer great time-saving advantage, as it may take at least that amount of time to locate the ultrasound machine. Fig. 1 shows a forest plot of the randomized controlled studies comparing failed catheter placement of 2D ultrasound versus the landmark technique at the internal jugular vein location.

Although not as extensively studied, the reviewers also supported ultrasound's role in the subclavian and femoral venous approaches despite small

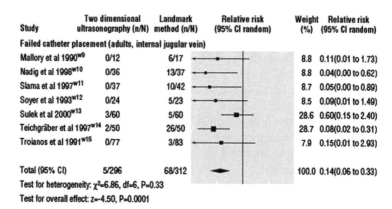

Fig. 1. Hind's meta-analysis of ultrasound versus landmark technique for central venous access shows a success advantage for 2D ultrasound. (*Data from* Hind D, Calvert N, McWilliams R, et al. Ultrasonic locating devices for central venous cannulation: meta-analysis. BMJ 2003;327:361.)

sample sizes of 20 to 25 patients in each study arm. Similarly, ultrasound's use in pediatrics was advocated in the internal jugular region based on data compiled from 3 studies with about 80 patients in each division. Newer small studies and reports have continued to show favorable outcomes with ultrasound-guided femoral [10] and subclavian vein [11] catheterizations.

These often quoted meta-analyses along with growing public and medical awareness of central line complications prompted the Agency for Healthcare Research and Quality (AHRQ) of the US Department of Health & Human Services in 2001 to issue the following statement after their own investigation: "Real-time US guidance for CVC insertion...improves catheter insertion success rates, reduces the number of venipuncture attempts prior to successful placement, and reduces the number of complications associated with catheter insertion" [12]. The British Committee for Standards in Haematology issued their guidelines [13] for central venous access insertions in 2007, recommending the use of ultrasound "for *all* routes of central venous catheterization," and by 2008 the American College of Surgeons published guidelines that support the uniform use of real-time ultrasound guidance for the placement of CVCs in *all* patients [14]. A recent editorial has advocated that ultrasound for internal jugular central venous catheterization in the critical care setting should become the standard of care [15].

As practicing anesthesiologists, is there still a role for ultrasound? After all, the statements above did not deem it absolutely necessary for anesthesiologists to use this technology as the AHRQ wrote, "as experienced anesthesiologists can continue to place most CVCs without US guidance." In fact, surveys on use suggest ultrasound use is actually low among anesthesiologists. Bailey and colleagues [16] sent out an electronic survey to all members of the Society of Cardiovascular Anesthesiologists and with a response rate of 35% showed that two-thirds never or almost never use ultrasound guidance versus 15% who always or almost always use it. While ultrasound availability was absent in 18% of respondents, the most common reason (46%) for not using ultrasound is the perception that it is not needed, despite almost 75% of the respondents having experienced a previous carotid puncture, 16.7% a pneumothorax, and 1.1% a stroke due to CVC placement.

Other investigators have also found that ultrasound use is low despite having access to an ultrasound machine. After the United Kingdom's National Institute for Clinical Excellence recommended 2D ultrasound guidance, a survey of pediatric anesthetists in the United Kingdom also found lower than anticipated use. With a response rate of 63% and availability of ultrasound in 82% of the workplaces and 74% receiving 2D ultrasound training, only 26% of anesthetists with access to ultrasound used it on elective cases [17]. A separate postal survey in the United Kingdom found similar responses, with only 39% of pediatric anesthesiologists routinely using ultrasound guidance. The majority used either ultrasound or a landmark-based technique depending on the clinical circumstance, despite widespread access to and education in ultrasound [18]. However, the adaptation of this technology for central venous cannulation is taking place.

A large German survey of anesthesia departments in 2007 revealed ultrasound use at 40%, much improved from 2003 when it was at 19% [19]. Thus the majority of CVCs are still placed via the landmark-based technique, and studies comparing landmark-based approaches continue to be published [7].

Ultrasound use in specialties outside of radiology is already widespread, including cardiology (transesophageal or transthoracic echocardiography), regional anesthesia for peripheral nerve blocks [20], and critical care and emergency medicine [21]. For example, transesophageal echocardiography has supplanted pulmonary artery catheterization for hemodynamic assessment, ultrasound-guided pericardiocentesis is superior to blind, electrocardiographic-guided, or fluoroscopically-guided techniques, and the focused abdominal sonogram for trauma (FAST) is often considered superior to diagnostic peritoneal lavage. Ultrasound in vascular access may be more readily embraced by emergency and internal medicine than by anesthesia. Nomura and colleagues [22] revealed a remarkable 90% ultrasound use among internal medicine and emergency medicine residents at a tertiary hospital, with most (88%) believing it to be easier than a landmark-based technique and 74% of respondents believing it should be used for all CVC placements. The investigators' rationale for such high ultrasound use was attributed to increased adoption by the physicians-in-training versus those who have finished postgraduate training and, in addition, the presence of an emergency medicine ultrasound fellowship program.

Like many other great "discoveries" in medicine, it often takes many years before evidence-based practices are integrated at an institutional level. An editorial response to one of the surveys showing low ultrasound use suggested the implementation of hospital-wide clinical protocols for the routine use of ultrasound, as was successfully employed in the Veteran Affairs system [23]. Fig. 2 depicts the major steps in integrating evidence-based medicine in daily practice. The 2 arrows point to the adaptation points where most of medicine stands on ultrasound's role in central venous access. Minimal new evidence from prospective randomized studies has been published on ultrasound for CVC placement in the last few years. Many local and national levels are developing the evidence-based clinical policies, on the plethora of existing data, and applying ultrasound in routine CVC placements. Of note, the American Society of Anesthesiologists (ASA) (Rupp, personal communication, 2010), National Institutes of Health, and the Cochrane Collaboration [24] are expected to release guidelines on ultrasound's importance in central venous catheterization. It is very likely that their statements will further accelerate ultrasound adoption.

What really is, then, the incidence of complications of central venous catheterization? After all, complications [25] are often unnoticed unless severe, and more often than not they are underreported or not surveyed. Prior to ultrasound, the ASA Closed Claims project in 1996 gave some insight as to what constitutes complications [26] (Table 1). By self-reporting without an actual denominator, the registry helped promote awareness but did not create

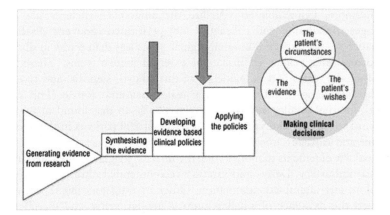

Fig. 2. Practicing evidence-based medicine requires much time and organization. The solid arrows point at the current state of ultrasound in CVC placement at many local and national levels. (*Data from* Haynes B, Haines A. Barriers and bridges to evidence-based clinical practice. BMJ 1998;317:273.)

urgency despite the report of deaths associated with central venous cannulation, because these numbers appear small compared with the perceived number of central venous lines placed. In one of the earliest articles comparing ultrasound to landmark anatomy [27], carotid artery puncture occurred in 8.3% of patients and brachial plexus irritation occurred in 1.7% of patients in the traditional landmark-based technique versus 1.7% and 0.4% with ultrasound, respectively, in the "experienced" hands of cardiology fellows and attending physicians.

Table 1
The ASA Closed Claims project provides some of the dangers associated with central venous catheterization

Complication	Total	Fatalities
Cardiac tamponade	11	10
Wire or catheter embolism	12	0
Vascular injuries (nonpulmonary artery):	13	5
Hemothorax	6	4
Hydrothorax	3	1
Carotid artery injury	3	0
Subclavian artery aneurysm	1	0
Pulmonary artery rupture	2	2
Pneumothorax	7	1
Air embolism	2	2
Fluid extravasation in neck	1	0
Total	48	20

Data from Bowdle T. Central line complications from the ASA Closed Claims Project. ASA Newsl 1996;60:22.

Furthermore, being able to visualize the anatomic structures has other advantages. Asouhidou and colleagues [28] performed cadaveric dissections in 93 patients, and showed 3 internal jugular veins less than 6 mm in diameter with corresponding enlarged ipsilateral external jugular veins. These small internal jugular veins had no evidence of thrombosis, stenosis, and recent or previous cannulation, and traveled the usual anatomic course. This 3% of "absent" internal jugular veins was similar (2.5%) to that found in the 1991 ultrasound survey by Denys and Uretsky [29] of 200 patients in the intensive care unit and cardiac catheterization laboratory. With that discovery and an additional 2% of patients demonstrating the internal jugular vein located medial to the carotid artery, Denys and Uretsky recommended ultrasound examination before any attempted cannulation. Other investigators [30,31] have also confirmed the existence of smaller internal jugular veins, and consider this a "powerful predictor" for prolonged procedure time and carotid puncture. Mey and colleagues [30] concluded that an internal jugular vein smaller than or equal to 7 mm, when normally averaging 1.0 cm (range 0.46–3.6 cm), is an independent predictor of catheterization failure ($P = .001$).

Ultrasound also has benefit in reducing complications in children. In a 4-year retrospective study, Tercan and colleagues [32] compared pediatric (average age 3.3 years) with adult (56.3 years) patients and found similarly low complication rates (2.3% vs 2.4%) when ultrasound was used. No major mechanical complications such as pneumothorax or hemothorax were noted in 859 adult and 247 pediatric catheterization attempts.

Normal anatomic variations, probe position, and head rotation all influence the relationship of the internal jugular vein and carotid artery. For example, internal jugular vein duplication is estimated at 4 in 1000 patients [33]. As expected, the internal jugular vein is not always immediately anterior and lateral to the carotid artery as previously described [2]. Lin and colleagues [34] described variations in the position of the internal jugular vein in as many as 17.3% in 104 consecutive uremic patients for dialysis catheters. Another similar study in 450 nonuremic patients also noted that the "classic" anterior lateral position is found only in 79.3% on the right side and 83.5% on the left [35].

Head rotation (as is commonly used to help facilitate the classic surface landmark-based techniques in internal jugular venous cannulation) may potentially increase the risk of carotid injury. In a large ultrasound study, Troianos and colleagues [36] recorded the images of 1136 patients with normal surface anatomy for central venous placement to determine the relationship of the right internal jugular vein relative to the carotid artery. All patients were in the supine position without a pillow, with their heads rotated as far to the left as was comfortable. After independent scoring into 5 segments (completely lateral, up to 25% overlap, 25%–50%, 50%–75%, and >75% overlap) by 3 investigators, they concluded that the internal jugular vein overlies the carotid artery by 75% or more in 54% of all patients. Arai and colleagues [37] demonstrated in infants and children that head rotation to 45° as opposed to 0° at the cricoid level increases the overlap of the internal jugular vein to the carotid artery. Lieberman and colleagues [38] further investigated the influence of head rotation by comparing rotations at 0°, 15°, 30°, 45°, and 60° left of the midline in simulated catheterization of volunteer adults. This group found that the occurrence of carotid artery contact with the internal jugular vein is increased with excessive head rotation. Recommendations for optimal rotation in patients with body mass index (BMI) greater than 25 kg/m^2 is 30° and 45° to 60° for patients with BMI <25 kg/m^2. Fujiki and colleagues [39] also found a much higher degree of vessel overlap in obese patients when the head was rotated away from the neutral position. Thus, ultrasound may allow the operator to decide on the optimal approach, and the optimal neck positioning may indeed be neutral, contrary to prior practices for landmark-based approaches.

Of course, this would lead to the question, how often does carotid puncture occur and does it matter? The likely answer is it happens more frequently than reported. The Mayo Clinic answered this with a prospective study of 1011 consecutive cardiothoracic and vascular surgery patients, and found the incidence of carotid puncture with a "finder" needle at 9.3% with a landmark-based technique for internal jugular vein cannulation [40]. Damen and Bolton [41], in another large prospective study of 1400 patients scheduled for cardiac surgery, found an incidence of 4.8%, and in the pediatric population the reported incidence is 7% to 8% [42,43].

The adverse consequences of arterial punctures with a "finder" needle are likely less than that of dilation and placement of a large-bore catheter. Because of successful early detection of arterial puncture by pressure transduction or manometry in the Mayo study [40], actual carotid artery catheterization was avoided, with no neurologic or vascular complications noted within the first 24 hours. Thus, arterial puncture with a "small" needle, at least in this large study, did not have immediate obvious consequences of hematoma or neurologic events. However, once a large-bore (7–12F) introducer or catheter has been inserted, stroke or death is a potential complication, especially if the catheter is removed without repair by vascular surgery or interventional radiology. The Canadian Society for Vascular Surgery proposed an algorithm after retrospectively reviewing the management of catheter-related carotid injury at 3 Montreal centers in patients with inadvertent placement of large caliber (≥7F) catheters [44]. Because of its rarity, they also performed a literature review and, on evaluation together with the multicenter data, they discovered that patients who underwent open or endovascular repair had no complications versus a 47% complication rate, including death and stroke, if the catheter was removed and only direct external pressure then applied ($P = .004$). This prompted a letter to the editors [45] not congratulating the proposed action plan but stressing the importance of prevention and achieving competency in ultrasound-guided central venous cannulation via a rigorous education curriculum (composed of basic ultrasound physics, development of psychomotor skills, and simulation training), such that these algorithms would not have to be used.

Ultrasound by itself does not equate to increased safety. It is a tool that requires training and practice to understand its limitations. Misidentification of anatomic structures, a lack of understanding of applied ultrasound physics, and inadequate psychomotor skills to properly guide the needle to the intended target while avoiding nontarget structures can lead to complications even with ultrasound. The use of ultrasound for regional anesthesia, for example, is moving toward standardization of training processes in ultrasound [46], and whether this will promote or restrict ultrasound use is not known. Although there are no learning curve studies for central venous access, landmark or ultrasound, the increased adoption of ultrasound in regional anesthesia has given some insights on the learning curve of the psychomotor skills needed to guide a needle under ultrasound [47]. Novices quickly improved their speed and accuracy in a breast cyst aspiration model, with the most commonly committed error in 7 of 10 subjects being the failure to accurately image the needle while advancing, resulting in excessive depth and potential harm. Blaivas and Adhikari [48] designed a prospective observational study to measure the frequency of posterior vessel wall penetration for CVC for the internal jugular vein. In a vascular access mannequin, 16 of 25 residents (64%) who underwent a 2-day ultrasound course that included hands-on sessions inadvertently penetrated the posterior wall of the vein. Five of the residents (20%) mistakenly punctured the carotid artery. Most surprising, however, is that these residents had a median number of 8 previous ultrasound-guided cannulation attempts and their mean self-reported confidence of accurate placement was 8.0 out of 10 [48]. This study highlights that ultrasound use with inexperienced operators may contribute to a false sense of security and lack of self-awareness with regard to the limitations of their psychomotor skills and risk of injury to target and nontarget structures.

With ultrasound, physicians in multiple specialties all want to become proficient, yet there are no binding standards for education and training [49–51]. Short of a ban on ultrasound use by the national or local credentialing agencies, multiple specialties will continue to expand their use of ultrasound. Fortunately, many concepts, target identifications, and physical skills are now effectively taught in didactics and medical simulations [52,53] rather than by initial "practice" on actual patients, as was the case not too long ago [54].

The common assumption is that experience plays an important factor in success rate and complications, but proper education and training is likely more important because of the ability to recognize preventable dangers and incorrect placements [30]. Case reports on complications [55,56] while using ultrasound exist, and it may be useful to review Blaivas' [56] compilations of videos on accidental arterial cannulation as an education module. The ability to interpret ultrasound images led to changes in management in 14% of the small series of patients studied by Gann and Sardi [57] undergoing port placement. Similarly, ultrasound detected asymptomatic thromboses in the internal jugular vein in 4 of 55 obese patients, and allowed for early detection and correction of malpositioned catheters [58]. The ability to visualize the guidewire in the lumen of the target venous structure before subsequent dilation and cannulation may serve to be a useful confirmatory and complementary step to pressure manometry in order to avoid unintended arterial cannulation [59].

As technology improves and the expense of machines decreases, cost analyses should strongly favor ultrasound in addition to the other evidence for use presented earlier. As early as 2003 Hind and colleagues [9] calculated a hypothetical cost saving of £2000 for every 1000 procedures even after incorporating machine acquisition and education costs. With Medicare and Medicaid no longer paying for complications, hospitals have refocused their efforts and budgets on prevention.

The investigators of the Third Sonography Outcomes Assessment Program (SOAP-3) Trial [60] compared the overall success rate of internal jugular venous cannulation with the use of anatomic landmark-based techniques (LM), ultrasound-guided static (S) techniques (quick-look visualization of the target vessels to evaluate the optimal approach and mark the skin over the intended needle insertion site), and dynamic (D) techniques (direct real-time visualization of needle advancement and entrance into the target vessel). The results, controlled for pretest difficulty assessment, were reported as odds improvement (95% CIs) over LM for D and S. D was shown to have an odds 53.5 (95% CI 6.6–440) times higher success than LM, and S had an odds 3 (95% CI 1.3–7) times higher success than LM, with an unadjusted success rate of cannulation of 98% (D), 82% (S), and 64% (LM). In addition, for first-attempt success, D had an odds of 5.8 (95% CI 2.7–13) times higher success compared with LM, and S had an odds of 3.4 (95% CI 1.6–7.2) times higher success compared with LM, with an unadjusted first-attempt success of 62% (D), 50% (S), and 23% (LM). The investigators concluded that both ultrasound techniques were superior to landmark-based techniques and that D was superior to S, but may require more training (Table 2). The second part of this article describes many of the technical skills needed to help employ ultrasound in CVC placement.

TECHNICAL CONSIDERATIONS

Short-axis (SAX) and long-axis (LAX) views may be used to visualize and guide cannulation of the target vessel. The SAX view provides visualization of the target vessel in the transverse (axial) plane, and is obtained by placing the long axis of the transducer perpendicular to the long axis of the vessel. To obtain a SAX view of a vessel, the probe is positioned on the patient (Fig. 3) so that the target vessel is viewed as a dark, anechoic circular structure (Fig. 4). When the transducer is centered over the target vessel, the midpoint of the transducer serves as the reference point for introduction of the access needle. The LAX view provides visualization of the target vessel in the longitudinal (sagittal) plane and is obtained by placing the long axis of the transducer parallel to the long axis of the vessel, producing a sonographic image along the length of the vessel. For a long-axis view of a vessel, the probe is rotated 90° from the short-axis view (Fig. 5). The vessel will now appear as

Table 2
Comparison of Static versus Dynamic versus Landmark from SOAP-3

	Patients (N)	Mean number of attempts	Mean time to cannulation (s)	Complication rate (%)	Success rate for cannulation (%)
Landmark	69	5.2	250	13	64
Static	72	2.9	126	3	82
Dynamic	60	2.3	109	3	98

Both static and dynamic use of ultrasound decreased the number of attempts and the duration of procedure, and improved success. An attempt is a single pass of the 18-gauge locator needle without redirection or withdrawal and with subsequent forward motion. Complication is any carotid artery puncture.

Data from Milling TJ Jr, Rose J, Briggs WM, et al. Randomized, controlled clinical trial of point-of-care limited ultrasonography assistance of central venous cannulation: the Third Sonography Outcomes Assessment Program (SOAP-3) Trial. Crit Care Med 2005;33:1764.

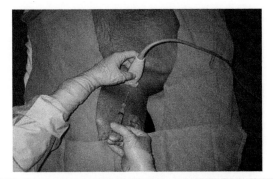

Fig. 3. Short-axis (vessel), out-of-plane (needle) internal jugular cannulation technique with linear array ultrasound transducer. Note: To better illustrate the probe position, the ultrasound probe cover has been removed. For actual placement of a central line, a complete sterile field is required, including a sterile ultrasound probe cover.

a dark, anechoic structure extending across the ultrasound screen (Fig. 6). The transducer is then oriented to view the vessel at widest anterior-posterior diameter. In contrast to the SAX view, the LAX view allows only a single vessel to be maintained in the imaging plane (field of view) and is not suitable to define the anatomic relationships between vessels.

As with landmark-based techniques, Trendelenburg (head-down) positioning for internal jugular or subclavian line insertion is recommended for

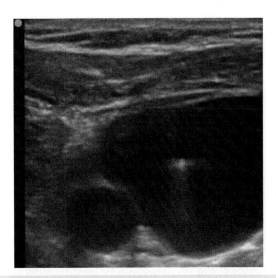

Fig. 4. Ultrasound image of a short-axis (vessel), out-of-plane (needle) internal jugular cannulation with a linear array transducer. Left side of image is medial, right side is lateral. Small anechoic (dark) circle in bottom left (medial) = carotid artery. Large anechoic (dark) area (internal jugular vein) has a hyperechoic (bright) dot (needle) in the vessel lumen.

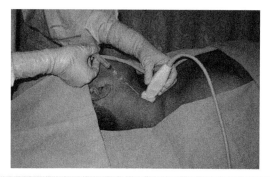

Fig. 5. Long-axis (vessel), in-plane (needle) internal jugular cannulation technique using a linear array transducer. The transducer is positioned to obtain an appropriate long-axis view of the target vessel.

ultrasound-guided procedures. Increasing venous pressure from proper positioning results in larger vein targets, and the increased venous pressure may also limit the compression of the vein during needle entry [61].

As previously noted, ultrasound may be used for guidance to a central vein in 2 ways: static and dynamic. Static ultrasound uses the image to locate the vein. Once the vein is located, a mark is made on the patient. After the mark is made, the ultrasound is removed from the field and the procedure continues in a similar fashion to landmark techniques, but using the mark for the initial needle entry site. Dynamic ultrasound, sometimes referred to as real-time

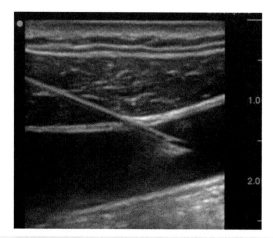

Fig. 6. Ultrasound image of long-axis (vessel), in-plane (needle) internal jugular cannulation technique using a linear array transducer. Cranial linear needle entry (right side of image) with tip of needle within lumen of internal jugular vein (dark, anechoic area). The needle tip is advanced in-plane aligned with the long axis of the transducer. Imaging the needle entry into the lumen of the vessel and aspiration of venous blood confirm access of the target vessel.

ultrasound, uses ultrasound during needle insertion to visualize the needle and the vessel together. Both of these techniques, static and dynamic, have been shown to improve initial success rates [60,62,63] as well as to decrease access time and arterial puncture [63–65]. Recent evidence indicates that ultrasound guidance also significantly improves the success rate and decreases the number of attempts and complications for related femoral vein dialysis catheter insertion [10].

Appropriate target vessels for central venous cannulation with ultrasound include the internal jugular vein, subclavian vein, and femoral vein. The internal jugular vein can be located on either side of the neck, in close proximity to the carotid artery. The internal jugular vein, though classically described as being superficial and lateral to the artery, can be found in various orientations to the carotid artery, even medial [66]. The subclavian vein is adjacent, caudal, and anterior to the subclavian artery. The subclavian vein can be located more easily with ultrasound laterally and then traced medially (Fig. 7). As the vein is traced medially, it will become shallower and then ultimately course underneath the clavicle (Fig. 8). Because the ultrasound beam cannot penetrate though bone, the needle entry site for the subclavian vein using ultrasound will likely be more lateral than with landmark approaches to the same vein without ultrasound. The femoral vein is a direct continuation of the popliteal vein and becomes the external iliac vein at the level of the inguinal ligament. The femoral vein is found medial to the artery in the inguinal region. The optimal cannulation site for femoral vein cannulation will be 2–3 cm distal to the inguinal ligament, ensuring that venipuncture occurs caudal to the inguinal ligament, which decreases the risk of a retroperitoneal hematoma in the event of puncture of the external iliac artery. As the femoral vein runs cranially, it will course deep into the pelvis along the anterior surface of the iliopsoas muscle to become the external iliac vein.

Selection of a catheter insertion site should ultimately depend on the indication catheter insertion and the characteristics of the patient. Although femoral

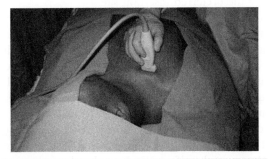

Fig. 7. Subclavian long-axis (vessel) ultrasound probe position just caudal to the clavicle, with linear array transducer.

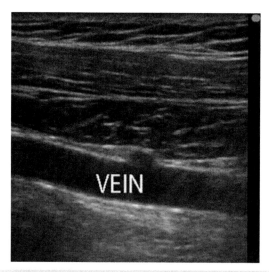

Fig. 8. Ultrasound image corresponding to transducer position illustrated in Fig. 7. The subclavian vein in long axis is anechoic (dark). The location of the subclavian vein on the left side of image is proximal and shallower (anterior) than the location on the right side (distal aspect of subclavian vein) of the image.

venous cannulation has several practical advantages (directly compressible, away from the airway and pleura, does not typically require Trendelenburg position), it is associated with the higher catheter infection rates and more frequent thrombotic complications [67]. Therefore, in most controlled settings, selection of an internal jugular or subclavian central venous line is usually preferred. Ultrasound guidance for internal jugular cannulation is easier because the internal jugular vein is much shallower than the subclavian vein. However, if the practitioner has more experience with subclavian line placement, that may be the preferred insertion site.

Before cannulation, target vessels must be identified properly, especially to distinguish artery from vein. Using a SAX imaging plane, the artery and vein can be imaged simultaneously so each can be positively identified. Ultrasound characteristics of arteries include pulsatility, resistance to compression, and imaged walls that are often thicker than veins. Veins may also be pulsatile, especially if imaged proximally, but are often easy to compress with pressure exerted on the ultrasound transducer.

Color flow Doppler (CFD) allows for the identification and quantification of blood flow and can be helpful to distinguish an artery from a vein. The Doppler principle states that if an ultrasound pulse is sent out and strikes moving red blood cells, the ultrasound that is reflected back to the transducer will have a frequency that is different from the original emitted frequency. This change in frequency is known as the Doppler shift. The Doppler equation states that:

Frequency shift $= (2 \times V \times F_1)(\text{cosine } \theta)/c$

where V is the velocity of the red blood cells, F_1 is the transmitted frequency, θ is the angle incidence of the ultrasound beam and the direction of blood flow, and c is the speed of the ultrasound in the media. It is this change in frequency that can be used to calculate (and subsequently displayed on the ultrasound screen) the presence (or absence) of blood flow and velocity. CFD on ultrasound is usually represented on the ultrasound screen as either red or blue. The red or blue color on the ultrasound image does not signify oxygenated (arterial) blood or deoxygenated (venous) blood. Rather, the color on the ultrasound image represents flow coming toward or away from the ultrasound transducer based on the Doppler principle. The brightness of the color, either red or blue, relates to the velocity of the blood flow. A brighter color represents a higher velocity of blood flow in that given direction. If a structure appears red when using CFD, this signifies that the blood flow is moving toward the transducer (the frequency of the returning signal is higher than the original emitted frequency). If a structure appears blue when using CFD, blood flow is moving away from the transducer (the frequency of the returning signal is lower than the original emitted frequency). A mix of color may signify turbulent blood flow, or flow that surpasses the maximum setting of the flow that can be measured (Nyquist limit). Sometimes there will be no color on the ultrasound image in a structure that may be a blood vessel. The angle between the flow of blood and the ultrasound beam must be either greater or less than 90°, as the cosine of 90° is 0; this means that the probe must be tilted in one direction or the other (away from perpendicular) to detect blood flow with CFD. A useful method to detect flow in blood vessels that are not identified by CFD is to use color power Doppler mode (CPD, which has a higher sensitivity for detecting low flow and is not dependent on θ). A useful clinical pearl to detect flow in the subclavian vein or femoral vein is to squeeze the distal extremity (arm or thigh, respectively) to increase venous return to the central venous system. Often, this will help identify a venous structure using color Doppler.

If dynamic needle visualization with ultrasound is used, it is important to visualize the needle image as best as possible as the needle approaches the target vessel, whether in-plane or out-of-plane. The ultrasound waves must contact the needle and be reflected back at the ultrasound transducer. If the needle is advanced to the target with a trajectory that is more parallel to the ultrasound beam, the ultrasound waves will not be reflected by needle well. The ultrasound image in this situation will result in a needle with low visibility. Therefore, clinically, it is important to advance the needle as perpendicular to the oncoming ultrasound beam as possible to image the needle well in both out-of-plane (single dot representing a cross section of the needle) or in-plane (entire needle shaft and tip). To keep the needle's angle of incidence flat, start the needle entry site 1 to 3 cm away from the ultrasound probe for vessel cannulation (see Fig. 3).

In-plane techniques have the needle advancing to the target in the plane of the ultrasound beam. If performed correctly, in-plane approaches allow the entire needle (shaft and tip) to be visualized as it approaches and enters the target vessel. However, in-plane techniques can be difficult because keeping the needle and/or vessel in-plane throughout the procedure can be difficult. Also, arteries and veins often lie in close proximity. Any slight dislocation or tilt of the ultrasound transducer may inappropriately target the nearby artery, resulting in arterial cannulation, possibly leading to significant mechanical complications. In addition, not all vessels continue in a straight line. If vessels are tortuous, it may be difficult to keep the target in a long-axis view for an in-plane approach.

The out-of-plane needle technique most closely resembles needle insertion techniques used for vessel cannulation with landmark-based techniques. Some clinicians prefer out-of-plane needle technique because they are more comfortable with the traditional techniques to cannulate blood vessels (peripheral intravenous and arterial cannulation). However, out-of-plane needle techniques may not allow visualization of the tip of the needle at all times and therefore, potentially do not offer the same level of confidence that comes with always knowing where the needle tip is located. Robust technique is required to localize the needle tip with out-of-plane approaches. Two such techniques are described in the following paragraphs.

The out-of-plane technique to needle insertion appears simple, but can be difficult. The major disadvantage with the out-of-plane technique is that a needle will appear as a hyperechoic, bright dot on the ultrasound screen. This bright dot simply represents a cross section of the long axis of the needle (and is often assumed to be the tip of the needle). However, the dot can also be the shaft of the needle, and the tip can be much deeper than the bright dot on the ultrasound screen, giving the user a false belief that the tip is shallower than it actually is.

Optimal out-of-plane needle technique follows the tip of the needle as it is advanced through tissue toward the target vessel. There are 2 recommended techniques to follow the needle tip:

1. Sliding the probe
2. Tilting the probe.

These 2 techniques require one important quality when looking for the bright (hyperechoic) dot of the needle: the bright dot must appear (as it crosses the plane of the ultrasound beam), then disappear, then appear again as it is advanced through the tissue. If the dot does not disappear, there is no way to rigorously confirm the dot is the needle tip.

Sliding Probe Technique

The needle is advanced out-of-plane until a bright dot is visualized above (shallow) the target. Once this dot is visualized, needle movement stops. The probe is then advanced forward (away from the needle) until the dot disappears. The needle is then advanced again, until the dot reappears. The dot should now be deeper and closer to the target. The probe is advanced until the dot disappears. The needle is then re-advanced. These steps are repeated until the dot is near the target vessel and subsequently enters the lumen of the target vessel (accompanied by presence of blood in the syringe while exerting continuous application of negative pressure). The dot must appear and disappear as the needle and probe are alternately advanced. This way, the tip is confirmed as it approaches the nerve or vessel target.

Tilting Probe Technique

Very similar to the sliding technique, this allows the probe to stay in one spot and may be useful in tighter areas where the probe cannot slide very far. The needle is advanced out-of-plane until a bright dot is visualized above (shallow) the target. Once this dot is visualized, needle movement stops. The ultrasound beam is then tilted forward (away from the needle) until the dot disappears. The needle is then advanced again, until the dot reappears. The dot should now be deeper and closer to the target. The ultrasound beam is again tilted forward until the dot disappears. The needle is then re-advanced. These steps are repeated until the dot is near the target. The dot must appear and disappear as the needle and probe are alternately moved. This way, the tip is confirmed as it approaches the nerve or vessel target.

As mentioned previously, despite all the advantages ultrasound confers to central line placement, morbidity and mortality persists. Therefore, confirmatory methods of accurate needle placement in a vein should be used including pressure measurement (waveform or manometry), continuous electrocardiography (ectopy), and/or ultrasound visualization of the guidewire, fluoroscopy, or venous blood gas.

SUMMARY

Anesthesiology trains for the unexpected. Malignant hyperthermia, intraoperative awareness, and permanent neurologic injuries are examples where emphasis and education has taken place to decrease mortality and morbidity of infrequent but serious complications.

Complications exist for central venous catheterization, likely a few magnitudes more common than those mentioned earlier, and the evidence for the routine use of ultrasound-guided central venous access to decrease, though not necessarily eliminate complications is strong. The various techniques for ultrasound-guided central venous cannulation should be systematically taught within a structured educational curriculum along with hands-on simulation (in the form of phantom gels or specially designed mannequins) to optimize both procedural success and patient safety. Based on the increasing applications of ultrasound technology in the perioperative setting and the emerging evidence for its benefits, ultrasound-guided central venous cannulation will likely increase and potentially become the standard of care in the future.

References

[1] McGee D, Gould M. Preventing complications of central venous catheterization. N Engl J Med 2003;348:1123.

[2] Metz S, Horrow JC, Balcar I. A controlled comparison of techniques for locating the internal jugular vein using ultrasonography. Anesth Analg 1984;63:673.

[3] Tryba M, Kleine P, Zenz M. [Sonographic studies for optimizing the cannulation of the internal jugular vein]. Anaesthesist 1982;31:626 [in German].

[4] Hosokawa K, Shime N, Kato Y, et al. A randomized trial of ultrasound image-based skin surface marking versus real-time ultrasound-guided internal jugular vein catheterization in infants. Anesthesiology 2007;107:720.

[5] Pittiruti M, LaGreca A, Scoppettuolo G, et al. Ultrasound-guided vs ultrasound-assisted central venous catheterization. In: 27th International Symposium on Intensive Care and Emergency Medicine. Brussels (Belgium): 2007. p. 158.

[6] Pittiruti M, Malerba M, Carriero C, et al. Which is the easiest and safest technique for central venous access? A retrospective survey of more than 5,400 cases. J Vasc Access 2000;1:100.

[7] Xiao W, Yan F, Ji H, et al. A randomized study of a new landmark-guided vs traditional para-carotid approach in internal jugular venous cannulation in infants. Paediatr Anaesth 2009;19:481.

[8] Randolph AG, Cook DJ, Gonzales CA, et al. Ultrasound guidance for placement of central venous catheters: a meta-analysis of the literature. Crit Care Med 1996;24:2053.

[9] Hind D, Calvert N, McWilliams R, et al. Ultrasonic locating devices for central venous cannulation: meta-analysis. BMJ 2003;327:361.

[10] Prabhu MV, Juneja D, Gopal PB, et al. Ultrasound-guided femoral dialysis access placement: a single-center randomized trial. Clin J Am Soc Nephrol 2010;5:235.

[11] Sakamoto N, Arai Y, Takeuchi Y, et al. Ultrasound-guided radiological placement of central venous port via the subclavian vein: a retrospective analysis of 500 cases at a single institute. Cardiovasc Intervent Radiol 2010 [online].

[12] Rothschild J. In: Shojania KG, Duncan BW, McDonald KM, et al, editors. Making health care safer: a critical analysis of patient safety practices [AHRQ Evidence Reports no. 43]. Rockville, MD: Association for Healthcare Research and Quality (AHRQ); 2001.

[13] Bishop L, Dougherty L, Bodenham A, et al. Guidelines on the insertion and management of central venous access devices in adults. Int J Lab Hematol 2007;29:261.

[14] Surgeons ACo: College's Committee on Perioperative Care. Statement on recommendations for uniform use of real-time ultrasound guidance for placement of central venous catheters. Bull Am Coll Surg 2008;93:35.

[15] Feller-Kopman D. Ultrasound-guided central venous catheter placement: the new standard of care? Crit Care Med 1875;33:2005.

[16] Bailey PL, Glance LG, Eaton MP, et al. A survey of the use of ultrasound during central venous catheterization. Anesth Analg 2007;104:491.

[17] Tovey G, Stokes M. A survey of the use of 2D ultrasound guidance for insertion of central venous catheters by UK consultant paediatric anaesthetists. Eur J Anaesthesiol 2007;24:71.

[18] Bosman M, Kavanagh RJ. Two dimensional ultrasound guidance in central venous catheter placement; a postal survey of the practice and opinions of consultant pediatric anesthetists in the United Kingdom. Paediatr Anaesth 2006;16:530.

[19] Schummer W, Sakka SG, Huttemann E, et al. [Ultrasound guidance for placement control of central venous catheterization. Survey of 802 anesthesia departments for 2007 in Germany]. Anaesthesist 2009;58:677 [in German].

[20] Marhofer P, Harrop-Griffiths W, Kettner SC, et al. Fifteen years of ultrasound guidance in regional anaesthesia: Part 1. Br J Anaesth 2010;104:538–46.

[21] Johnson MA, McKenzie L, Tussey S, et al. Portable ultrasound: a cost-effective process improvement tool for PICC placement. Nurs Manage 2009;40:47.

[22] Nomura JT, Sierzenski PR, Nace JE, et al. Cross sectional survey of ultrasound use for central venous catheter insertion among resident physicians. Del Med J 2008;80:255.

[23] Bjerke R. Survey of specialists shows we are not special. Anesth Analg 2007;105:879 [author reply 879].

[24] Brass P, Hellmich M, Kolodziej L, et al. Traditional landmark versus ultrasound guidance for central vein catheterization (Protocol). The Cochrane Library; 2009 [online].

[25] Defalque RJ, Fletcher MV. Neurological complications of central venous cannulation. JPEN J Parenter Enteral Nutr 1988;12:406.

[26] Bowdle T. Central line complications from the ASA Closed Claims Project. ASA Newsl 1996;60:22.

[27] Denys BG, Uretsky BF, Reddy PS. Ultrasound-assisted cannulation of the internal jugular vein. A prospective comparison to the external landmark-guided technique. Circulation 1993;87:1557.

[28] Asouhidou I, Natsis K, Asteri T, et al. Anatomical variation of left internal jugular vein: clinical significance for an anaesthesiologist. Eur J Anaesthesiol 2008;25:314.

[29] Denys BG, Uretsky BF. Anatomical variations of internal jugular vein location: impact on central venous access. Crit Care Med 1991;19:1516.

[30] Mey U, Glasmacher A, Hahn C, et al. Evaluation of an ultrasound-guided technique for central venous access via the internal jugular vein in 493 patients. Support Care Cancer 2003;11:148.

[31] Sibai AN, Loutfi E, Itani M, et al. Ultrasound evaluation of the anatomical characteristics of the internal jugular vein and carotid artery—facilitation of internal jugular vein cannulation. Middle East J Anesthesiol 2008;19:1305.

[32] Tercan F, Oguzkurt L, Ozkan U, et al. Comparison of ultrasonography-guided central venous catheterization between adult and pediatric populations. Cardiovasc Intervent Radiol 2008;31:575.

[33] Prades JM, Timoshenko A, Dumollard JM, et al. High duplication of the internal jugular vein: clinical incidence in the adult and surgical consequences, a report of three clinical cases. Surg Radiol Anat 2002;24:129.

[34] Lin BS, Kong CW, Tarng DC, et al. Anatomical variation of the internal jugular vein and its impact on temporary haemodialysis vascular access: an ultrasonographic survey in uraemic patients. Nephrol Dial Transplant 1998;13:134.

[35] Dolla D, Cavatorta F, Galli S, et al. Anatomical variations of the internal jugular vein in non-uremic outpatients. J Vasc Access 2001;2:60.

[36] Troianos CA, Kuwik RJ, Pasqual JR, et al. Internal jugular vein and carotid artery anatomic relation as determined by ultrasonography. Anesthesiology 1996;85:43.

[37] Arai T, Matsuda Y, Koizuka K, et al. Rotation of the head might not be recommended for internal jugular puncture in infants and children. Paediatr Anaesth 2009;19:844.

[38] Lieberman JA, Williams KA, Rosenberg AL. Optimal head rotation for internal jugular vein cannulation when relying on external landmarks. Anesth Analg 2004;99:982.

[39] Fujiki M, Guta CG, Lemmens HJ, et al. Is it more difficult to cannulate the right internal jugular vein in morbidly obese patients than in nonobese patients? Obes Surg 2008;18:1157.

[40] Oliver WC Jr, Nuttall GA, Beynen FM, et al. The incidence of artery puncture with central venous cannulation using a modified technique for detection and prevention of arterial cannulation. J Cardiothorac Vasc Anesth 1997;11:851.

[41] Damen J, Bolton D. A prospective analysis of 1,400 pulmonary artery catheterizations in patients undergoing cardiac surgery. Acta Anaesthesiol Scand 1986;30:386.

[42] Rey C, Alvarez F, De La Rua V, et al. Mechanical complications during central venous cannulations in pediatric patients. Intensive Care Med 2009;35:1438.

[43] Nicolson SC, Sweeney MF, Moore RA, et al. Comparison of internal and external jugular cannulation of the central circulation in the pediatric patient. Crit Care Med 1985;13:747.

[44] Guilbert MC, Elkouri S, Bracco D, et al. Arterial trauma during central venous catheter insertion: case series, review and proposed algorithm. J Vasc Surg 2008;48:918.

[45] Smith J. Regarding "Arterial trauma during central venous catheter insertion: case series, review, and proposed algorithm". J Vasc Surg 2009;49:1363 [discussion: 1363].

[46] Sites BD, Chan VW, Neal JM, et al. The American Society of Regional Anesthesia and Pain Medicine and the European Society of Regional Anaesthesia and Pain Therapy Joint Committee recommendations for education and training in ultrasound-guided regional anesthesia. Reg Anesth Pain Med 2010;35:S74.

[47] Sites BD, Gallagher JD, Cravero J, et al. The learning curve associated with a simulated ultrasound-guided interventional task by inexperienced anesthesia residents. Reg Anesth Pain Med 2004;29:544.

[48] Blaivas M, Adhikari S. An unseen danger: frequency of posterior vessel wall penetration by needles during attempts to place internal jugular vein central catheters using ultrasound guidance. Crit Care Med 2009;37:2345.

[49] Price S, Via G, Sloth E, et al. Echocardiography practice, training and accreditation in the intensive care: document for the World Interactive Network Focused on Critical Ultrasound (WINFOCUS). Cardiovasc Ultrasound 2008;6:49.

[50] Thys D, Abel M, Brooker R, et al. Practice guidelines for perioperative transesophageal echocardiography. An updated report by the American Society of Anesthesiologists and the Society of Cardiovascular Anesthesiologists Task Force on Transesophageal Echocardiography. Anesthesiology 2010;112:1084.

[51] Lee AC, Thompson C, Frank J, et al. Effectiveness of a novel training program for emergency medicine residents in ultrasound-guided insertion of central venous catheters. CJEM 2009;11:343.

[52] Ursino M, Tasto JL, Nguyen BH, et al. CathSim: an intravascular catheterization simulator on a PC. Stud Health Technol Inform 1999;62:360.

[53] Barsuk JH, McGaghie WC, Cohen ER, et al. Simulation-based mastery learning reduces complications during central venous catheter insertion in a medical intensive care unit. Crit Care Med 2009;37:2697.

[54] Gawande A. The learning curve: like everyone else, surgeons need practice. That's where you come in. New York: The New Yorker Magazine; 2002.

[55] Parsons AJ, Alfa J. Carotid dissection: a complication of internal jugular vein cannulation with the use of ultrasound. Anesth Analg 2009;109:135.

[56] Blaivas M. Video analysis of accidental arterial cannulation with dynamic ultrasound guidance for central venous access. J Ultrasound Med 2009;28:1239.

[57] Gann M Jr, Sardi A. Improved results using ultrasound guidance for central venous access. Am Surg 2003;69:1104.

[58] Brusasco C, Corradi F, Zattoni PL, et al. Ultrasound-guided central venous cannulation in bariatric patients. Obes Surg 2009;19:1365.

[59] Stone MB, Nagdev A, Murphy MC, et al. Ultrasound detection of guidewire position during central venous catheterization. Am J Emerg Med 2010;28:82.

[60] Milling TJ Jr, Rose J, Briggs WM, et al. Randomized, controlled clinical trial of point-of-care limited ultrasonography assistance of central venous cannulation: the Third Sonography Outcomes Assessment Program (SOAP-3) Trial. Crit Care Med 2005;33:1764.

[61] Samy Modeliar S, Sevestre MA, de Cagny B, et al. Ultrasound evaluation of central veins in the intensive care unit: effects of dynamic manoeuvres. Intensive Care Med 2008;34:333.

[62] Legler D, Nugent M. Doppler localization of the internal jugular vein facilitates central venous cannulation. Anesthesiology 1984;60:481.

[63] Bansal R, Agarwal SK, Tiwari SC, et al. A prospective randomized study to compare ultrasound-guided with nonultrasound-guided double lumen internal jugular catheter insertion as a temporary hemodialysis access. Ren Fail 2005;27:561.

[64] Mallory DL, McGee WT, Shawker TH, et al. Ultrasound guidance improves the success rate of internal jugular vein cannulation. A prospective, randomized trial. Chest 1990;98:157.

[65] Karakitsos D, Labropoulos N, De Groot E, et al. Real-time ultrasound-guided catheterisation of the internal jugular vein: a prospective comparison with the landmark technique in critical care patients. Crit Care 2006;10:R162.

[66] Gordon AC, Saliken JC, Johns D, et al. US-guided puncture of the internal jugular vein: complications and anatomic considerations. J Vasc Interv Radiol 1998;9:333.

[67] Merrer J, De Jonghe B, Golliot F, et al. Complications of femoral and subclavian venous catheterization in critically ill patients: a randomized controlled trial. JAMA 2001;286:700.

Advances in Anesthesia 28 (2010) 81–109

ADVANCES IN ANESTHESIA

Peripheral Blocks of the Chest and Abdomen

Matthew S. Abrahams, MD*, Jean-Louis Horn, MD

Department of Anesthesiology and Perioperative Medicine, Oregon Health and Science
University, 3181 SW Sam Jackson Park Road, Portland, OR, USA

Peripheral blocks of the chest and abdomen, such as the thoracic paravertebral and transversus abdominis plane (TAP) blocks, are versatile and useful techniques. This article reviews the history of the blocks, their indications, specific associated risks, relevant anatomy, and outcomes data. Various techniques for performing each block are described, and the pros and cons of each discussed.

THORACIC PARAVERTEBRAL BLOCK

History

Pioneered by Sellheim in 1905 [1], the technique for thoracic paravertebral blockade (TPVB) commonly used today was originally described by Kappis in 1919 [2]. During the early part of the 20th century, the TPVB was used as a diagnostic tool to differentiate between different causes of abdominal pain [3,4], as well as to treat conditions including angina pectoris, supraventricular tachycardias, and bronchial asthma in addition to providing relief from pain associated with surgery, traumatic injuries, herpes zoster, malignancy, and sympathetic dystrophies [5]. Despite the versatility and early enthusiasm for the TPVB, it became less frequently used during the mid-twentieth century as refinements in general anesthetic agents and monitoring techniques outpaced developments in local/regional anesthesia.

More recently, there has been renewed interest in regional techniques to overcome persistent limitations of general anesthesia (GA) and systemic opioid-based analgesic techniques. Eason and Wyatt [6] renewed interest in the TPVB specifically with their 1979 description of a technique for placing catheters within the thoracic paravertebral space (TPVS). At present, developments in ultrasound (US) imaging technology and increasing operator experience with interventional US techniques are contributing to increased TPVB

This research was funded internally by the Department of Anesthesiology and Perioperative Medicine, Oregon Health and Sciences University.

*Corresponding author. E-mail address: abrahama@ohsu.edu.

0737-6146/10/$ – see front matter
doi:10.1016/j.aan.2010.07.005

use. In addition, intriguing preliminary data suggesting that TPVBs may be associated with a reduction in the recurrence rate of breast cancer following surgical excision [7] may potentially increase surgeons' requests for TPVBs in their patients.

Indications

The TPVB has been used to provide surgical anesthesia for superficial procedures of the chest or abdomen. It is most commonly used to provide surgical anesthesia for breast surgery, including radical mastectomy procedures [8–10]. The TPVB can serve as an alternative to systemic or epidural analgesia following thoracotomy, thoracoscopy, laparotomy, open cholecystectomy, and liver or kidney surgery [11–16]. It may be especially useful in situations where epidural techniques may not be possible (such as in patients with spinal trauma [17,18] or previous posterior fusion of the thoracic spine). A paravertebral catheter can be used to provide and extend the duration of analgesia after such procedures or for painful conditions including multiple traumatic rib fractures [19–21] or herpes zoster [5,22].

Contraindications

Specific contraindications for TPVB are few. TVPB should be avoided in patients with ipsilateral empyema or severe disease of the contralateral lung. Contraindications to any regional anesthetic/analgesic technique (overlying infection or neoplasm, allergy to local anesthetics, patient or surgeon refusal, inability to obtain informed consent) apply to the TVPB as well. Patients who have significantly abnormal anatomy may be at an increased risk for complications such as inadvertent pleural or dural puncture. The use of TPVBs in patients with coagulopathy or receiving anticoagulant medications is controversial, and the TPVB currently is not considered safer than neuraxial techniques [23]. It is possible that that there is less potential for neurologic injury than with central neuraxial techniques. That a hematoma confined to the central neuraxial space could lead to spinal cord injury is well known. However, a hematoma in the TPVS could possibly extend to the adjoining epidural space through the intervertebral foramina and subsequently cause compression of the spinal cord. In addition, because the TPVS is within the thoracic cage (deep to the ribs/transverse processes), applying external pressure may not control bleeding, and significant blood loss into the pleural cavity could occur.

Specific Risks

Risks specific to the TPVB include hemothorax/pneumothorax [24–26], epidural or intrathecal injection [27–30], mediastinal puncture [31,32] and systemic local anesthetic toxicity [33]. Of importance, it is possible that pneumothoraces resulting from pleural puncture during TPVB placement may be subclinical before patient discharge and develop slowly (more likely for single-injection techniques using small-gauge needles). Thus, patients should be advised to seek medical care immediately should they experience shortness of breath, and to avoid air travel or other significant changes in atmospheric pressure soon after TPVB placement.

Performing bilateral blocks could theoretically increase the risks for several reasons: bilateral sympathetic blockade can produce hemodynamic effects (bradycardia and hypotension) similar to epidural techniques [34], the increased doses of local anesthetics used to achieve bilateral blockade may increase the risk of systemic local anesthetic toxicity [33,35], and there is a risk of bilateral hemothorax/pneumothorax. Rostral or caudal spread of anesthetic within the paravertebral space can produce a block of cervical or lumbar nerve roots causing a motor, sensory, or sympathetic block of the arm (cervical plexus or stellate ganglion block) or leg [36,37]. The inferior boundary of the TPVS is controversial, however, as the origin of the psoas muscle may prevent spread below T12. In addition, anesthetic fluid injected in the lower part of the TPVS could spread via the epidural space to effect a lumbar plexus block [38], or via the transversalis fascia to the celiac ganglion, and produce splanchnic vasodilation and hypotension [39].

Anatomy
The TPVS is a wedge-shaped triangular space located on both sides of the thoracic vertebral column. The anterolateral boundary is formed by the parietal pleura and the base (medial boundary) is formed by the posterolateral aspect of the vertebral body, intervertebral disc, and the intervertebral foramina. The posterior border is formed by the superior costotransverse ligament, which extends from the lower border of the transverse process above to the upper border of the transverse process below. The TPVS communicates with the epidural space medially via the intervertebral foramina, and at the tips of the transverse processes the TPVS is continuous with the intercostal space laterally. The TPVS contains the proximal intercostal nerves (as continuation of the ventral rami), the dorsal rami, the sympathetic chain, the intercostal vessels, the endothoracic fascia, and adipose tissue (Fig. 1A) [37,40].

For anesthesia and/or analgesia of the chest and/or abdominal wall, blocks can be performed from the first thoracic to the first lumbar spinal level. Local anesthetics spread easily to adjacent levels and occasionally spread to the contralateral space via the prevertebral fascia or to the epidural space medially [41–43]. The extent of rostral/caudad spread of local anesthetic is determined by the volume of fluid injected for single-injection techniques as well as the number of levels blocked for multiple-injection techniques [44,45]. Local anesthetics placed within the TPVS act on somatic fibers as well as the sympathetic chain. As a result, TPVBs can have greater hemodynamic effects (such as vasodilation or bradycardia) than more peripheral truncal blocks, such as those of individual intercostal nerves [46].

Techniques
Landmarks
After determining the appropriate level(s) to be blocked based on the surgical procedure, the midline is marked, and a line parallel to the midline is marked

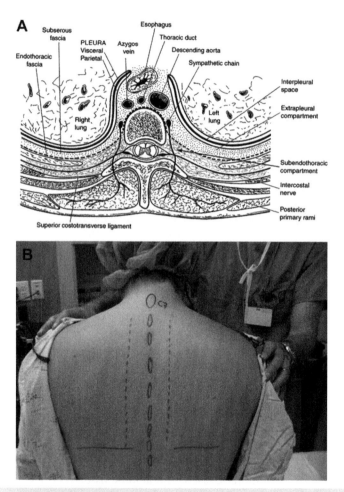

Fig. 1. Anatomy of the thoracic paravertebral space (TPVS). (A) Diagram showing the anatomy of the TPVS. (*Reprinted from* Karmakar MK. Thoracic paravertebral block. Anesthesiology 2001;95(3):771–80; with permission.) (B) Surface anatomy for thoracic paravertebral block (TPVB). Spinous processes are outlined. Dotted lines are 2.5 cm lateral to the midline. The prominent spinous process of C7 (marked C7) is a consistent surface landmark. The angle of the scapula corresponds roughly to the T7/8 interspace (marked with a *horizontal line*).

2.5 cm lateral on the side(s) to be blocked (Fig. 1B). After sterile preparation of the skin, subcutaneous infiltration of local anesthetic is performed along the paramedian line. Infiltration may be performed with chloroprocaine to minimize the risk of systemic local anesthetic toxicity while allowing infiltration of the entire area. The block needle is then introduced along this line at the level of the respective spinous processes and perpendicular to all skin planes, and it is advanced until its tip contacts the posterior surface of the transverse process. The depth to the transverse process varies with patient size and block level [47,48]. In an adult patient of normal body habitus, the needle should not be advanced past 4 cm without bony contact. If no bony contact is made, the needle should be reoriented cephalad or caudad to seek bony contact. After contact, the depth of contact is noted, the needle is partially withdrawn slightly, and oriented slightly more cephalad or caudad to "walk off" the transverse process. The needle is advanced 1 to 1.5 cm past the depth of bony contact, and local anesthetic is injected. Using a needle with depth markings on the shaft, or placing a "depth guard" on the needle may be helpful. A distinct "pop" may be felt as the needle tip enters the paravertebral space (through the costotransverse ligament), though this is not consistent.

It is important to not advance the needle more than 1.5 cm past the depth of bony contact, as this could lead to pleural puncture. The needle should not be redirected medially, as this can increase the risk of epidural or intrathecal injection [40]. Whether it is better to perform multiple small-volume injections or a single large-volume injection remains controversial. Multiple-injection techniques may be associated with an increased likelihood of block success [44,49], though each needle pass carries a risk of puncturing the pleura. Single-injection techniques may decrease this risk, although injecting a large volume of local anesthetic in a single paravertebral space may promote contralateral or epidural spread of anesthetic and produce more severe hemodynamic effects [50].

Surgical placement of catheters within the paravertebral space under direct vision [51], and video assistance during thoracoscopic procedures [52] have also been described.

Loss of resistance
The technique is identical to that described for the landmark-based approach, except that loss of resistance (LOR) is used to confirm positioning of the needle tip within the paravertebral space [17]. The LOR technique generally uses larger-gauge needles, and is especially well suited to placing catheters within the paravertebral space for continuous blocks [6]. A "pressure measurement technique" has been advocated as an objective and reproducible means to identify the TPVS [53]. This technique relies on measuring pressure changes during phases of the respiratory cycle, with a classic "pressure inversion" (pressure during expiration higher than during inspiration) indicating needle tip position within the TPVS. Fluoroscopy [42] may be used as a supplementary method of confirming correct needle or catheter placement within the TPVS.

Nerve stimulation
The technique is essentially identical to that described for landmark-based and LOR techniques, with the addition of electrical neurostimulation as an additional confirmatory end point [54]. High stimulating currents (5 mA, 2 Hz, 0.3 ms pulse width) may be used initially, and contraction of the paraspinal muscles may be observed before the needle tip makes contact with the transverse process. Stimulation can be used to confirm positioning of the needle tip within the TPVS, as contractions of appropriate intercostal/abdominal

muscles may be observed at low stimulating currents (0.4–0.6 mA). Because these contractions may be subtle and difficult to see (especially in obese patients) it may be helpful to have an assistant palpate the patient's intercostal muscles during block placement. Slight movements of the needle tip within the TPVS may help elicit contractions by moving the needle tip closer to nerve roots. It is important that these movements should not be "in-and-out" as this could increase the risk or pleural puncture. Rather, "side-to-side," "up-and-down," or rotational maneuvers should be used. It is also helpful to use insulated needles designed for use with a nerve stimulator.

Ultrasonography

Because US guidance is a relatively new technique for aiding the placement of TPVBs, a standard technique does not yet exist. Several different techniques are possible. Each technique has specific advantages and risks that should be taken into consideration before deciding which one to use in a particular clinical situation. Because US imaging of the TPVS may be challenging and because there is a significant risk of pleural puncture or injection of anesthetic directly into a nerve root, the subarachnoid space, and even the spinal cord itself, this technique should not be attempted by practitioners without significant experience in performing US-guided procedures and TPVBs. For those who do have a sufficient amount of training and experience, use of ultrasonography can be helpful as an adjunct to traditional techniques, or as a stand-alone method of guiding block placement.

As an aid to traditional techniques, ultrasonography can be helpful for measuring the depth to the transverse process and pleura as well as planning the trajectory of the needle, which may be especially helpful in patients with abnormal anatomy. Jamieson and Mariano [55] published a case report of 2 TPVBs placed using a nerve-stimulator guided technique after a US prescan. Pusch and colleagues [56] reported a series of 22 patients who had TPVBs placed using a landmark-based technique after measuring the depth to the transverse process and pleura at the T4 level. These studies found that the US prescan reliably measured the depth to the transverse process. Hara and colleagues [57] reported a series of 25 patients with TPVBs placed at the T4 and T1 level using an LOR technique in combination with real-time US guidance, using ultrasonography to guide the needle to make contact with the transverse process. After contact was made, the needle was advanced without US visualization and LOR was used to confirm entry of the needle tip into the TPVS.

Several techniques have been described using ultrasonography as a stand-alone technique for placing single-injection and continuous TPVBs. US-guided procedures can be performed by imaging the target structure(s) in the long or short axis. Needle guidance can be performed using the in-plane or out-of-plane technique. Although any combination of transducer orientation and needle guidance technique can be used to perform a block, the in-plane needle approach is generally preferred for TPVBs as it allows more consistent identification of the needle's tip. For the out-of-plane approach, practitioners should use surrogate methods such as hydrolocalization to locate the needle's tip.

To obtain a long-axis view of the TPVS, the US transducer is placed in a sagittal orientation (parallel to the long axis of the spine, Fig. 2A) and moved medially and laterally to identify the spinous processes, the transverse processes, the ribs, and the pleura (Fig. 2B). By scanning medially and laterally, the transverse process and rib (Fig. 2C) can be identified, and the spatial relationship of the rib and transverse process can be delineated (Fig. 2D). This parasagittal view has the advantage of allowing simultaneous visualization of multiple levels. Use of a curved-array US transducer may provide a "wider" field of view (more levels). It may be difficult to use an in-plane needling technique with this view as the transducer's "footprint" (50 mm) may make it difficult to pass the needle's tip between the transverse processes (Fig. 2E). Use of a transducer with a smaller "footprint" (20–25 mm) may eliminate this problem, however. Alternatively, this technique can be used to guide the needle to contact the transverse process, and it can then be "walked off" using needle depth or LOR to confirm entry of the needle's tip into the TPVS. This long-axis view can also be helpful to determine the extent of spread of local anesthetic within the TPVS. After the block is performed, the anesthetic fluid can be seen as a hypoechoic (dark) stripe superficial to the pleura. Scanning rostrally and caudally, the superior and inferior limits of local anesthetic spread can be determined.

O'Riain and colleagues [58] described a similar parasagittal long-axis in-plane technique and reported block success in 8 of 9 patients undergoing breast surgery. All patients received a continuous TPVB placed at the T3 level on the operative side. The TPVS was expanded with saline and a catheter was then passed 3 cm past the needle's tip. If there was no hemodynamic response to a standard test dose, 10 mL of 0.25% bupivacaine was injected through the catheter. The number of dermatomes blocked using this technique was not formally assessed. All patients had GA for the surgical procedure. No complications were reported. The investigators stated that needle visualization may be challenging using this approach due to the "acute angle the needle must take to enter between adjacent transverse processes." Although the reported block success rate was high in this series, the small number of patients, the fact that blocks were not used for surgical anesthesia, and the lack of a control group (TPVBs performed without US guidance) make it difficult to make definitive statements regarding the efficacy of this approach. Confirmation with larger series and prospective comparisons with standard approaches are still needed.

To obtain a short-axis view of the TPVS, the transducer is placed in an axial orientation (perpendicular to the long axis of the spine, Fig. 3A). With the transducer in this orientation, the spinous processes, laminae, transverse processes, ribs, and pleura can be seen simultaneously (Fig. 3B). Because these structures cannot be seen simultaneously using the long-axis view, this type of imaging may allow better appreciation of the TPVS. The TPVS can be imaged using this view by scanning in a rostral or caudal orientation until the rib is not in view (Fig. 3C). The rib and pleura may appear similar on the US image, and must be distinguished from one another for the block to be performed safely. The rib can usually be identified by the characteristic acoustic dropout "shadowing" seen during US imaging of bone (hyperechoic surface, US waves unable to penetrate past the surface, see Fig. 3C). In contrast, the parenchyma of the lung can usually be visualized deep to the hyperechoic pleura. In addition, the "sliding lung sign" can help confirm the identity of the pleura. By having the patient take a deep breath, the sliding of the parietal and visceral pleura can be seen. After confirmation of the relevant anatomic relationships, the needle tip can then be positioned in the TVPS using an in-plane needling

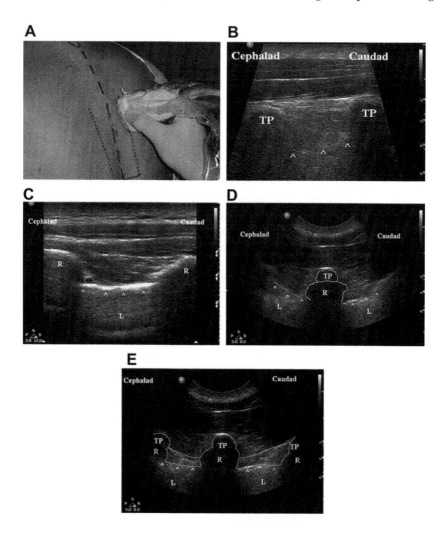

technique by inserting the needle from the lateral edge of the transducer (see Fig. 3A). This short-axis in-plane technique has the advantage of consistently allowing visualization of the needle as it is advanced toward the paravertebral space. However, this approach should be used with great caution, as failure to maintain visualization of the needle's tip could allow the needle tip to pass through the intervertebral foramen into the central neuraxial space or the spinal cord itself.

Luyet and colleagues [59], using the short-axis in-plane technique, placed styleted catheters in the TPVS of 20 cadavers. In all cases, the relevant anatomy and needle were easily visualized, and the catheters were easy to pass. However, during the subsequent anatomic dissection, a mixture of local anesthetic and contrast dye injected through 9 of the 20 catheters was seen in the epidural space, the pleural cavity, or the mediastinum. Although it is not clear how this could impact blocks performed in clinical situations, the high incidence of concerning patterns of local anesthetic spread in this study highlight that caution should be exercised using this technique.

Fig. 2. Sonoanatomy of the TPVS in the long-axis view. (A) US transducer position for long-axis imaging of the TPVS. After determining the appropriate level(s) to be blocked, a high-frequency curved or linear-array transducer is placed vertically along a paramedian line 2 to 3 cm lateral to the midline. Other types of transducers may be helpful in specific clinical situations such as deeper blocks (low-frequency, wide-footprint, curved-array) or pediatrics (very high-frequency, small-footprint, linear-array "hockey sticks"). (B) Long-axis US image of the TPVS. Cephalad and caudad aspects of the US image are labeled. The top of the image is superficial (posterior) and the bottom deep (anterior). The transverse processes (TP) typically have hyperechoic flat posterior surfaces with acoustic shadowing below. The pleura (arrowhead) is below (anterior) and the deeper lung parenchyma can be seen. Note that the distance between the posterior surface of the transverse process and the pleura is approximately 1.5 cm (depth markings on right-hand side of image). Movement between the visceral and parietal pleura can be observed during inspiration and expiration (the "sliding lung sign"), allowing identification of the pleura (more difficult on still images than real-time). (C) By moving the US transducer laterally (maintaining parasagittal orientation) the ribs (R) can be demonstrated, and the pleura (arrowhead) and lung (L) can be seen below. Cephalad and caudad aspects of the image are labeled. The ribs typically have a rounded posterior surface with shadowing below, and are wider than the transverse processes. An intercostals artery is circled on the inferior aspect of the cephalad rib. Note that the distance from the superficial surface of the rib and the pleura is approximately 1 cm (depth markings on right-hand side of image). (D) Simultaneous long-axis US image of the transverse process (TP) and rib (R). Both are outlined. Cephalad and caudad aspects of the image are labeled. Note that the rib is anterior (deep) to the transverse process. The pleura is marked with arrows (arrowhead) and the lung (L) is seen below. (E) Curved-array US image of the TPVS in the "long-axis" view. Cephalad and caudad aspects of the image are labeled. Because the probe is narrow but allows a wide field of view, multiple levels can be imaged simultaneously and the needle can be directed almost vertically anterior (deep) using an in-plane technique to pass between the transverse processes (TP, outlined) and enter the TPVS (outlined). The ribs (R, outlined) can be seen below the transverse processes. The pleura (arrowhead) and lung parenchyma (L) can also be seen between the acoustic shadows created by the bony structures.

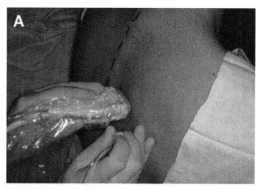

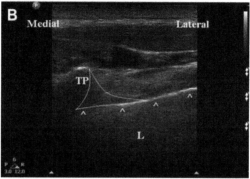

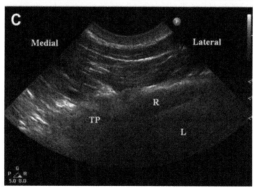

Fig. 3. Sonoanatomy of the TPVS in the short-axis view. (*A*) US transducer position for short-axis US imaging of the TPVS. To perform an in-plane TPVB using this type of imaging, the needle is inserted from the lateral edge of the probe and directed medially. (*B*) Short-axis US image of the TPVS. Medial and lateral aspects of the Image are labeled. The posteromedial surface of the transverse process (TP) is well seen, but the anterior aspect is not due to acoustic shadowing. The pleura can be seen as a curved hyperechoic line with lung parenchyma beneath. Use of the sliding lung sign can be helpful to differentiate pleura from rib. To perform an in-plane TPVB using this view, the needle is directed from lateral to medial so that its tip is positioned within the TPVS (outlined). Constant visualization of the needle's tip is essential to prevent injury to the pleura or entry into the spinal column through the intervertebral foramen (*arrowheads*). (*C*) Short-axis US image of the TPVS showing the transverse process (TP), lung (L) and rib (R) simultaneously. The pleura and lung can be distinguished from the rib as the parenchyma of the lung is visible, while structures deep to the rib's surface are not well seen due to acoustic shadowing.

Renes and colleagues [60] recently described a similar technique in a series of 36 patients undergoing various surgical procedures of the chest or abdomen. Each block was placed at a level deemed appropriate for the surgical procedure. Under real-time US guidance, the needle's tip was positioned within the TVPS. Fifteen milliliters of 0.75% ropivacaine was then injected through the needle and a catheter passed 2 cm past the needle's tip. Placement of the catheter was confirmed by injecting an additional 5 mL of 0.75% ropivacaine with US visualization of spread within the TPVS. A blinded observer assessed block success, and catheter placement was confirmed radiographically by injecting contrast dye through the catheter tip. Renes and colleagues reported a block success rate of 100% with reduced cold sensation in a median of 6 dermatomal segments, and all catheters were radiographically well -positioned. One patient had evidence of epidural spread of contrast dye, but had no sensory changes on the contralateral side. All patients in this series reported adequate pain relief, and no complications were reported. No control group was included for comparison.

When we (the authors of this article) use this short-axis, in-plane technique to place a catheter in the TPVS, we inject saline (3–5 mL) through the needle to create a "pocket" within the TVPS for the catheter to pass into. Because of the high rate of apparently malpositioned styleted catheters in the aforementioned cadaver study by Luyet and colleagues, we do not use catheters with stylets. We prefer to use wire-reinforced flexible single-orifice epidural catheters (such as the Arrow Flextip Plus: Teleflex Medical, Research Triangle Park, NC. USA). Occasionally we will use a styleted stimulating peripheral nerve catheter (such as the Arrow StimuCath: Teleflex Medical), as these catheters may be easier than the epidural catheters to visualize with ultrasonography. If we are using one of these stimulating catheters, we remove the stylet before passing the catheter past the needle's tip. Once we have passed the catheter 3 to 4 cm past the needle tip (we do not recommend passing the catheter more than this to minimize the risk of the catheter advancing into the epidural space), we inject saline (3–5 mL) through the catheter using real-time US visualization to confirm proper spread of fluid within the TPVS. We prefer to confirm appropriate spread of fluid injected through the needle and catheter with saline in order to avoid potential inadvertent subarachnoid or epidural injection of local anesthetic. We inject local anesthetic under low pressure, slowly and incrementally, to decrease the risk of epidural spread and minimize hemodynamic consequences if the catheter is malpositioned within the epidural or subarachnoid space.

Outcomes Data

Several studies have shown improved early recovery for patients undergoing breast surgery with TPVBs with sedation as compared with patients undergoing similar procedures under GA [8–10,61–63]. Patients in the TPVB/sedation groups had significantly less rest and/or dynamic pain, nausea, and sedation. In addition, patients in the TPVB/sedation groups were able to be discharged home earlier than patients who had received GA. Although the risk of complications from the TPVB was generally low in these studies, one pneumothorax was reported (in a series of 100 patients) [61], so caution is warranted in settings where surgical backup may not be available if urgent thoracostomy is necessary. A 1% risk of pneumothorax may be unacceptably high for elective minor procedures, especially in an ambulatory setting.

TPVB/sedation has also been compared with GA for other types of surgical procedures including inguinal hernia repair [64,65], ventral hernia repair [11], and endovascular abdominal aortic aneurysm (AAA) repair [66]. For these procedures, patients had similar improvements in pain control and early recovery. In addition, TPVB/sedation was associated with a reduced risk of hypotension in patients undergoing endovascular AAA repair compared with GA, suggesting that this type of anesthetic may be a good alternative for patients who may not tolerate GA.

Two studies have compared TPVBs to spinal anesthesia (SA) for inguinal hernia repair [67,68]. Both studies found that patients in the TPVB group had longer anesthesia-related times and block onset times. The TPVB groups required higher doses of propofol for sedation during surgery, but these differences were not clinically significant. Both studies also found that patients in the TPVB group had lower postoperative pain scores, longer times to first-rescue analgesic dose, shorter time to recovery of ambulation, and faster discharge from the postanesthesia care unit (PACU). In the study that reported rates of urinary retention [68], no patients in the TPVB group (30 patients) required bladder catheterization, compared with 5 patients (of 30) in the SA group.

Several studies have shown that TPVBs provide better pain control than systemic opioid-based analgesics following many types of surgical procedures of the chest and abdomen, including breast surgery [69,70], thoracotomy or thoracoscopy [13,71,72], laparoscopic or open cholecystectomy [12,73], open hepatic resection [16] or radiofrequency ablation of liver masses [74], transhepatic biliary drainage procedures [75], and major kidney surgery [15]. These studies all showed that compared with patients receiving systemic opioid-based analgesics alone, patients who received TPVBs had lower pain scores, decreased opioid consumption, and a lower incidence of postoperative nausea and vomiting (PONV). The duration of analgesia from single-injection techniques may be short-lived, however, as one study found no differences in pain scores between groups following patient discharge from the PACU [70]. This result suggests that continuous techniques may be more effective [76], but there have been no comparisons of single-injection with continuous techniques to date.

Few trials have compared TPVBs and local infiltration of local anesthetic or more selective peripheral nerve blocks. One trial found that compared with continuous wound infusions of ropivacaine, single-injection ropivacaine TPVBs provided superior early pain control and a lower incidence of PONV following modified radical mastectomy, but patients with wound infusions had lower pain scores 16 and 24 hours after surgery [77]. A continuous

TPVB group was not included for comparison. Two studies have compared TPVBs with ilioinguinal/iliohypogastric (II/IH) blocks for pain control following inguinal hernia repair under GA [78,79]. In both studies TPVBs were performed before surgery and II/IH blocks were performed during surgery. Both of the studies found that patients in the TPVB group had lower pain scores and required fewer opioid analgesics, and neither study reported any complications in either group.

Numerous trials have compared TPVBs with thoracic epidural analgesia (TEA) following major thoracic surgery. In a recent meta-analysis, Davies and colleagues [80] pooled data from 10 trials involving a total of 520 patients, and found no significant differences between study groups' pain scores from 4 to 8, 24, or 48 hours postoperatively with similar doses of supplemental morphine usage between groups at all time points. The TPVB groups had lower risks of pulmonary complications (odds ratio [OR] 0.36), urinary retention (OR 0.23), nausea and vomiting (OR 0.47), and hypotension (OR 0.23). In addition, the TPVB groups had lower block failure rates (OR 0.28). All differences were highly statistically significant (P values .03 to <.0001). It was concluded that TPVBs provided similar pain relief compared with TEA but have a more favorable side effect profile. These findings are in agreement with those of an earlier systematic review of regional techniques for post-thoracotomy analgesia by Joshi and colleagues [81], which found that TPVBs provided similar pain relief to TEA but was associated with a lower risk of pulmonary complications and hypotension. Of note, this study found that TPVBs were associated with lower rates of pulmonary complications than systemic analgesic regimens, whereas TEA was not. In another systematic review, Scarci and colleagues [82] reported that compared with TEA, TPVBs were associated with improved pulmonary function, lower plasma cortisol concentrations, shorter operative times, lower rates of technical failure or catheter displacement, and a reduction in the incidence and severity of hypotension. In a recent meta-regression analysis of different TPVB techniques for post-thoracotomy analgesia, Kotze and colleagues [45] analyzed 25 trials involving a total of 763 patients, and found that higher doses of local anesthetic were associated with improved pain control and faster recovery of pulmonary function. These investigators also found that compared with intermittent bolus dosing, regimens involving continuous infusions of local anesthetic provided better pain relief, whereas the addition of adjuvants such as clonidine or fentanyl did not improve the analgesic effect of the TPVB.

In a prospective trial of 20 patients undergoing open cholecystectomy, patients were randomly assigned to receive either a continuous TPVB or TEA for postoperative pain control [83]. There were no differences between groups with regard to postoperative hemodynamic stability or pulmonary function; however, patients in the TPVB group had higher pain scores and required more opioid analgesics than patients in the TEA group. One trial compared left-sided TPVB with TEA for pain control following elective robotic-assisted coronary artery bypass grafting via a left-sided minithoracotomy approach [84]. There were no differences in outcomes between groups with regard to pain control, hemodynamic stability, or complications. There was a trend toward improved pulmonary function in the TPVB group, but this did not reach statistical significance.

Additional studies have also suggested that TPVBs may reduce the risk of chronic postsurgical pain (CPSP) following breast surgery. In a 1-year follow-up study of patients enrolled in a previous study comparing TPVB/sedation to GA for surgical anesthesia for breast surgery, Kairaluoma and colleagues [85] found that patients who had received TPVBs had significantly decreased prevalence of pain symptoms as well as a decreased intensity of pain with movement and at rest. Iohom and colleagues [86] studied the effect of TPVB on acute and chronic pain following breast surgery with axillary clearance; they followed patients for 10 weeks postoperatively and found that patients who received GA and TPVBs were less likely to develop CPSP than patients who received GA and systemic analgesics alone (0/14 in the TPVB group, 12/14 in the GA group, $P = .009$). This study also investigated the role that nitric oxide production could play in the development of CPSP, but no correlation between perioperative plasma nitric oxide levels and risk of subsequent CPSP was demonstrated. However, the results of this study could be confounded by the fact that patients in the TPVB group also received parecoxib after induction of GA and celecoxib for up to 5 days postoperatively, whereas patients in the GA group did not.

One of the most intriguing outcomes examined recently is the potential effect TPVBs may have on the rates of breast cancer recurrence. A recent retrospective analysis [7] of patients undergoing surgical excision of malignant breast lesions showed a significant reduction in the rates of local recurrence during a 36-month follow-up period (6% vs 24%, $P = .007$). This effect could be caused by a blunted stress response to surgery, as patients undergoing breast cancer surgery with TPVBs have been shown to have lower serum concentrations of glucose, cortisol, and C-reactive protein than patients treated with systemic opioids [87]. However, in this study TPVBs did not reduce the serum levels of the vascular endothelial growth factor (VEGF) or prostaglandin-E2 (PGE2). Others have proposed that the TPVB leads to a reduction in substance P production with decreased tumor cell proliferation and neoangiogenesis via activation of tumor neurokinin-1 receptors [88], though they have not yet tested these hypotheses in vitro or in vivo. It does appear that the TPVB may indeed contribute to the lower rates of recurrence, as serum from patients with TPVBs undergoing excision of malignant breast lesions inhibited proliferation of estrogen-receptor negative breast cancer cells in vitro [89]. The authors wish to emphasize that although these findings are very intriguing, confirmation with large-scale prospective studies is necessary. The design of these studies has been proposed [90], and patient recruitment is currently under way.

Future Directions

Although there are good data supporting the use of TPVBs over TEA for pain relief after thoracic surgery and the use of TPVBs over systemic analgesics following abdominal surgery, additional studies comparing bilateral TPVBs with TEA for abdominal procedures could be valuable. Comparisons of continuous TPVBs and continuous wound infusion techniques could also help determine the relative efficacy and efficiency, as well as the risks of these modalities. The use of single- or multiple-injection techniques for performing TPVBs remains controversial, and additional studies comparing these may help clarify the advantages and risks of the two. Additional comparisons between TPVBs and more distal blocks such as TAP or II/IH blocks could also be helpful.

Comparisons between US-guided and traditional approaches (or combinations of the two) are needed before definitive conclusions regarding the relative merits and risks of either modality can be drawn. Improvements in US imaging technology and needle/catheter design may allow for more consistent visualization of anatomic structures and aid the correct placement of needles/catheters within the TVPS. Increasing operator experience may increase the understanding of relative advantages and disadvantages of various US-guided approaches, and lead to more standardization of techniques.

Prospective studies are needed to confirm the preliminary finding of decreased chronic pain as well as local recurrence rates following surgical excision of malignant breast lesions (a multicenter trial is currently under way), as well as to determine the underlying mechanisms for these potential beneficial effects.

TRANSVERSUS ABDOMINIS PLANE BLOCK
History
In 2001, Rafi [91] described a percutaneous technique to deposit local anesthetic solution via the iliolumbar triangle of Petit to produce an "abdominal field block." Based on their findings from cadaveric anatomic studies as well as clinical and imaging studies in volunteers, in 2007 McDonnell and Laffey [92] coined the term "transversus abdominis plane" block (commonly abbreviated as TAP block) to describe this novel block. Since that that time, the TAP block has been increasingly used by anesthesiologists as a means of providing postoperative somatic analgesia for adult and pediatric patients undergoing a wide array of abdominal surgical procedures (see later discussion).

Indications
The TAP block has been shown to be effective for reducing pain following many types of abdominal surgery including cesarean delivery [93], open retropubic prostatectomy [94], appendectomy [95], abdominal hysterectomy [96], vertical midline laparotomy with colon resection [97], and laparoscopic cholecystectomy [98]. To date, large series of prospective studies examining use of the TAP block for surgical anesthesia have not been published. The efficacy of the TAP block for providing analgesia after surgical procedures involving incisions above the umbilicus remains unclear (see Anatomy section).

Contraindications
There are no specific contraindications for the TAP block. Standard contraindications to any regional anesthetic technique (see TPVB section) also apply to

the TAP block. In theory, the TAP block would not be possible in patients with syndromes characterized by an absence of abdominal musculature such as the prune belly syndrome. Because it is a relatively superficial block, bleeding should be controlled by applying external pressure. For this reason, the TAP block could be performed in patients with bleeding disorders or who are taking anticoagulant medications. The risk of hematoma formation does exist, but is not associated with potential risk of the permanent spinal cord injury and paraplegia associated with a central neuraxial hematoma.

Specific Risks

Specific risks of the TAP block are predominantly related to intraperitoneal needle placement with injury to intra-abdominal organs. Jankovic and colleagues [99] reported a case of inadvertent intraperitoneal catheter placement without injury to viscera, and Farooq and Carey [100] reported a case of liver trauma during TAP block. Both cases involved blocks performed using a posterior, landmark-based "2-pop" technique.

Anatomy

The ventral rami of spinal nerve roots T6 to L1 give rise to the thoracolumbar nerves, which subsequently course through the lateral abdominal wall within a potential space defined superiorly by the costal margin, inferiorly by the iliac crest, medially by the lateral border of the rectus abdominis muscle (linea semilunaris), superficially by the internal oblique muscle, and deep by the transversus abdominis muscle (Fig. 4A). The lumbar triangle of Petit is defined by the posterior border of the external oblique muscle anteriorly, and the lateral border of the latissimus dorsi muscle posteriorly. The base of the triangle is defined by the iliac crest (Fig. 4B). Jankovic and colleagues [101] performed an anatomic study in cadavers to more precisely describe the position and size of the triangle. These investigators found that the triangle is more posterior than previous descriptions of McDonnell and Rafi (mean distance posterior to mid-axillary line 9.3 cm, range 4–15.1 cm). It was also noted that the thoracolumbar nerves were not in the TAP in this posterior location, but had entered the TAP at the level of the mid-axillary line. Small branches of the subcostal arteries within the triangle in 16 of 24 specimens were also noted. Rozen and colleagues [102] performed detailed dissections of the TAP in 20 cadaveric hemi-abdominal walls. These investigators demonstrated an extensive fascial layer between the internal oblique and transversus abdominis in all specimens. This layer was not adherent to the internal oblique, and bound down the thoracolumbar nerves on its deep surface to the transversus abdominis below. Segmental nerves T6 to T9 were observed to enter the TAP between the midline and anterior axillary line. At the level of the anterior axillary line, the segmental nerves of T9 to L1 had branched extensively, with every segmental origin contributing to at least 2 nerves within the TAP. Multiple locations were found where there was extensive communication between segmental nerves. Interconnections between subcostal and intercostal nerves (T6–T9) within the TAP form an "intercostal plexus," while T9 to L1

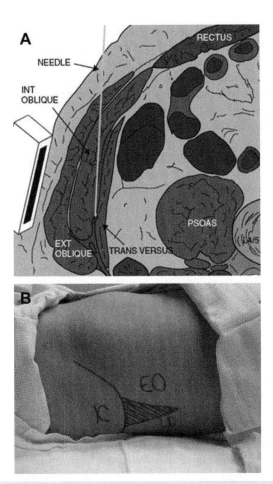

Fig. 4. Anatomy of the transversus abdominis plane (TAP). (A) Diagram shows anatomy of the TAP and needle trajectory in the TAP between the internal oblique and the transversus abdominis muscles. Ext Oblique, external oblique muscle; Int Oblique, internal oblique muscle; Transversus, transversus abdominis muscle. (*Data from* Ecole Polytechnique Fédérale de Lausanne, Switzerland, Visible Human Web Server. Available at: http://visiblehuman.epfl.ch) (*Reprinted from* Tran TM, Ivanusic JJ, Hebbard P, et al. Determination of spread of injectate after ultrasound-guided transversus abdominis plane block: a cadaveric study. Br J Anaesth 2009;102(1):123–7; with permission.) Note the location of the US transducer on the abdominal wall and the tangential (relative to the peritoneal cavity) trajectory of the needle inserted from the medial aspect of the transducer. (B) Surface anatomy for TAP block via the posterior approach. The lumbar triangle of Petit (shaded) is defined by the external oblique muscle (EO) anteriorly, the latissumus dorsi muscle (LD) posteriorly, and the iliac crest (IC) inferiorly. The needle insertion site is the center of the triangle.

contribute to plexi lateral to the deep circumflex iliac artery ("TAP plexus") and alongside the deep inferior epigastric artery located within the rectus abdominis muscle ("rectus sheath plexus").

McDonnell and colleagues [103] evaluated the spread of injectate within the TAP both in a cadaver model and using radiographic imaging in healthy volunteers. These investigators reported a sensory block extending from T7 to L1 dermatomes in the volunteers, and have reported satisfactory analgesia with this technique even for surgical procedures using a vertical midline incision extending above the umbilicus [97]. However, Hebbard [104] and Shibata and colleagues [105] performed separate retrospective audits and, based on their experiences, suggested that the TAP block performed just above the iliac crest does not reliably provide sensory analgesia above the umbilicus. Hebbard described a new "oblique subcostal" approach to the TAP, and reported that this modified approach resulted in a more cephalad distribution of the block [106]. Tran and colleagues [107] and Barrington and colleagues [108] confirmed these findings in separate studies examining the distribution of dye injected into the TAP of cadavers. These studies found that the spread of dye was limited to the T10-L1 nerve roots with the originally described US-guided posterior TAP approach, but from T9 to T11 if a US-guided subcostal approach was used. Multiple-injection techniques within the TAP (as the needle was advanced from medial to lateral) were found to be more likely to involve the T7 and T8 segmental nerves.

Lee and colleagues [109] recently published an observational study of patients receiving bilateral US-guided TAP blocks for analgesia following major abdominal surgery. Patients received the TAP blocks via either a posterior or oblique subcostal approach. This study found that patients in the oblique subcostal group had a larger number of affected dermatomal segments, and that the oblique subcostal approach was more likely to block more cephalad segments (median block height T8 vs T10 in the posterior-approach group, $P = .001$).

Techniques

The TAP block is a compartment or field block, and the end points for all of the techniques described in this section are not determined by placing the needle's tip in close proximity to the individual thoracolumbar nerves themselves. For this reason (and because it is predominantly used for postoperative analgesia rather than surgical anesthesia), the TAP block can be performed in patients under GA or SA. The TAP block is a unilateral block extending from the mid-axillary line to the ipsilateral rectus abdominis muscle, and procedures involving midline or bilateral incisions require a TAP block on each side.

Landmark-based loss-of-resistance technique

The lumbar triangle of Petit is marked following identification of muscular and bony landmarks by palpation. A short-bevel needle is inserted in the center of the triangle perpendicular to all skin planes. A classic "2-pop" end point is used to determine correct placement of the needle's tip within the TAP. The "pops" indicate the fascia under the external oblique (first) and internal oblique (second). Typically, large volumes of local anesthetic (up to 20 mL in adults, 0.2 mL/kg in children) are then injected incrementally in the TAP. Caution should be used with injection of large volumes of anesthetic, and doses of local anesthetic should be kept below recommended maximum dosing guidelines (eg, 2.5 mg/kg for bupivacaine, and so forth) especially in the case of bilateral blocks. Kato and colleagues [110] have shown that the US-guided TAP blocks in patients under GA resulted in significant increases in the plasma levels of local anesthetic (peak plasma lidocaine levels above therapeutic range for anti-arrhythmic effect), though it is not known if similar levels are encountered in patients who are awake at the time of block placement.

If a continuous technique is planned, a catheter can be passed through the needle into the pocket created by the local anesthetic in the TAP at that time. To prevent secondary block failure, the potential space of the TAP can be distended with saline, water, or D5W (dextrose 5% in water) to facilitate placement of the catheter, and the block can then be "loaded" with local anesthetic injected through the catheter.

Ultrasound-guided technique

With a linear-array, high-frequency transducer placed in an axial orientation on the lateral abdominal wall (Fig. 5A), the US image can show the subcutaneous tissues, the internal and external oblique muscles, the transversus abdominis muscle, and the peritoneum and viscera (Fig. 5B). The muscular layers of the lateral abdominal normally have a characteristic "3-stripe" appearance. The internal and external oblique muscles usually have a characteristic striated appearance, whereas the transversus abdominis usually appears relatively hypoechoic (dark) and homogeneous. Walter and colleagues [111] reported variability of the layers of the abdominal wall in Petit's area, and the best US image may be obtained with the transducer somewhat more anterior than directly over the triangle. The implications of injecting anesthetic anterior to the triangle remain unclear.

For the posterior approach to the TAP block, the US transducer is positioned axially over the iliac crest along the mid-axillary line (see Fig. 5A). The transducer's position is adjusted as necessary until the classic 3-stripe image of the muscular layers of the abdominal wall is obtained (see Fig. 5B). This 3-stripe image may be more difficult to find in obese patients, as the muscles are deeper due to abundant overlying adipose tissue, and the muscles may be atrophic and as a result relatively thin. If the 3-stripe image is difficult to obtain, the transversus abdominis muscle can often be identified by first locating the peritoneal cavity, then looking superficially. Peristaltic movements of the intestine can be seen within the peritoneal cavity, and the transversus abdominis is the muscular layer directly overlying the parietal peritoneum, though in very obese patients a thick layer of preperitoneal fat can be mistaken for the transversus abdominis muscle. Alternatively, the transducer can initially be placed more medially over the rectus abdominis muscle. By scanning

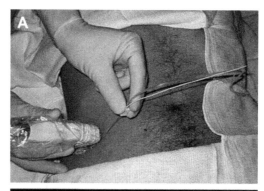

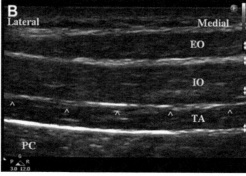

Fig. 5. Sonoanatomy for posterior-approach TAP block. (A) US transducer placement for posterior-approach TAP block. A high-frequency, linear-array probe is placed transversely on the anterolateral abdominal wall. To perform the block using an in-plane technique, the needle is usually inserted from the medial aspect of the transducer and directed laterally. (B) US image of the muscular layers of the anterolateral abdominal wall below the level of the umbilicus. EO, external oblique muscle; IO, internal oblique muscle; TA, transversus abdominis muscle; PC, peritoneal cavity. The medial and lateral aspects of the image are labeled. Local anesthetic should be injected below the fascia overlying the transversus abdominis muscle (marked with *arrowheads*) to act on the nerves traveling within the TAP.

laterally, the posterior capsule of the rectus sheath can be demonstrated, dividing to envelop the transversus abdominis and internal oblique muscles. The anterior capsule can be seen splitting to envelop the external and internal oblique muscles (the internal oblique muscle's fascial aponeurosis contributes to both the anterior and posterior capsules of the rectus sheath above the level of the arcuate line).

An in-plane needle approach is typically used, and the needle is usually inserted from the medial aspect of the transducer (see Figs. 4 and 5); this results in a tangential needle trajectory that may decrease the likelihood of puncturing the peritoneum (see Fig. 4A). Once the needle's tip penetrates the fascia (seen as a hyperechoic line) between the internal oblique and transversus abdominis muscles, local anesthetic is injected incrementally into the TAP. The local anesthetic may initially be seen spreading into the substance of the transversus abdominis muscle itself. In this case, the needle should be withdrawn slightly so that the local anesthetic spreads in the TAP. The local anesthetic must be deposited deep to the fascia that binds the thoracolumbar nerves onto to the transversus abdominis muscle, which will lift off from the transversus abdominis as more fluid is injected. The key to a successful block is not to accept anesthetic spread above this fascial layer, as the thoracolumbar nerves are below it. The needle should under no circumstances be advanced through the transversus abdominis, as injury to intraperitoneal structures could result.

Because this is a compartment block, reducing the volume of local anesthetic could theoretically decrease the extent of local anesthetic distribution within the TAP. Indeed, most of the studies that have investigated the spread of fluid within the TAP have used injectate volumes of 15 to 20 mL. (see earlier discussion). If bilateral blocks are planned or if there is concern over the potential risk of systemic local anesthetic toxicity, larger volumes of anesthetic fluid with lower concentrations can be used rather than smaller volumes with higher concentrations.

A catheter can be placed within the space created by the fluid in the TAP if a continuous block is planned. For continuous blocks, the authors prefer to distend the space with a small volume of saline first, then dose the block through the catheter, thus ensuring that the resulting block derives from the correct placement of the catheter, minimizing the risk of secondary block failure.

The sonoanatomy of the abdominal wall in the subcostal region is usually similar. However, local anesthetic can be deposited between the posterior capsule and the belly of the rectus abdominis muscle (similar to the rectus sheath block, see later discussion) if the transversus abdominis muscle (normally posterior to the rectus abdominis muscle at this level) cannot be identified in this location. For the subcostal approach, the US transducer is placed obliquely below the costal margin (Fig. 6A) along the lateral border of the rectus muscle (linea semilunaris). The muscular layers are again demonstrated (Fig. 6B). The transversus muscle may be located more medially at this level. Usually it is demonstrated posterior to the belly of the rectus abdominis muscle. If the transversus cannot be identified, local anesthetic can be injected between the belly of the rectus and the posterior capsule of the rectus sheath. A multiple-injection technique with injections both in this location and in the TAP along the costal margin described above may result in more extensive spread of local anesthetic [108]. This spread may be due to the injections being both medial and lateral to the anterior axillary line (see Anatomy section). Catheter placement may be performed in a manner similar to that described earlier for the posterior TAP block. The location of the catheter should be selected based on the dermatomal levels involved in the surgical incision.

Outcomes Data

In several small prospective randomized controlled trials, the TAP block has been shown to improve pain control and decrease opioid consumption

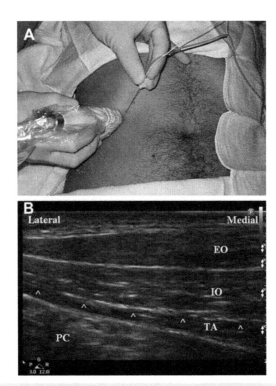

Fig. 6. Sonoanatomy for oblique subcostal-approach TAP block. (*A*) Oblique US transducer position for US imaging of the subcostal TAP. The transducer is placed on the anterior abdominal wall along the inferior costal margin, medial to the anterior axillary line. As for the posterior-approach TAP block, an in-plane technique is usually used and the needle is inserted from the medial aspect of the transducer and directed laterally. (*B*) US image of the muscular layers of the subcostal anterolateral abdominal wall. EO, external oblique muscle; IO, internal oblique muscle; TA, transversus abdominis muscle; PC, peritoneal cavity. The medial and lateral aspects of the image are labeled. Local anesthetic should be injected below the fascia overlying the transversus abdominis muscle (marked with *arrowheads*) to act on the nerves traveling within the TAP.

following several abdominal surgical procedures, including large bowel resection via a vertical midline incision [97], cesarean delivery through a Pfannenstiel incision [93], abdominal hysterectomy through a low transverse incision [96], open appendectomy [95], and laparoscopic cholecystectomy with all port sites at or below the umbilicus [98,112]. Several other case reports and case series have reported reduced pain scores and decreased morphine consumption compared with historical controls for other abdominal procedures such as retropubic prostatectomy [94].

Petersen and colleagues [113] recently conducted a systematic review of studies that have examined the effect of the TAP block on postoperative pain. These investigators identified 7 prospective studies involving a total of

364 patients. The studies overall had good methodological quality (median score 5/5, range 2–5) and validity (median score 14/16, range 2–15) as evaluated by the Oxford Quality and Oxford Pain Validity Scales. Three studies involved blocks performed using the traditional landmark-based technique. Four studies involved US-guided blocks. In 6 studies, bilateral blocks were performed. Meta-analysis of patient outcomes was performed, and significant reductions in pain scores at rest and with movement, as well as morphine consumption during the first 24 hours postoperatively, were demonstrated for patients in the TAP block groups. Of note, subgroup analysis revealed a significant difference in reduction of morphine consumption between landmark-based and US-guided blocks. Landmark-based blocks resulted in a greater reduction in mean morphine consumption (−38 mg vs −11 mg). It is not clear if this difference was due to a difference in the location of injection with the 2 techniques, or if it reflects specific differences related to the surgical procedures included in these trials.

Future Directions

The TAP block has not been used extensively for surgical anesthesia, and comparisons with GA or SA for suitable surgical procedures such as inguinal or umbilical hernia repair could be helpful. To date, no study has formally compared the various approaches for the TAP block (eg, posterior vs subcostal). Studies comparing different techniques (eg, landmark-based with LOR vs ultrasonography) could help define their relative efficacy, success rates, and other advantages and/or limitations. Direct comparisons between TAP blocks and TPVBs or neuraxial techniques such as TEA are also needed [114] to evaluate their relative success rates, analgesic effects, side effect profiles, the incidence of complications or side effects, and to reveal any additional advantages of efficiency into daily clinical practice. Although one study has shown increased plasma levels of local anesthetic following US-guided TAP blocks [110], the pharmacokinetics of various local anesthetics within the TAP remains unclear. The effect of adding epinephrine to local anesthetics on plasma levels has not been investigated. No study to date has evaluated the effects of adding adjuvants such as opioids, bicarbonate, or clonidine to the local anesthetic solution.

SUMMARY

TPVBs are a useful technique for providing anesthesia/analgesia for surgical procedures or painful conditions of the chest or upper abdomen. TPVBs may provide excellent surgical conditions or postoperative pain relief, with fewer adverse effects than central neuraxial blocks. Traditional techniques for performing TPVBs involving use of anatomic landmarks, nerve stimulation, or LOR may be aided by use of US guidance. US guidance can also be used as the sole technique to determine correct placement of needles or catheters within the TPVS. Preliminary data suggest that TPVBs may be associated with decreased recurrent rates of surgically excised breast tumors. TPVBs may also decrease the risk of chronic pain following breast surgery. Additional research may clarify risks and benefits of TPVBs relative to alternative anesthetic and analgesic techniques.

Although relatively new by comparison, the TAP block has proven to be a versatile and valuable technique for postoperative pain control. It is a relatively simple block, and is easy to learn and perform. Use of ultrasonography may improve success rates for those without experience using landmark-based techniques, and theoretically could decrease the risk of complications. Additional research comparing landmark-based and US-guided approaches, TAP blocks to GA or SA for surgical anesthesia for appropriate procedures, and TAP blocks to TEA or TPVBs for postoperative analgesia following abdominal surgery will help clarify the indications and limitations of the TAP block.

References

[1] Bonica J. The management of pain with analgesic block. In: The management of pain. London: Henry Kimpton; 1953. p. 166.

[2] Mandl F. Paravertebral block. New York: Grune and Stratton; 1946.

[3] Lawen A. Ueber segmentare schmerzaufhebung durch paravertebrale novokaininjektion zur differentialdiagnose intrabdominaler erkrangkungen. Mediziniche Wochenschrift 1922;69:1423.

[4] Scheinin TM. Use of paravertebral block in diseases of the abdominal viscera. Ann Chir Gynaecol Fenn 1954;43(3):170–7.

[5] Rosenak SS. Paravertebral procaine block for the treatment of herpes zoster. N Y State J Med 1956;56(17):2684–7.

[6] Eason MJ, Wyatt R. Paravertebral thoracic block-a reappraisal. Anaesthesia 1979;34(7): 638–42.

[7] Exadaktylos AK, Buggy DJ, Moriarty DC, et al. Can anesthetic technique for primary breast cancer surgery affect recurrence or metastasis? Anesthesiology 2006;105(4):660–4.

[8] Pusch F, Freitag H, Weinstabl C, et al. Single-injection paravertebral block compared to general anaesthesia in breast surgery. Acta Anaesthesiol Scand 1999;43(7):770–4.

[9] Klein SM, Bergh A, Steele SM, et al. Thoracic paravertebral block for breast surgery. Anesth Analg 2000;90(6):1402–5.

[10] Najarian MM, Johnson JM, Landercasper J, et al. Paravertebral block: an alternative to general anesthesia in breast cancer surgery. Am Surg 2003;69(3):213–8 [discussion: 218].

[11] Naja Z, Ziade MF, Lonnqvist PA. Bilateral paravertebral somatic nerve block for ventral hernia repair. Eur J Anaesthesiol 2002;19(3):197–202.

[12] Naja MZ, Ziade MF, Lonnqvist PA. General anaesthesia combined with bilateral paravertebral blockade (T5-6) vs. general anaesthesia for laparoscopic cholecystectomy: a prospective, randomized clinical trial. Eur J Anaesthesiol 2004;21(6):489–95.

[13] Marret E, Bazelly B, Taylor G, et al. Paravertebral block with ropivacaine 0.5% versus systemic analgesia for pain relief after thoracotomy. Ann Thorac Surg 2005;79(6): 2109–13.

[14] Vogt A, Stieger DS, Theurillat C, et al. Single-injection thoracic paravertebral block for postoperative pain treatment after thoracoscopic surgery. Br J Anaesth 2005;95(6):816–21.

[15] Berta E, Spanhel J, Smakal O, et al. Single injection paravertebral block for renal surgery in children. Paediatr Anaesth 2008;18(7):593–7.

[16] Moussa AA. Opioid saving strategy: bilateral single-site thoracic paravertebral block in right lobe donor hepatectomy. Middle East J Anesthesiol 2008;19(4):789–801.

[17] Karmakar MK, Chui PT, Joynt GM, et al. Thoracic paravertebral block for management of pain associated with multiple fractured ribs in patients with concomitant lumbar spinal trauma. Reg Anesth Pain Med 2001;26(2):169–73.

[18] Williamson S, Kumar CM. Paravertebral block in head injured patient with chest trauma. Anaesthesia 1997;52(3):284–5.

[19] Karmakar MK, Critchley LA, Ho AM, et al. Continuous thoracic paravertebral infusion of bupivacaine for pain management in patients with multiple fractured ribs. Chest 2003;123(2):424–31.

[20] Karmakar MK, Ho AM. Acute pain management of patients with multiple fractured ribs. J Trauma 2003;54(3):615–25.

[21] Flashman FL, Lundy JS. Relief of pain by paravertebral block in complicated fractures of the ribs; report of case. Mayo Clin Proc 1948;23(19):446.

[22] Johnson LR, Rocco AG, Ferrante FM. Continuous subpleural-paravertebral block in acute thoracic herpes zoster. Anesth Analg 1988;67(11):1105–8.

[23] Horlocker TT, Wedel DJ, Rowlingson JC, et al. Regional anesthesia in the patient receiving antithrombotic or thrombolytic therapy: American society of regional anesthesia and pain medicine evidence-based guidelines (third edition). Reg Anesth Pain Med 2010;35(1): 64–101.

[24] Lall NG, Sharma SR. "Clicking" pneumothorax following thoracic paravertebral block. Case report. Br J Anaesth 1971;43(4):415–7.

[25] Thomas PW, Sanders DJ, Berrisford RG. Pulmonary haemorrhage after percutaneous paravertebral block. Br J Anaesth 1999;83(4):668–9.

[26] Hill RP, Greengrass R. Pulmonary haemorrhage after percutaneous paravertebral block. Br J Anaesth 2000;84(3):423–4.

[27] Bogacki E, Pielowski J. Transient cessation of the spinal cord function as a complication of paravertebral blockade with lignocaine. Neurol Neurochir Pol 1970;4(6):717–9.

[28] Gay GR, Evans JA. Total spinal anesthesia following lumbar paravertebral block: a potentially lethal complication. Anesth Analg 1971;50(3):344–8.

[29] Sharrock NE. Postural headache following thoracic somatic paravertebral nerve block. Anesthesiology 1980;52(4):360–2.

[30] Brittingham TE, Berlin LN, Wolff HG. Nervous system damage following paravertebral block with efocaine: report of three cases. J Am Med Assoc 1954;154(4):329–30.

[31] Naja Z, Lonnqvist PA. Somatic paravertebral nerve blockade. incidence of failed block and complications. Anaesthesia 2001;56(12):1184–8.

[32] Wyatt SS, Price RA. Complications of paravertebral block. Br J Anaesth 2000;84(3):424.

[33] Cheung SL, Booker PD, Franks R, et al. Serum concentrations of bupivacaine during prolonged continuous paravertebral infusion in young infants. Br J Anaesth 1997;79(1):9–13.

[34] Garutti I, Olmedilla L, Perez-Pena JM, et al. Hemodynamic effects of lidocaine in the thoracic paravertebral space during one-lung ventilation for thoracic surgery. J Cardiothorac Vasc Anesth 2006;20(5):648–51.

[35] Catala E, Casas JI, Galan J, et al. Thoracic paravertebral blockade: postoperative analgesic effectiveness and plasma concentrations of bupivacaine. Rev Esp Anestesiol Reanim 1993;40(3):125–8.

[36] Saito T, Gallagher ET, Yamada K, et al. Broad unilateral analgesia. Reg Anesth 1994; 19(5):360–1.

[37] Richardson J, Lonnqvist PA. Thoracic paravertebral block. Br J Anaesth 1998;81(2): 230–8.

[38] Saito T, Den S, Tanuma K, et al. Anatomical bases for paravertebral anesthetic block: fluid communication between the thoracic and lumbar paravertebral regions. Surg Radiol Anat 1999;21(6):359–63.

[39] Saito T, Tanuma K, Den S, et al. Pathways of anesthetic from the thoracic paravertebral region to the celiac ganglion. Clin Anat 2002;15(5):340–4.

[40] Karmakar MK. Thoracic paravertebral block. Anesthesiology 2001;95(3):771–80.

[41] Karmakar MK, Kwok WH, Kew J. Thoracic paravertebral block: radiological evidence of contralateral spread anterior to the vertebral bodies. Br J Anaesth 2000;84(2): 263–5.

[42] Purcell-Jones G, Pither CE, Justins DM. Paravertebral somatic nerve block: a clinical, radiographic, and computed tomographic study in chronic pain patients. Anesth Analg 1989;68(1):32–9.

[43] Garutti I, Hervias M, Barrio JM, et al. Subdural spread of local anesthetic agent following thoracic paravertebral block and cannulation. Anesthesiology 2003;98(4):1005–7.

[44] Naja ZM, El-Rajab M, Al-Tannir MA, et al. Thoracic paravertebral block: Influence of the number of injections. Reg Anesth Pain Med 2006;31(3):196–201.

[45] Kotze A, Scally A, Howell S. Efficacy and safety of different techniques of paravertebral block for analgesia after thoracotomy: a systematic review and metaregression. Br J Anaesth 2009;103(5):626–36.

[46] Cheema SP, Ilsley D, Richardson J, et al. A thermographic study of paravertebral analgesia. Anaesthesia 1995;50(2):118–21.

[47] Chelly JE, Uskova A, Merman R, et al. A multifactorial approach to the factors influencing determination of paravertebral depth. Can J Anaesth 2008;55(9):587–94.

[48] Naja MZ, Gustafsson AC, Ziade MF, et al. Distance between the skin and the thoracic paravertebral space. Anaesthesia 2005;60(7):680–4.

[49] Lemay E, Guay J, Cote C, et al. The number of injections does not influence local anesthetic absorption after paravertebral blockade. Can J Anaesth 2003;50(6):562–7.

[50] Baumgarten RK, Greengrass RA. Thoracic paravertebral block: Is single-injection really safer? Reg Anesth Pain Med 2006;31(6):584–5, author reply 585.

[51] Sabanathan S, Smith PJ, Pradhan GN, et al. Continuous intercostal nerve block for pain relief after thoracotomy. Ann Thorac Surg 1988;46(4):425–6.

[52] Soni AK, Conacher ID, Waller DA, et al. Video-assisted thoracoscopic placement of paravertebral catheters: a technique for postoperative analgesia for bilateral thoracoscopic surgery. Br J Anaesth 1994;72(4):462–4.

[53] Richardson J, Cheema SP, Hawkins J, et al. Thoracic paravertebral space location. A new method using pressure measurement. Anaesthesia 1996;51(2):137–9.

[54] Wheeler LJ. Peripheral nerve stimulation end-point for thoracic paravertebral block. Br J Anaesth 2001;86(4):598–9.

[55] Jamieson BD, Mariano ER. Thoracic and lumbar paravertebral blocks for outpatient lithotripsy. J Clin Anesth 2007;19(2):149–51.

[56] Pusch F, Wildling E, Klimscha W, et al. Sonographic measurement of needle insertion depth in paravertebral blocks in women. Br J Anaesth 2000;85(6):841–3.

[57] Hara K, Sakura S, Nomura T. Use of ultrasound for thoracic paravertebral block. Masui 2007;56(8):925–31.

[58] O'Riain SC, Donnell BO, Cuffe T, et al. Thoracic paravertebral block using real-time ultrasound guidance. Anesth Analg 2010;110(1):248–51.

[59] Luyet C, Eichenberger U, Greif R, et al. Ultrasound-guided paravertebral puncture and placement of catheters in human cadavers: an imaging study. Br J Anaesth 2009;102 (4):534–9.

[60] Renes SH, Bruhn J, Gielen MJ, et al. In-plane ultrasound-guided thoracic paravertebral block: a preliminary report of 36 cases with radiologic confirmation of catheter position. Reg Anesth Pain Med 2010;35(2):212–6.

[61] Cooter RD, Rudkin GE, Gardiner SE. Day case breast augmentation under paravertebral blockade: a prospective study of 100 consecutive patients. Aesthetic Plast Surg 2007; 31(6):666–73.

[62] Moller JF, Nikolajsen L, Rodt SA, et al. Thoracic paravertebral block for breast cancer surgery: a randomized double-blind study. Anesth Analg 2007;105(6):1848–51, table of contents.

[63] Oguz S, Kucuk C, Eskicirak E, et al. Thoracic paravertebral block for breast surgery in a patient with myasthenia gravis. J Anesth 2007;21(3):449.

[64] Hadzic A, Kerimoglu B, Loreio D, et al. Paravertebral blocks provide superior same-day recovery over general anesthesia for patients undergoing inguinal hernia repair. Anesth Analg 2006;102(4):1076–81.

[65] Naja ZM, Raf M, El Rajab M, et al. Nerve stimulator-guided paravertebral blockade combined with sevoflurane sedation versus general anesthesia with systemic analgesia for postherniorrhaphy pain relief in children: a prospective randomized trial. Anesthesiology 2005;103(3):600–5.

[66] Falkensammer J, Hakaim AG, Klocker J, et al. Paravertebral blockade with propofol sedation versus general anesthesia for elective endovascular abdominal aortic aneurysm repair. Vascular 2006;14(1):17–22.

[67] Akcaboy EY, Akcaboy ZN, Gogus N. Ambulatory inguinal herniorrhaphy: paravertebral block versus spinal anesthesia. Minerva Anestesiol 2009;75(12):684–91.

[68] Bhattacharya P, Mandal MC, Mukhopadhyay S, et al. Unilateral paravertebral block: an alternative to conventional spinal anaesthesia for inguinal hernia repair. Acta Anaesthesiol Scand 2010;54(2):246–51.

[69] Boezaart AP, Raw RM. Continuous thoracic paravertebral block for major breast surgery. Reg Anesth Pain Med 2006;31(5):470–6.

[70] Dabbagh A, Elyasi H. The role of paravertebral block in decreasing postoperative pain in elective breast surgeries. Med Sci Monit 2007;13(10):CR464–7.

[71] Hill SE, Keller RA, Stafford-Smith M, et al. Efficacy of single-dose, multilevel paravertebral nerve blockade for analgesia after thoracoscopic procedures. Anesthesiology 2006;104 (5):1047–53.

[72] Kaya FN, Turker G, Basagan-Mogol E, et al. Preoperative multiple-injection thoracic paravertebral blocks reduce postoperative pain and analgesic requirements after video-assisted thoracic surgery. J Cardiothorac Vasc Anesth 2006;20(5):639–43.

[73] Kumar CM. Paravertebral block for post-cholecystectomy pain relief. Br J Anaesth 1989;63(1):129.

[74] Culp WC, Payne MN, Montgomery ML. Thoracic paravertebral block for analgesia following liver mass radiofrequency ablation. Br J Radiol 2008;81(961):e23–5.

[75] Culp WC, McCowan TC, DeValdenebro M, et al. Paravertebral block: an improved method of pain control in percutaneous transhepatic biliary drainage. Cardiovasc Intervent Radiol 2006;29(6):1015–21.

[76] Ben-David B, Merman R, Chelly JE. Paravertebral blocks in thoracoscopy: single no, continuous yes. Anesthesiology 2007;106(2):398 [author reply: 398–9].

[77] Sidiropoulou T, Buonomo O, Fabbi E, et al. A prospective comparison of continuous wound infiltration with ropivacaine versus single-injection paravertebral block after modified radical mastectomy. Anesth Analg 2008;106(3):997–1001, table of contents.

[78] Naja ZM, Raf M, El-Rajab M, et al. A comparison of nerve stimulator guided paravertebral block and ilio-inguinal nerve block for analgesia after inguinal herniorrhaphy in children. Anaesthesia 2006;61(11):1064–8.

[79] Klein SM, Pietrobon R, Nielsen KC, et al. Paravertebral somatic nerve block compared with peripheral nerve blocks for outpatient inguinal herniorrhaphy. Reg Anesth Pain Med 2002;27(5):476–80.

[80] Davies RG, Myles PS, Graham JM. A comparison of the analgesic efficacy and side-effects of paravertebral vs epidural blockade for thoracotomy—a systematic review and meta-analysis of randomized trials. Br J Anaesth 2006;96(4):418–26.

[81] Joshi GP, Bonnet F, Shah R, et al. A systematic review of randomized trials evaluating regional techniques for postthoracotomy analgesia. Anesth Analg 2008;107(3):1026–40.

[82] Scarci M, Joshi A, Attia R. In patients undergoing thoracic surgery is paravertebral block as effective as epidural analgesia for pain management? Interact Cardiovasc Thorac Surg 2010;10(1):92–6.

[83] Bigler D, Dirkes W, Hansen R, et al. Effects of thoracic paravertebral block with bupivacaine versus combined thoracic epidural block with bupivacaine and morphine on pain and pulmonary function after cholecystectomy. Acta Anaesthesiol Scand 1989;33(7): 561–4.

[84] Mehta Y, Arora D, Sharma KK, et al. Comparison of continuous thoracic epidural and paravertebral block for postoperative analgesia after robotic-assisted coronary artery bypass surgery. Ann Card Anaesth 2008;11(2):91–6.

[85] Kairaluoma PM, Bachmann MS, Rosenberg PH, et al. Preincisional paravertebral block reduces the prevalence of chronic pain after breast surgery. Anesth Analg 2006; 103(3):703–8.

[86] Iohom G, Abdalla H, O'Brien J, et al. The associations between severity of early postoperative pain, chronic postsurgical pain and plasma concentration of stable nitric oxide products after breast surgery. Anesth Analg 2006;103(4):995–1000.

[87] O'Riain SC, Buggy DJ, Kerin MJ, et al. Inhibition of the stress response to breast cancer surgery by regional anesthesia and analgesia does not affect vascular endothelial growth factor and prostaglandin E2. Anesth Analg 2005;100(1):244–9.

[88] Munoz M, Rosso M, Casinello F, et al. Paravertebral anesthesia: how substance P and the NK-1 receptor could be involved in regional block and breast cancer recurrence. Breast Cancer Res Treat 2010;122:601–3.

[89] Deegan CA, Murray D, Doran P, et al. Effect of anaesthetic technique on oestrogen receptor-negative breast cancer cell function in vitro. Br J Anaesth 2009;103(5):685–90.

[90] Sessler DI, Ben-Eliyahu S, Mascha EJ, et al. Can regional analgesia reduce the risk of recurrence after breast cancer? Methodology of a multicenter randomized trial. Contemp Clin Trials 2008;29(4):517–26.

[91] Rafi AN. Abdominal field block: a new approach via the lumbar triangle. Anaesthesia 2001;56(10):1024–6.

[92] McDonnell JG, Laffey JG. Transversus abdominis plane block. Anesth Analg 2007;105(3): 883.

[93] McDonnell JG, Curley G, Carney J, et al. The analgesic efficacy of transversus abdominis plane block after cesarean delivery: a randomized controlled trial. Anesth Analg 2008;106(1):186–91, table of contents.

[94] O'Donnell BD, McDonnell JG, McShane AJ. The transversus abdominis plane (TAP) block in open retropubic prostatectomy. Reg Anesth Pain Med 2006;31(1):91.

[95] Niraj G, Searle A, Mathews M, et al. Analgesic efficacy of ultrasound-guided transversus abdominis plane block in patients undergoing open appendicectomy. Br J Anaesth 2009;103(4):601–5.

[96] Carney J, McDonnell JG, Ochana A, et al. The transversus abdominis plane block provides effective postoperative analgesia in patients undergoing total abdominal hysterectomy. Anesth Analg 2008;107(6):2056–60.

[97] McDonnell JG, O'Donnell B, Curley G, et al. The analgesic efficacy of transversus abdominis plane block after abdominal surgery: a prospective randomized controlled trial. Anesth Analg 2007;104(1):193–7.

[98] El-Dawlatly AA, Turkistani A, Kettner SC, et al. Ultrasound-guided transversus abdominis plane block: description of a new technique and comparison with conventional systemic analgesia during laparoscopic cholecystectomy. Br J Anaesth 2009; 102(6):763–7.

[99] Jankovic Z, Ahmad N, Ravishankar N, et al. Transversus abdominis plane block: how safe is it? Anesth Analg 2008;107(5):1758–9.

[100] Farooq M, Carey M. A case of liver trauma with a blunt regional anesthesia needle while performing transversus abdominis plane block. Reg Anesth Pain Med 2008;33(3):274–5.

[101] Jankovic ZB, du Feu FM, McConnell P. An anatomical study of the transversus abdominis plane block: location of the lumbar triangle of petit and adjacent nerves. Anesth Analg 2009;109(3):981–5.

[102] Rozen WM, Tran TM, Ashton MW, et al. Refining the course of the thoracolumbar nerves: a new understanding of the innervation of the anterior abdominal wall. Clin Anat 2008; 21(4):325–33.

[103] McDonnell JG, O'Donnell BD, Farrell T, et al. Transversus abdominis plane block: a cadaveric and radiological evaluation. Reg Anesth Pain Med 2007;32(5):399–404.

[104] Hebbard P. Audit of "rescue" analgesia using TAP block. Anaesth Intensive Care 2007; 35(4):617–8.

[105] Shibata Y, Sato Y, Fujiwara Y, et al. Transversus abdominis plane block. Anesth Analg 2007;105(3):883 [author reply: 883].

[106] Hebbard P. Subcostal transversus abdominis plane block under ultrasound guidance. Anesth Analg 2008;106(2):674–5, author reply 675.

[107] Tran TM, Ivanusic JJ, Hebbard P, et al. Determination of spread of injectate after ultrasound-guided transversus abdominis plane block: a cadaveric study. Br J Anaesth 2009;102(1): 123–7.

[108] Barrington MJ, Ivanusic JJ, Rozen WM, et al. Spread of injectate after ultrasound-guided subcostal transversus abdominis plane block: a cadaveric study. Anaesthesia 2009; 64(7):745–50.

[109] Lee TH, Barrington MJ, Tran TM, et al. Comparison of extent of sensory block following posterior and subcostal approaches to ultrasound-guided transversus abdominis plane block. Anaesth Intensive Care 2010;38(3):452–60.

[110] Kato N, Fujiwara Y, Harato M, et al. Serum concentration of lidocaine after transversus abdominis plane block. J Anesth 2009;23(2):298–300.

[111] Walter EJ, Smith P, Albertyn R, et al. Ultrasound imaging for transversus abdominis blocks. Anaesthesia 2008;63(2):211.

[112] Ra YS, Kim CH, Lee GY, et al. The analgesic effect of the ultrasound-guided transverse abdominis plane block after laparoscopic cholecystectomy. Korean J Anesthesiol 2010; 58(4):362–8.

[113] Petersen PL, Mathiesen O, Torup H, et al. The transversus abdominis plane block: a valuable option for postoperative analgesia? A topical review. Acta Anaesthesiol Scand 2010;54(5):529–35.

[114] Tornero-Campello G. Transversus abdominis plane block should be compared with epidural for postoperative analgesia after abdominal surgery. Anesth Analg 2007; 105(1):281–2 [author reply: 282–3].

Advances in Anesthesia 28 (2010) 111–146

ADVANCES IN ANESTHESIA

Postdural Puncture Headache

Brian E. Harrington, MD

Billings Clinic Hospital, PO Box 1837, Billings, MT 59103, USA

Practitioners of anesthesia are universally aware of postdural puncture headache (PDPH), yet our understanding of this serious complication remains surprisingly incomplete. This review summarizes the current state of knowledge regarding this familiar iatrogenic problem as well as the closely related topics of accidental dural puncture (ADP) and the epidural blood patch (EBP).

HISTORY AND CURRENT RELEVANCE

As one of the earliest recognized complications of regional anesthesia, PDPH has a long and colorful history [1]. Dr August Bier noted this adverse effect in the first patient to undergo successful spinal anesthesia on August 16, 1898. Bier observed: "Two hours after the operation his back and left leg became painful and the patient vomited and complained of severe headache. The pain and vomiting soon ceased, but *headache was still present the next day*" (italics added) [2]. The following week, Bier and his assistant, Dr August Hildebrandt, performed experiments with cocainization of the spinal cord on themselves. In a description scarcely improved upon in an intervening century, Bier later reported first-hand his experience in the days to follow: "I had a feeling of very strong pressure on my skull and became rather dizzy when I stood up rapidly from my chair. All these symptoms vanished at once when I lay down flat, but returned when I stood up... I was forced to take to bed and remained there for nine days, because all the manifestations recurred as soon as I got up... The symptoms finally resolved nine days after the lumbar puncture" [2]. In medical history, few complications have come to be considered as closely linked to a specific technique as PDPH with spinal anesthesia.

Employing the methods of the early twentieth century, spinal anesthesia was frequently followed by severe and prolonged headache, casting a long shadow over the development and acceptance of this modality. Investigations into the cause of these troubling symptoms eventually led to the conclusion that they were due to persistent cerebrospinal fluid (CSF) loss through the rent created in the meninges. The most notable successful efforts to minimize the loss of

E-mail address: bhbillings@aol.com

0737-6146/10/$ – see front matter
doi:10.1016/j.aan.2010.07.006

CSF were through the use of smaller gauge and "noncutting" needles (as convincingly demonstrated by Vandam and Dripps [3] and Hart and Whitacre [4], respectively, in the 1950s). Despite these significant advances in prevention, PDPH remained a frustratingly common occurrence.

The extensive search for effective treatments for PDPH dates to Bier's time. Yet efforts through the first half of the 20th century, while often intensive and creative, were questionably worthwhile. In a monograph intended to be a comprehensive review of PDPH from the 1800s through 1960, Dr Wallace Tourette and colleagues [5] cite dozens of separate and far-ranging treatment recommendations, including such interventions as intravenous ethanol, x-rays to the skull, sympathetic blocks, and manipulation of the spine. Unfortunately, before the introduction of the EBP there were no treatment measures that could be described as significant improvements over the simple passage of time. In his 1955 textbook, *Complications of Regional Anesthesia,* Dr Daniel Moore describes in detail a full 3-day treatment protocol for PDPH. He concludes by noting that 3 days is the usual duration of untreated mild to moderate headaches, but that "nevertheless, the patient feels an attempt to help his problem is being made" [6].

The EBP, a startlingly unique medical procedure, proved to be the breakthrough in the treatment of PDPH. The concept of using autologous blood to "patch" a hole in the meninges was introduced in late 1960 by Dr James Gormley, a general surgeon [7]. Yet Gormley's brief report went largely unnoticed for nearly a decade because, to the practitioners of the day, an iatrogenic epidural hematoma raised serious concerns of scarring, infection, and nerve damage. The procedure was only later popularized in anesthesia circles, and performed as a true epidural injection, largely through the work of Drs Anthony DiGiovanni and Burdett Dunbar [8]. The EBP procedure was further refined through the 1970s as the volume of blood commonly used increased to 20 mL [9]. Today, the EBP is nearly universally employed as the cornerstone of treatment for severe PDPH [10].

PDPH remains a prominent clinical concern to the present day. Largely due to modifications in practice that followed the identification of risk factors, rates of PDPH following spinal anesthesia have steadily declined; from an incidence exceeding 50% in Bier's time, to around 10% in the 1950s [3], until currently a rate of 1% or less can be reasonably expected. However, as perhaps the highest risk group, an unfortunate 1.7% of obstetric patients continue to experience PDPH after spinal anesthesia using 27-gauge Whitacre needles [11]. Since epidural techniques intend to avoid meningeal puncture, they are attractive alternatives to spinal anesthesia. Yet occasional ADP, with either the needle or catheter, is unavoidable (or may be unrecognized at the time in more than 25% of patients who eventually develop PDPH) [12]. In nonobstetric situations (eg, interlaminar epidural steroid injections), the rate of ADP should be considerably less than 0.5%. However, ADP is of greatest concern in the obstetric anesthesia setting, where the incidence of this adverse event is around 1.5% [11]. Over half of all patients who experience an ADP will eventually develop headache symptoms, and many studies in obstetric populations report PDPH rates exceeding 75%. In addition to anesthesia interventions, PDPH remains a too-common iatrogenic complication following myelography and diagnostic/therapeutic lumbar puncture (LP). In these situations, rates of PDPH around 10% are commonly cited, as practitioners often continue to use Quincke needles, and large-gauge needles are considered necessary because of the viscosity of contrast material as well as to facilitate the timely collection of CSF. Consequently, there is evidence to suggest that the majority of instances of PDPH now have a nonanesthesia origin [13].

The practical significance of PDPH is illustrated in being noted in the American Society of Anesthesiologists Closed Claims Project database as one of the most frequent claims for malpractice involving obstetric anesthesia [14], regional anesthesia [15], and chronic pain management [16]. Justifiably, headache is the most commonly disclosed risk when obtaining consent for spinal and epidural anesthesia [17]. The potentially serious nature of this complication necessitates inclusion in informed consent involving any procedure that may result in PDPH. As part of this discussion, patients should also be apprised of the normal delayed onset of symptoms and given clear instructions for the timely provision of advice or management should they experience adverse effects.

PATHOPHYSIOLOGY

It has long been accepted that PDPH results from a disruption of normal CSF homeostasis. However, despite a great deal of research and observational data, the pathophysiology of PDPH remains incompletely understood [18].

CSF is produced primarily in the choroid plexus at a rate of approximately 0.35 mL/min and reabsorbed through the arachnoid villa. The total CSF volume in adults is maintained around 150 mL, of which approximately half is extracranial, and gives rise to normal lumbar opening pressures of 5 to 15 cm H_2O in the horizontal position (40–50 cm H_2O in the upright position). It has been shown experimentally that the loss of approximately 10% of total CSF volume predictably results in the development of typical PDPH symptoms, which resolve promptly with reconstitution of this deficit [19]. It is agreed that PDPH is caused by the loss of CSF through a persistent leak in the meninges. In this regard, it has been postulated that the cellular arachnoid mater (containing frequent tight junctions and occluding junctions) is perhaps more important than the more permeable and acellular dura mater in the genesis of PDPH [20]. This tenet has led some, including this author, to advocate the term "meningeal puncture headache" (MPH) as more accurate and descriptive than PDPH [21,22]. However, "postdural puncture headache" is used in this review as it is the more common terminology at the present time. Regardless of nomenclature, it is also important to acknowledge that references to "dural puncture" throughout the medical literature (including this article) actually describe puncture of the dura-arachnoid and are more correctly termed "meningeal puncture." Furthermore, the apparent role of the arachnoid mater calls into question the significance of the many published studies concerning PDPH of isolated in vitro dura mater.

The actual means by which CSF hypotension generates headache is controversial and is currently ascribed to a bimodal mechanism involving both loss of intracranial support and cerebral vasodilation (predominantly venous). Diminished buoyant support is thought to allow the brain to sag in the upright position, resulting in traction and pressure on pain-sensitive structures within the cranium (dura, cranial nerves, bridging veins, and venous sinuses). Adenosine-mediated vasodilation may occur secondary to diminished intracranial CSF (in accordance with the Monro-Kellie hypothesis, which states that intracranial volume must remain constant) and reflexively secondary to traction on intracranial vessels.

Multiple neural pathways are involved in generating the symptoms of PDPH. These pathways include the ophthalmic branch of the trigeminal nerve (CN V_1) in frontal head pain, cranial nerves IX and X in occipital pain, and cervical nerves C1 to C3 in neck and shoulder pain [23]. Nausea is attributed to vagal stimulation (CN X). Auditory and vestibular symptoms are secondary to the direct communication between the CSF and the perilymph via the cochlear aqueduct, which results in decreased perilymphatic pressures in the inner ear and an imbalance between the endolymph and perilymph [24]. Significant visual disturbances may represent a transient palsy of the nerves supplying the extraocular muscles of the eye (CN III, IV, and, VI). Here, the lateral rectus muscle is most often involved, which is attributed to the long, vulnerable intracranial course of the abducens nerve (CN VI) [25]. Other, much less frequent cranial nerve palsies of the trigeminal (CN V), facial (CN VII), and auditory (CN VIII) nerves have also been reported [26].

CLINICAL PRESENTATION AND CHARACTERISTICS
Although many clinical variations have been described, most cases of PDPH are characterized by their typical onset, presentation, and associated symptoms.

Onset
Onset of symptoms is generally delayed, with headache usually beginning 12 to 48 hours and rarely more than 5 days following meningeal puncture. In their landmark observational study, Vandam and Dripps reported onset of headache symptoms within 3 days of spinal anesthesia in 84.8% of patients for whom such data were available [3]. More recently, Lybecker and colleagues [27] performed a detailed analysis of 75 consecutive patients with PDPH following spinal anesthesia (primarily using 25-gauge cutting-point needles). Although none of their patients noted the onset of symptoms during the first hour following meningeal puncture, 65% experienced symptoms within 24 hours and 92% within 48 hours. An onset of symptoms within 1 hour of neuraxial procedures is suspicious for pneumocephalus, especially in the setting of an epidural loss-of-resistance technique using air [28]. Occasional reports of unusually delayed onset of PDPH highlight the importance of seeking a history

of central neuraxial instrumentation whenever positional headaches are evaluated [29].

Presentation

The cardinal feature of PDPH is a postural nature, with headache symptoms worsening in the upright position and relieved, or at least improved, with recumbency. The International Classification of Headache Disorders further describes this positional quality as worsening within 15 minutes of sitting or standing, and improving within 15 minutes after lying [30]. Headache is always bilateral, with a distribution that is frontal (25%), occipital (27%), or both (45%) [27]. Headaches are typically described as "dull/aching", "throbbing", or "pressure-type".

The severity of headache symptoms, a feature with important ramifications for treatment, varies considerably among patients. Although there is no widely accepted severity scale, one practical approach is to have patients simply rate their headache intensity using a 10-point analog scale, with 1 to 3 classified as "mild," 4 to 6 "moderate," and 7 to 10 "severe." Lybecker and colleagues [27] further categorized patients according to restriction in physical activity, degree of confinement to bed, and presence of associated symptoms (Fig. 1). A prospective analysis of PDPH after spinal anesthesia using the Lybecker classification system demonstrated that 11% were mild, 23% moderate, and 67% severe.

Associated Symptoms

If headaches are severe, they are more likely to be accompanied by a variety of other symptoms. Pain and stiffness in the neck and shoulders is common, and seen in nearly half of all patients experiencing PDPH [31]. With questioning, nausea may be reported by a majority of patients and can lead to vomiting [27].

Patients uncommonly may experience auditory or visual symptoms [24], and the risk for either appears to be directly related to needle size [25,32]. In the large study of PDPH by Vandam and Dripps [3], each was seen to a clinically apparent degree in 0.4% of patients. Auditory symptoms include hearing loss, tinnitus, and even hyperacousis, and can be unilateral. It is interesting to note that subclinical hearing loss, especially in the lower frequencies, has been found to be common following spinal anesthesia, even in the absence of PDPH [32]. Closely associated with auditory function, vestibular disturbances (dizziness or vertigo) may also occur. Visual problems include blurred vision, difficulties with accommodation, mild photophobia, and diplopia [25]. In contrast to headache complaints, which are consistently bilateral, nearly 80% of episodes of diplopia secondary to meningeal puncture involve unilateral cranial nerve palsies.

RISK FACTORS

Risk factors for PDPH can be broadly categorized into patient characteristics and procedural details.

Severity of PDPH

Mild	Postural headache slightly restricting daily activities	
	Patient is not bedridden at any time during the day	
	No associated symptoms	
Moderate	Postural headache that significantly restricts daily activities	
	Patient is bedridden part of the day	
	Associated symptoms may or may not be present	
Severe	Postural headache severe enough to stay in bed all day	
	Associated symptoms always present	

Associated Symptoms of PDPH

Vestibular	Nausea, vomiting, dizziness
Cochlear	Hearing loss, hyperacousis, tinnitus
Ocular	Photophobia, teichopsia, diplopia, difficulty with accommodation
Musculoskeletal	Neck stiffness, scapular pain

Fig. 1. Classification of severity of postdural puncture headache (PDPH). (*Adapted from* Lybecker H, Djernes M, Schmidt JF. Postdural puncture headache (PDPH): onset, duration, severity, and associated symptoms. An analysis of 75 consecutive patients with PDPH. Acta Anaesthesiol Scand 1995;39:606; with permission.)

Patient Characteristics

The patient characteristic having the greatest impact on risk of PDPH is age. Uncommonly reported in children younger than 10 years, PDPH has a peak incidence in the teens and early 20s [33]. The incidence then declines over time, becoming much less frequent in patients older than 50 years (Fig. 2). Females have long been recognized as being at increased risk for PDPH, and a systematic review of published studies found the odds of developing PDPH were significantly lower for male than age-matched nonpregnant female subjects (odds ratio = 0.55; 95% confidence interval, 0.44–0.67) [34]. The etiology behind this gender difference is not clear. Body mass index (BMI; calculated as the weight in kilograms divided by height in meters, squared) appears to be a mixed risk factor. Morbid obesity presents obvious technical difficulties for central neuraxial procedures, increasing the likelihood of multiple needle passes and ADP [35]. However, low BMI has been reported as an independent risk factor for PDPH [36] and high BMI (ie, obesity) may actually decrease risk, possibly due to a beneficial effect of increased intra-abdominal pressure [37].

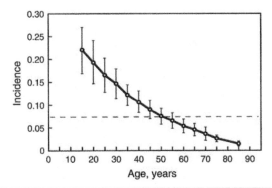

Fig. 2. Logistic regression of the incidence of PDPH as a function of age: Pa = [1 + exp (0.633 + 0.039 × age)]$^{-1}$. Age-specific incidence means and 95% confidence limits are shown as vertical lines. Overall incidence of PDPH for this study, which used cutting needles only, was 7.3% (*dashed horizontal line*). (*Data from* Lybecker H, Moller JT, May O, et al. Incidence and prediction of postdural puncture headache: a prospective study of 1021 spinal anesthesias. Anesth Analg 1990;70:389–94.)

Pregnancy has traditionally been regarded as a risk factor for PDPH [3], but this consideration partially reflects the young age as well as the high incidence of ADP in the gravid population. Although controversial, pushing during the second stage of labor, thought to promote the loss of CSF through a hole in the meninges, has been reported to influence the risk of PDPH following ADP. Angle and colleagues [38] noted that the cumulative duration of bearing down correlated with the risk of developing PDPH in patients who had experienced an ADP. These investigators also found that patients who avoided pushing altogether (proceeded to cesarean delivery before reaching second stage of labor) had a much lower incidence of PDPH (10%) than those who pushed (74%).

PDPHs appear to have an interesting association with other headaches. Patients who report having had a headache within the week prior to LP have been observed to have a higher incidence of PDPH [36]. On further analysis, only those with chronic bilateral tension-type headaches were found to be at increased risk [39]. A history of unilateral headache [39] or migraine [40] has not been linked to an increased risk of PDPH. Menstrual cycle, a factor in migraine headaches, did not influence the rate of PDPH in one small pilot study [41]. Patients with a history of previous PDPH, particularly women, appear to have an increased risk for new PDPH after spinal anesthesia [42]. With epidural procedures, patients with a history of ADP have been shown to be at slightly increased risk for another ADP (and subsequent PDPH) [43].

Procedural Details
Needle size and tip design are the most important procedural factors related to PDPH (Fig. 3) [44]. Needle size is directly related to the risk of PDPH. Meningeal puncture with larger needles is associated with a higher incidence of PDPH

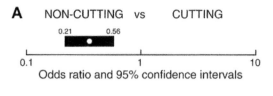

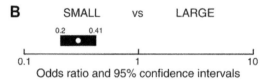

Fig. 3. Pooled odds ratios and 95% confidence intervals (from meta-analysis of nonheterogeneous studies) for risk of PDPH based on (A) needle type and (B) needle size. (*Data from* Halpern S, Preston R. Postdural puncture headache and spinal needle design. Meta-analysis. Anesthesiology 1994;81:1376–83.)

[3], more severe headache and associated symptoms [44], a longer duration of symptoms [45], and a greater need for definitive treatment measures [46]. Needle tip design is also a major influence, with "noncutting" needles clearly associated with a reduced incidence of PDPH compared with "cutting" (usually Quincke) needles of the same gauge. In general, noncutting needles have an opening set back from a tapered ("pencil-point") tip and include the Whitacre, Sprotte, European, Pencan, and Gertie Marx needles. Adding to this somewhat confusing terminology, noncutting needles are sometimes still incorrectly referred to as "atraumatic" needles, despite being shown with electron microscopy to produce a more traumatic rent in the dura than cutting needles (perhaps resulting in a better inflammatory healing response) [47]. The influence of needle size on risk of PDPH appears to be greatest for cutting needles (for example, the reduction seen in the incidence of PDPH between 22- and 26-gauge sizes is greater for cutting than noncutting needles). Insertion of cutting needles with the bevel parallel to the long axis of the spine significantly reduces the incidence of PDPH [48]. This observation was for many years attributed to a spreading rather than cutting of longitudinal-oriented dural fibers. However, scanning electron microscopy reveals the dura to be made of many layers of concentrically directed fibers [49], and the importance of needle bevel insertion is now thought to be related to longitudinal tension on the meninges, particularly in the upright position, and its influence on CSF leakage through holes having differing orientations.

Not surprisingly, a greater number of meningeal punctures have been shown to increase the rate of PDPH [50]. The degree of experience/comfort/skill of the operator is clearly associated with the incidence of ADP during epidural procedures, with higher ADP rates consistently reported when procedures are performed by residents [51,52]. The risk of ADP also appears to be higher for procedures done at night, strongly suggesting a significant contribution of operator fatigue [53].

Several procedural details do not appear to influence the rate of development of PDPH, including patient position at the time of meningeal puncture, "bloody tap" during spinal anesthesia, addition of opiates to spinal block, and volume of CSF removed (for diagnostic purposes) [1].

PREVENTION

Although prophylaxis is most simply thought of as preventing any symptoms of PDPH, in the clinical context this issue is deceptively complex. It is important to appreciate that significant "prevention" may encompass several other end points, such as a reduced incidence of severe PDPH, a shorter duration of symptoms, or decreased need for EBP. Unfortunately, despite the clear relevance of this issue, the overall quality of evidence for preventive measures is generally weak [54,55].

General Measures

As with all regional techniques, appropriate patient selection is crucial in minimizing complications. In this regard, anesthesiologists should take pause when caring for patients having known risk factors for PDPH. As age is a major risk factor, spinal anesthesia is perhaps best avoided in patients younger than 40 years unless the benefits are sufficiently compelling (such as in the obstetric population). Practitioners (and patients alike) may also wish to avoid central neuraxial techniques in those with a previous history of ADP or PDPH (particularly females). Other patient-related factors (eg, obesity) should be considered on a case-by-case basis, weighing the risks of PDPH with the benefits of regional anesthesia.

Central neuraxial procedures should be performed with needles having the smallest gauge possible. However, extremely small spinal needles are more difficult to place, have a slow return of CSF, may be associated with multiple punctures of the dura, and can result in a higher rate of unsuccessful block. The ideal choice for spinal anesthesia is generally a 24- to 27-gauge noncutting needle. Epidural options are limited, especially with catheter techniques, but the risk of PDPH following ADP can probably also be reduced by always using the smallest feasible epidural needles.

Though only recently used for neuraxial techniques, the use of ultrasonography for regional anesthesia holds some promise in reducing the risk of PDPH. Ultrasonography can decrease the number of needle passes required for regional procedures and has been shown to accurately predict the depth of the epidural space [56]. Further study is ongoing to define this potential for ultrasonography to reduce the incidence of ADP and PDPH.

Pharmacologic measures, notably caffeine, continue to be widely used in hopes of decreasing the incidence of PDPH following meningeal puncture [10]. In support of this practice, one small study (n = 60) found that intravenous caffeine (500 mg caffeine sodium benzoate within 90 minutes after spinal anesthesia) significantly reduced the incidence of moderate to severe headache [57]. However, generalizing these results to other clinical settings is difficult, as this investigation involved the use of 22-gauge Quincke needles in a relatively young patient population. In another study, oral caffeine (75 or 125 mg) administered every 6 hours during the first 3 days following spinal anesthesia failed to influence the rate of PDPH [58]. A critical review of the available evidence fails to support the use of caffeine in prevention of PDPH [59]. More recently, a small pilot study raised the possibility of using the long-acting 5-HT receptor agonist frovatriptan (2.5 mg/d orally for 5 days) in the prevention of PDPH [60]. At present, however, there is no proven pharmacologic prophylaxis for PDPH.

A recent survey of United States anesthesiologists reported that bed rest and aggressive oral and intravenous hydration continue to be employed by a sizable majority as prophylactic measures against PDPH [10]. However, a systematic review of the literature regarding bed rest versus early mobilization after dural puncture failed to show any evidence of benefit from bed rest, and suggested that the risk of PDPH may actually be decreased by early mobilization [61]. It is notable that the practice of United States anesthesiologists regarding bed rest is in direct contrast to that seen in United Kingdom maternity units, where 75% encourage mobilization as early as possible following ADP as prophylaxis against PDPH [62]. Likewise, a randomized prospective trial of increased oral hydration following LP failed to decrease the incidence or duration of PDPH [61]. In summary, at this time there is no evidence to support the common recommendations of bed rest or aggressive hydration in the prevention of PDPH.

Spinal Technique

Attention to needle tip design is an important technical means of reducing the risk of PDPH with spinal anesthesia. If available, noncutting needles should be employed. If cutting-tip needles are used, the bevel should be directed parallel to the long axis of the spine.

Replacing the stylet after CSF collection but before needle withdrawal is an effective means of lowering the incidence of PDPH after LP. This recommendation is based on a prospective, randomized study of 600 patients using 21-gauge Sprotte needles. In this setting, replacing the stylet reduced the incidence of PDPH from 16.3% to 5.0% ($P < .005$). This safe and simple maneuver is theorized to decrease the possibility of a wicking strand of arachnoid mater from extending across the dura (Fig. 4) [63].

Continuous spinal anesthesia (CSA) has been reported by some to be associated with surprisingly low incidences of PDPH compared with single-dose spinal techniques using similar gauge needles [64]. This observation has been attributed to reaction to the catheter, which may promote better sealing of a breach in the meninges. Continuous spinal anesthesia with small-gauge needles and catheters ("microcatheters") is an appealing option when titration of

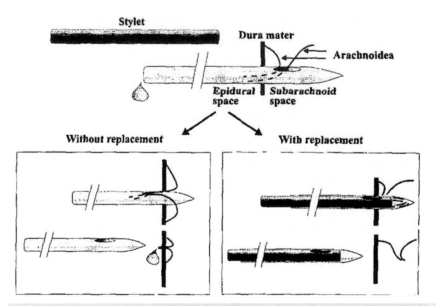

Fig. 4. Proposed mechanism of decreased incidence of PDPH seen with stylet replacement. (*Upper*) Flow of CSF from the subarachnoid space may draw strands of arachnoid mater into the needle. (*Lower left*) Removal of the needle without stylet replacement results in threading of arachnoid across the dura, promoting prolonged CSF leak. (*Lower right*) Replacing the stylet fully before needle removal either pushes out or cuts the arachnoid mater, reducing the risk of CSF loss into the epidural space. (*From* Strupp M, Brandt T, Muller A. Incidence of post-lumbar puncture syndrome reduced by reinserting the stylet: a randomized prospective study of 600 patients. J Neurol 1998;245:591; with permission.)

spinal drug is desirable and duration of surgery is uncertain, but is currently unavailable in the United States, where the risk of PDPH with CSA remains concerning when using "macrocatheters" of approximately 20-gauge. For this reason, deliberate CSA may be underutilized and has been investigated almost exclusively in low-risk populations.

Epidural Technique

The issue of air versus liquid for identification of the epidural space with the loss-of-resistance technique has long been a source of controversy. Each method has acknowledged advantages and disadvantages, but neither has been convincingly shown to result in a lower risk of ADP [65]. In this case, operator preference and experience would be expected to strongly influence performance, and the overriding significance of this factor is illustrated in fewer instances of ADP noted when the medium is chosen at the anesthesiologist's discretion [66].

Bevel orientation for epidural needle insertion remains a matter of debate. Norris and colleagues [67] found the incidence of moderate to severe PDPH after ADP was only 24% when the needle bevel was oriented parallel to the long axis of the spine (compared with 70% with perpendicular insertion). This orientation resulted in fewer therapeutic EBPs administered to patients in the parallel group ($P<.05$). However, this technique necessitates a controversial 90° rotation of the needle for catheter placement [68]. It seems that several factors regarding parallel needle insertion (lateral needle deviation, difficulties with catheter insertion, and dural trauma with needle rotation) are of greater concern to practitioners. Most respondents (71.3%) to a survey of United States anesthesiologists preferred to insert epidural needles with the bevel perpendicular to the long axis of the spine (consistent with the intended direction of catheter travel) [10].

Combined spinal-epidural (CSE) techniques have been reported to be associated with a low incidence of PDPH. While providing the advantages of a spinal anesthetic, CSE appears to have no increased incidence of PDPH or need for EBP when compared with plain epidural analgesia [69]. This observation may be due to several factors, including the ability to successfully use extremely small (eg, 27-gauge) noncutting spinal needles and tamponade provided by epidural infusions.

Measures to Reduce the Risk of PDPH after ADP

The risk-to-benefit ratio of prophylaxis should be most favorable in situations having the greatest likelihood of developing severe PDPH. Therefore, most efforts to reduce the risk of PDPH after ADP have been in the obstetric patient population. Several prophylactic measures, discussed below, are worthy of consideration and have been used alone or in combination [70]. However, because not all patients who experience an ADP will develop PDPH, and only a portion of those who do will require definitive treatment (ie, an EBP), a cautious approach in this regard is still generally warranted.

Stylet replacement

Although there have not been any studies to support the use of this technique in the setting of ADP, replacing the stylet is a simple and effective means of lowering the incidence of PDPH after LP [63]. Given the innocuous nature of this maneuver, if no other prophylactic measures are taken, there seems to be little reason not to replace the stylet before epidural needle removal in the event of ADP.

Subarachnoid saline

Limited evidence indicates that the subarachnoid injection of sterile preservative-free saline following ADP may be associated with a significant reduction in the incidence of PDPH and need for EBP. In one small study (n = 43), immediate injection of 10 mL saline through the epidural needle substantially reduced the incidence of PDPH (32%, compared with 62% in a matched control group) and resulted in a significant reduction in the need for EBP ($P = .004$) [71]. The injection of saline and the reinjection of CSF have been speculated as important in the prevention of PDPH by maintaining CSF volume [70]. However, given the relatively rapid rate of CSF regeneration, it may be that the benefit of fluid injection following ADP is actually in preventing a wicking strand of arachnoid (as proposed for stylet replacement). Further investigation into this issue is clearly needed.

Intrathecal catheters
Immediately placing an intrathecal catheter (ITC) after ADP has the advantages of being able to rapidly provide spinal analgesia as well as eliminate the possibility of another ADP under challenging clinical circumstances. However, the potential benefits of ITC use must be weighed against the readily appreciated risks involved (accidental use, misuse, and infection). Although evidence is extremely limited, ITC use has also been proposed to reduce the risk of PDPH after ADP [55]. Ayad and colleagues [72] placed and maintained an ITC for 24 hours following ADP. In their obstetric population, catheter placement resulted in a PDPH rate of only 6.2%, with an expected incidence of greater than 50% in this setting. A similar reduction in the development of PDPH with 24-hour ITC maintenance after ADP has been noted in orthopedic patients [73]. This impressive reduction in the incidence of PDPH has generally not been reported from studies where catheters have been left in place for less than 24 hours. It has been proposed that the mechanism of benefit from ITC maintenance may be due to reaction to the catheter, with inflammation or edema preventing further CSF loss after removal. There are also preliminary data to suggest that the incidence of PDPH may be further reduced by the injection of saline through an ITC immediately before removal [71]. With some accepted and other possible benefits, rates of ITC use following ADP have clearly increased during the past decade. Recent surveys of United States, United Kingdom, and Australian practice have noted rates of routine intrathecal catheterization following ADP in obstetric patients of 18%, 28%, and 35%, respectively [10,62,74].

Although ITC use has increased, reattempting an epidural at an adjacent interspace remains the preferred action following ADP [10]. Provided an epidural catheter can be successfully placed, several epidural approaches have been used in hope of reducing the incidence and severity of PDPH.

Epidural saline
Efforts have included both bolus (usually around 50 mL as a single or repeated injection) and continuous infusion techniques (commonly 600–1000 mL over 24 hours). As these measures are resource-intensive and may only serve to delay the inevitable onset of symptoms, they have generally not been continued beyond 36 hours. In one large analysis (n = 241), Stride and Cooper [75] reported a reduction in the incidence of PDPH from 86% in a conservatively treated control group to 70% with epidural saline infusion. Trivedi and colleagues [76] noted a similar reduction in PDPH (from 87% to 67%) in 30 patients who received a single prophylactic "saline patch" (40–60 mL) following completion of an obstetric procedure. Other studies of epidural saline have noted this modest decrease in the incidence of PDPH. Stride and Cooper also reported a lower incidence of severe headache (from 64% to 47%), but this

effect has been inconsistently seen by other investigators, and there is no convincing evidence that epidural saline reduces the eventual need for EBP.

Epidural opiates

Epidural opiates (especially morphine), while long used for the treatment of PDPH, have been thought unlikely to influence the natural history of the disorder. However, recently revisiting the issue of opiates as prophylaxis after ADP, Al-metwalli found that 2 epidural injections of morphine (3 mg in 10 mL), compared with epidural injections of an equal volume of saline, resulted in fewer episodes of PDPH ($P = .014$) and decreased the need for EBP ($P = .022$) [77]. Because of the small number of patients involved (n = 25), further prospective investigation is warranted.

Prophylactic epidural blood patch

The impressive efficacy of the EBP when used as treatment for PDPH has fueled interest in the technique for prophylaxis. Research into the efficacy of the EBP for prophylaxis has yielded mixed results, and closer scrutiny indicates that optimism should be guarded. The strongest investigation to date has been by Scavone and colleagues [78], who performed a prospective, randomized, double-blind study in 64 parturients comparing the prophylactic EBP (PEBP) to a sham EBP. In this study, an identical 56% of patients in each group went on to develop PDPH. Although there was a trend toward fewer therapeutic EBPs recommended and performed in the prophylactic group, the difference was not statistically significant ($P = .08$). The primary benefit of the PEBP was a shorter total duration of symptoms (from a median of approximately 5 days to 2 days) and, consequently, the overall pain burden (Fig. 5). While

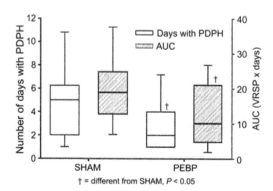

Fig. 5. Plot of the duration of PDPH (*open boxes*, with scale on left) and the pain intensity-duration (*shaded boxes*, with scale on right) for sham injection and prophylactic epidural blood patch (PEBP). Area under the curve (AUC) consists of the verbal rating score for pain (VRSP) multiplied by the number of days with PDPH. Boxes are the interquartile range, solid lines within the boxes represent the median value, and whiskers are the 10th and 90th percentiles. (*Data from* Al-metwalli RR. Epidural morphine injections for prevention of post dural puncture headache. Anaesthesia 2008;63:847–50.)

conferring some benefit, the PEBP is not currently recommended as a routine measure based on available evidence [55,79]. Due to concerns of exposing patients to a potentially unnecessary and marginally beneficial procedure, prophylactic application of the EBP has declined substantially in recent years [10,62]. If used for prophylaxis, the EBP should be performed only after any spinal or epidural local anesthetic has worn off, as premature administration has been associated with excessive cephalad displacement of local anesthetic [80]. Residual epidural local anesthetic may also inhibit coagulation of blood, further decreasing the efficacy of the EBP [81].

Limiting and avoiding pushing
In the event of ADP, limiting the duration of the second stage of labor (usually to 30–60 minutes) and avoiding pushing may reduce the risk of PDPH. Whereas these measures are not uncommonly recommended in United Kingdom maternity units [62], such management is rare in United States practice [10].

DIAGNOSTIC EVALUATION

PDPH remains a diagnosis of exclusion. Although headache following meningeal puncture will naturally be suspected to be PDPH, it remains critical to rule out other etiologies (Fig. 6). Fortunately, a careful history with a brief consideration of other possible diagnoses is usually all that is necessary to differentiate PDPH from other causes of headache. Although numerous clinical variations have been reported, most cases of PDPH will have (a) a history of known or possible meningeal puncture, (b) delayed onset of symptoms (but within 48 hours), and (c) bilateral postural headache (possibly accompanied by associated symptoms if moderate or severe). Of importance, most nonmeningeal puncture headaches will not have a strong positional nature. Laboratory studies are usually not necessary for the diagnosis of PDPH and, if obtained, are generally unremarkable (most commonly, magnetic resonance imaging [MRI] may show meningeal enhancement and LP may reveal low opening pressures and increased CSF protein).

Physical examination plays a limited role in the diagnosis of PDPH. Vital signs (normal blood pressure and absence of fever) and a basic neurologic examination (gross motor and sensory function plus ocular and facial movements) should be documented. Firm bilateral jugular venous pressure, applied briefly (10–15 seconds), tends to worsen headaches secondary to intracranial hypotension [19]. Conversely, the "sitting epigastric pressure test" may result in transient relief of PDPH symptoms [82]. For this test, the patient is placed in a sitting position until headache symptoms become manifest. Firm, continuous abdominal pressure is applied with one hand while the other hand is secure against the patient's back. In cases of PDPH, some improvement is usually noted within 15 to 30 seconds, with prompt return of symptoms on release of abdominal pressure.

Benign Etiologies

    Non-specific headache

    Exacerbation of chronic headache (e.g. tension-type headache)

    Hypertensive headache

    Pneumocephalus

    Sinusitis

    Drug side-effect

    Spontaneous intracranial hypotension

    Other

Serious Etiologies

    Meningitis

    Subdural hematoma (SDH)

    Subarachnoid hemorrhage

    Preeclampsia/eclampsia

    Intracranial venous thrombosis (ICVT)

    Other

Fig. 6. Differential diagnosis of postdural puncture headache.

It must be appreciated that benign headaches are frequently encountered in the perioperative setting, even in the absence of meningeal puncture, and have generally been noted to be less severe than PDPH (common causes include dehydration, hypoglycemia, anxiety, and caffeine withdrawal). With spinal anesthesia, the specific local anesthetic used, as well as the addition of dextrose or epinephrine, may influence the occurrence of nonspecific headache but do not affect the rate of true PDPH [83]. The majority of headaches following meningeal puncture will be benign nonspecific headaches. In a careful analysis of headache following spinal anesthesia using strict criteria for PDPH, Santanen and colleagues [84] found an incidence of nonmeningeal puncture headache of 18.5%, with an incidence of true PDPH of only 1.5%. Headaches and neck/shoulder pain are also common in the postpartum period [31]. In one study, 39% of postpartum patients were noted to be symptomatic, but more than 75% of these were determined to be primary headaches (migraine, tension-type, cervicogenic, and cluster) [52]. In this analysis, although 89% of patients received neuraxial anesthesia, only 4.7% of postpartum headaches were PDPH.

Benign headaches can often be differentiated from PDPH by characteristic features. Exacerbation of chronic headache (eg, tension-type, cluster, or migraine) is usually notable for a history of similar headaches. In the study cited above [52], a previous headache history was a significant risk factor for postpartum headache (adjusted odds ratio = 2.25, if >12 episodes per year). Significant hypertension may cause headaches and should be detected through routine vital sign assessment. Stella and colleagues [85] studied severe and unrelenting postpartum headaches with onset more than 24 hours from the time of delivery, and found that 39% were tension-type headaches, 24% were due to preeclampsia/eclampsia, and only 16% were PDPH (despite neuraxial anesthesia in 88% of patients). Based on this observation, they developed a treatment algorithm for severe postpartum headache that recommends treatment of tension/migraine headache before consideration of PDPH (Fig. 7). Pneumocephalus can produce a positional headache that can be difficult to distinguish from PDPH and does not respond to EBP, but is readily diagnosed with computed tomography (CT) [86]. Sinusitis may be associated with

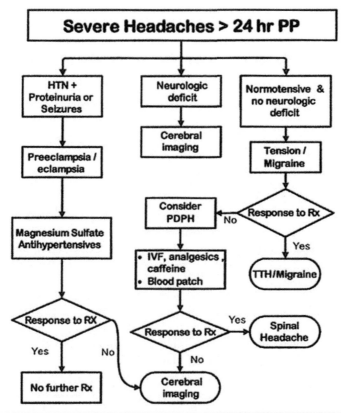

Fig. 7. Suggested treatment algorithm for management of severe postpartum headache present greater than 24 hours after delivery. PP, postpartum; HTN, hypertension; TTH, tension-type headache; IVF, intravenous fluid. (*From* Stella CL, Jodicke CD, How HY, et al. Postpartum headache: is your work-up complete? Am J Obstet Gynecol 2007;196:318e5; with permission.)

purulent nasal discharge and tenderness over the affected sinus, and is often improved with assuming an upright position. It should be kept in mind that headache is also a side-effect of some commonly used pharmacologic agents, such as ondansetron [87]. Although certainly unusual, classic PDPH symptoms may even conceivably represent a coincidental case of spontaneous intracranial hypotension. Several other benign etiologies are possible.

Serious causes of headache will be rare but must be excluded. It is important to remember that lateralizing neurologic signs, fever/chills, seizures, or changes in mental status are not consistent with a diagnosis of PDPH. Meningitis tends to be associated with fever, leukocytosis, changes in mental status, and meningeal signs (such as nuchal rigidity) [88]. Subdural hematoma (SDH) is a recognized complication of dural puncture, and is believed under these circumstances to be caused by intracranial hypotension resulting in excessive traction on cerebral vessels, leading to their disruption. Practitioners must maintain a high index of suspicion for SDH, which is often preceded by typical PDPH symptoms but progresses to lose its postural component, and may evolve to include disturbances in mentation and focal neurologic signs. It has been proposed that early definitive treatment of severe PDPH may serve to prevent SDH [89]. Subarachnoid hemorrhage, most commonly caused by rupture of a cerebral aneurysm or arteriovenous malformation, is usually associated with the sudden onset of excruciating headache followed by a decreased level of consciousness or coma [90]. Preeclampsia/eclampsia often presents with headache and may only become evident in the postpartum period [91]. Intracranial venous thrombosis (ICVT) is most often seen in the postpartum obstetric population, where headache symptoms are easily confused with PDPH but may progress to seizures, focal neurologic signs, and coma [92]. Predisposing factors for ICVT include hypercoagulability, dehydration, and inflammatory and infectious diseases. Reports of other intracranial pathology (intracranial tumor, intracerebral hemorrhage, and so forth) misdiagnosed as PDPH are rare, and such conditions will be detected only by a thorough neurologic evaluation [93].

Diagnosis of PDPH can be particularly challenging in patients who have undergone LP as part of a diagnostic workup for headache. In these situations a change in the quality of headache, most commonly a new postural nature, points toward PDPH. Occasionally, if the benign diagnostic possibilities cannot be narrowed down with certainty, a favorable response to EBP can provide definitive evidence for a diagnosis of PDPH.

TREATMENT

Once a diagnosis of PDPH has been made, patients should be provided a straightforward explanation of the presumed cause, anticipated natural course (factoring in the time from meningeal puncture), and a realistic assessment of treatment options (with consideration of needle gauge). A treatment algorithm, based primarily on the severity of symptoms, can serve as a useful guide for management (Fig. 8).

Time

As PDPH is a complication that tends to resolve spontaneously, the simple passage of time plays an important role in the appropriate management of this disorder. Before the introduction of the EBP as definitive therapy, the natural history of PDPH was documented by Vandam and Dripps [3] as they followed 1011 episodes of PDPH after spinal anesthesia using cutting needles of various sizes. Although their analysis is flawed by a lack of information regarding duration in 9% of patients, if one considers their observed data, spontaneous resolution of PDPH was seen in 59% of cases within 4 days and 80% within 1 week. More recently, Lybecker and colleagues [27] closely followed 75 episodes of PDPH and, while providing an EBP to 40% of their patients

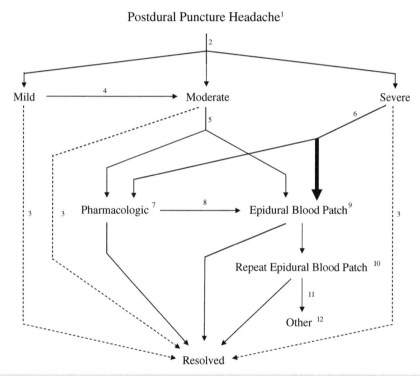

Postdural Puncture Headache[1]

Fig. 8. Treatment algorithm for established PDPH. See text for details. (1) Patient education, reassurance, and supportive measures. (2) Triage by severity of symptoms. (3) Resolution over time without further treatment. (4) Worsening symptoms or failure to substantially improve within 5 days. (5) Choice of EBP or less effective pharmacologic measures is based on patient preference. (6) Definitive treatment (EBP) is recommended (*bold arrow*). (7) Caffeine or other agents. (8) Failure, worsening of symptoms, or recurrence. (9) Patch materials other than blood remain preliminary. (10) Generally performed no sooner than 24 hours after a first EBP. (11) Serious reconsideration of diagnosis. (12) Radiologic guidance is recommended if another EBP is performed. (*From* Neal JM, Rathmell JP, editors. Complications in regional anesthesia & pain medicine. Philadelphia: Saunders; 2007. p. 82; with permission.)

(generally to those having the most severe symptoms), observed in the untreated patients a median duration of symptoms of 5 days with a range of 1 to 12 days. van Kooten and colleagues [94], in a small but prospective, randomized, blinded study of patients with moderate or severe PDPH, noted 18 of 21 patients (86%) in the control treatment group (24-hour bed rest, at least 2 L of fluids by mouth daily, and analgesics as needed) still having headache symptoms at 7 days, with over half of these still rating symptoms as moderate or severe (Fig. 9). These data serve to illustrate the unpredictable and occasionally prolonged duration of untreated PDPH. Indeed, Vandam and Dripps [3] reported 4% of patients still experiencing symptoms 7 to 12 months after spinal anesthesia. Given this reality, it is not surprising that there are several case reports of successful treatment of PDPH months and even years after known or occult meningeal puncture.

Largely due to the self-limited nature of PDPH, the optimal time course of treatment has not been well defined. Most practitioners currently advocate a trial, most commonly 24 to 48 hours, of conservative management [10]. However, the rationale behind this approach is questionable given the often severely disabling nature of symptoms, particularly in the postpartum period when newborn care may be significantly impaired. Clinically, the practical issue is how long definitive therapy (ie, the EBP) can appropriately be delayed, and is considered in comments regarding timing of the EBP.

Supportive Measures

Reassurance and measures directed toward minimizing symptoms, while not expected to alter the natural course of the disorder, are advised for all patients. By definition, the majority of patients with moderate to severe PDPH will naturally seek a recumbent position for symptomatic relief. Despite a lack of supportive evidence, aggressive hydration continues to be the most frequently

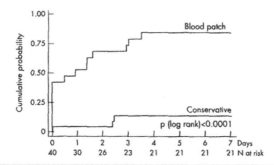

Fig. 9. Cumulative probability of recovery from moderate or severe PDPH. Full recovery was noted in 3.5 days, and unchanged by 7 days, in 16 of 19 patients (84%) in the blood patch group and 3 of 21 patients (14%) in the control treatment ("conservative") group. (*From* van Kooten F, Oedit R, Bakker SL, et al. Epidural blood patch in post dural puncture headache: a randomized, observer-blind, controlled clinical trial. J Neurol Neurosurg Psychiatry 2008;79:556; with permission.)

recommended practice used in treatment of PDPH [10]. Although aggressive hydration does not appear to influence the duration of symptoms [61], patients should and often must be encouraged to avoid dehydration.

Analgesics (acetaminophen, NSAIDS, opiates, and so forth.) may be administered by several different routes and are commonly used, yet the relief obtained is often unimpressive, especially with severe headaches. Antiemetics and stool softeners should be prescribed when indicated. Abdominal binders can provide some degree of relief, but are uncomfortable and seldom used in modern practice. Acupuncture has been suggested as an alternative measure in the management of PDPH [95].

Pharmacologic Therapies

Several pharmacologic agents have been advocated as treatments for PDPH [96]. While appealing, these options have generally been poorly studied and are of questionable value due to the small numbers of patients treated, methodological flaws in published reports, and the self-limited nature of the disorder.

Methylxanthines are used for their cerebral vasoconstrictive effect and include aminophylline, theophylline, and most familiar, caffeine. Experimentally, caffeine has been used intravenously (usually 500 mg caffeine sodium benzoate, which contains 250 mg caffeine) and orally (eg, 300 mg). Published studies of caffeine for PDPH consistently demonstrate improvement at 1 to 4 hours in more than 70% of patients treated [96]. However, a single oral dose of 300 mg caffeine for treatment of PDPH is statistically no better than placebo at 24 hours [97]. With a terminal half-life of generally less than 6 hours, repeated doses of caffeine would seem necessary for treatment of PDPH, yet few studies have evaluated more than 2 doses for efficacy or safety (of particular concern in the nursing parturient). Furthermore, there is no convincing evidence that any pharmacologic agents reduce the eventual need for EBP. Overall, the use of caffeine for PDPH does not appear to be supported by the available literature [59]. Nevertheless, surveys indicate that it continues to be widely used in the treatment of PDPH [10,62]. Clinically, encouraging unmonitored caffeine intake is of extremely uncertain value, especially considering the general lack of awareness of caffeine content in readily available beverages and medications (Fig. 10). The temporary benefit often observed with caffeine would indicate that, if used, it is perhaps most appropriate for the treatment of PDPH of moderate (and possibly mild or severe) intensity while awaiting spontaneous resolution of the condition. Although the familiarity of caffeine for nonmedical purposes would argue for its general safety, practitioners should note that its use is contraindicated in patients with seizure disorders, pregnancy-induced hypertension, or a history of supraventricular tachyarrhythmias.

In addition to the methylxanthines, experiences with other pharmacologic approaches to PDPH continue to be reported. Sumatriptan, a serotonin type-1d receptor agonist that causes cerebral vasoconstriction, is commonly used

	Amount	Caffeine Content
Beverages		
Coca Cola Classic	12 oz	35 mg
Diet Coke	12 oz	45 mg
Diet Pepsi	12 oz	36 mg
Espresso	single shot	75 mg
McDonald's Brewed Coffee	12 oz	109 mg
Monster	16 oz	160 mg
Mountain Dew (Diet or Regular)	12 oz	55 mg
Nestea Iced Tea	16 oz	34 mg
Pepsi-Cola	12 oz	38 mg
Red Bull	8.46 oz	80 mg
Rockstar	16 oz	160 mg
Snapple Tea	16 oz	42 mg
SoBe Green Tea	20 oz	35 mg
Starbucks Breakfast Blend Coffee	12 oz	260 mg
Sunkist Orange Soda	12 oz	41 mg
Over-the-Counter Medications		
Anacin Regular or Extra Strength	1 tablet	32 mg
Excedrin Extra Strength	1 tablet	65 mg
Goody's Extra Strength	1 powder	32.5 mg
Midol Menstrual Maximum Strength	1 caplet	60 mg
NoDoz Maximum Strength	1 caplet	200 mg
Prescription Medications		
Butalbital/aspirin or acetaminophen/caffeine		
(e.g. Fiorinal/Fioricet)	1 capsule	40 mg
Caffeine sodium benzoate	250 mg	125 mg
Ergotamine/caffeine (e.g. Cafergot)	1 tablet	100 mg
Orphenadrine/aspirin/caffeine		
(e.g. Norgesic Forte)	1 tablet	60 mg
Propoxyphene/aspirin/caffeine		
(e.g. Darvon Compound)	1 capsule	32.4 mg

Fig. 10. Caffeine content.

for migraine headache and has been used to treat PDPH. Corticosteroidogenics (corticotropin and its synthetic form, cosyntropin/tetracosactin) have long been proposed as treatments for PDPH. Although the mechanism of action remains speculative, corticotropin is known to have multiple physiologic effects that could theoretically improve symptoms of PDPH [98]. However, neither sumatriptan [99] nor a synthetic corticotropin analogue [100] were found to be effective in small randomized, prospective studies for treatment of severe PDPH. Hydrocortisone (100 mg intravenously every 8 hours for 6 doses) has been reported to be effective in treatment of severe PDPH following spinal anesthesia using a 25-gauge Quincke needle [101]. A small, uncontrolled pilot study of methylergonovine (0.25 mg orally 3 times daily for 24–48 hours) indicated that this vasoconstrictive agent may hasten resolution of PDPH [102]. A case report of gabapentin (400 mg orally every 8 hours for 3 days) suggests that this agent may also be useful in the setting of severe PDPH [103]. Reports of the successful use of these and other pharmacologic agents are intriguing, but their proper place in the management of PDPH awaits further study. However, given the initial optimism but eventually disproved role for so many pharmacologic agents through the years, practitioners are advised to have guarded expectations in this regard, especially when dealing with severe PDPH.

Epidural Therapies

Although not a contraindication to epidural treatments, a history of significant technical difficulties with attempted neuraxial techniques should naturally encourage a trial of less invasive measures. However, the appeal of epidural approaches is evident if access to the space is deemed reasonable or if the patient already has a correctly placed catheter in situ.

Epidural saline

Epidural saline, as bolus and infusion, has a long history of use for treatment of PDPH. Bolus injections of epidural saline (usually 20–30 mL, repeated as necessary if a catheter is present) have been reported to produce prompt and virtually universal relief of PDPH, yet the practice is plagued by an extremely high rate of headache recurrence. This transient effect is not surprising, as increases in epidural pressure following bolus administration of saline have been demonstrated to return to baseline within 10 minutes [104]. Favorable results achieved with this approach have been speculated to represent the mechanical reapproximation of a dural flap (the "tin-lid" phenomenon) [1]. However, bolus administration of saline for treatment of PDPH has been convincingly shown to be inferior to the EBP, especially when headaches are secondary to large-bore needle punctures [105]. Overall, epidural saline appears to be of limited value for established PDPH [55]. Nevertheless, the successful use of epidural saline, administered as bolus and/or infusion, continues to be reported occasionally under exceptional circumstances [106].

Epidural blood patch

During the past several decades, the EBP has emerged as the "gold standard" for treatment of PDPH [1]. A Cochrane review (a systematic assessment of the evidence) regarding the EBP recently concluded that the procedure now has proven benefit over more conservative treatment [79]. The mechanism of action of the EBP, while not entirely understood, appears to be related to the ability to stop further CSF loss by the formation of clot over the defect in the meninges as well as a tamponade effect with cephalad displacement of CSF (the "epidural pressure patch") [107]. The appropriate role of the EBP in individual situations will depend on multiple factors, including the duration and severity of headache and associated symptoms, type and gauge of original needle used, and patient wishes. The EBP should be encouraged in patients experiencing ADP with an epidural needle and those whose symptoms are categorized as severe (ie, pain score > 6 on a 1–10 scale). Informed consent for the EBP should include a discussion with the patient regarding the common as well as serious risks involved, anticipated side effects, and true success rate. Finally, patients should be provided clear instructions for the provision of timely medical attention should they experience a recurrence of symptoms.

Several controversies surround the EBP, reflecting the scarcity of adequately powered, randomized trials. The procedure itself has been well described and consists of the sterile injection of fresh autologous blood near the previous dural puncture (Fig. 11). An MRI study of the EBP in 5 young patients (age 31–44 years) using 20 mL blood noted a spread of 4.6 ± 0.9 intervertebral spaces (mean ± SD), averaging 3.5 levels above and 1 level below the site of injection [107]. This and other observations of a preferential cephalad spread of blood in the lumbar epidural space has led to the common recommendation to perform the EBP "at or below" the meningeal puncture level. However, the influence on efficacy of the level of placement and use of an epidural catheter (often situated considerably cephalad to a meningeal puncture) for EBP have never been clinically evaluated.

The optimal timing of the EBP is a matter of debate. After diagnosis, most practitioners prefer to delay performing the EBP, possibly to further confirm the diagnosis as well as to allow an opportunity for spontaneous resolution. A 1996 survey of United Kingdom neurologic departments found that only 8% would consider the EBP before 72 hours had passed following LP [108]. A recent survey of United Kingdom maternity units reported that 71% would perform the EBP only "after the failure of conservative measures" [62]. Likewise, the majority of respondents in a recent survey of United States practice usually waited at least 24 hours from the onset of symptoms before performing the EBP [10]. Several studies suggest that the EBP procedure may become more effective with the passage of time [109,110]. Safa-Tisseront and colleagues [110] found a delay of less than 4 days from meningeal puncture before performing an EBP to be an independent risk factor for failure of the procedure. Yet these investigators were careful to state that failure of the EBP may be primarily related to the severity of the CSF leak (with larger, harder to treat

* Obtain written informed consent.

* Establish intravenous access. An 18-gauge or larger saline lock is sufficient.

* Position the patient for epidural needle placement (mindful that a lateral decubitus position may be more comfortable for the patient).

* Using standard sterile technique, place an epidural needle into the epidural space at or below the level of previous meningeal puncture.

* Collect 20 ml fresh autologous venous blood using strict sterile technique (this is usually readily accomplished using the previously placed saline lock).

* Without delay, steadily inject blood through the epidural needle until the patient reports fullness or discomfort in the back, buttocks, or neck.

* Maintain the patient in a recumbent position for a period of time (1-2 hours may result in more complete resolution of symptoms). Intravenous infusion of 1 liter crystalloid during this interval is often helpful.

* Instructions for discharge:

    - Over-the-counter analgesics as needed (patient preference).

    - Avoid lifting, straining, or air travel for 24 hours.

    - Contact anesthesia for inadequate relief or recurrence of symptoms.

Fig. 11. The epidural blood patch procedure.

situations demanding earlier attention) and that their study should not be grounds for delaying the EBP. Sandesc and colleagues [111] performed a prospective, randomized, double-blind study of the EBP versus conservative management (intravenous/oral fluids up to 3 L/d, nonsteroidal anti-inflammatory drugs, and caffeine sodium benzoate 500 mg intravenously every 6 hours) in 32 patients with severe PDPH symptoms (mean pain intensity = 8.1). At the time treatment was initiated, none of these patients had experienced symptoms for longer than 24 hours. Whereas all patients in the EBP group had satisfactory resolution of symptoms at 24-hour follow-up, the control group was essentially unchanged (mean pain intensity = 7.8). Of note, 14 of 16 patients in the conservatively treated group then elected for EBP treatment. The investigators concluded that there was no reason to delay the EBP for more than 24 hours after making a diagnosis of severe PDPH. This recommendation is further supported by a prospective analysis of 79 patients with PDPH, which determined that early EBP in those with moderate to severe symptoms minimized patient suffering [112].

The ideal volume of blood for EBP is unclear. Conceptually, the volume of blood used should be sufficient to form an organized clot over the meningeal defect as well as produce some degree of epidural tamponade [107]. When performing the EBP, anesthesiologists commonly inject as much blood as was drawn (usually around 20 mL), stopping when the patient complains of discomfort or fullness in the back, buttocks, or neck. There appear to be regional preferences regarding blood volume. The largest analysis of the EBP to date (n = 504) used a blood volume of 23 ± 5 mL (mean ± SD) [110]. Of importance, this French study found no significant difference in blood volumes between successful and failed EBP. The investigators noted "discomfort" in 78% of injections with 19 ± 5 mL and "pain" in 54% with 21 ± 5 mL, with the only independent risk factor for pain during EBP being age less than 35 years. A recent survey of United States anesthesiologists reported general unanimity for a smaller blood volume, with two-thirds (66.8%) most commonly using between 16 and 20 mL [10]. As previously mentioned, there may be some experimental support for using a blood volume of 15 to 20 mL, as early studies of CSF drainage in volunteers reported consistently producing positional headache symptoms with loss of 10% of total CSF volume (approximately 15 mL) [19]. Furthermore, the reduction in CSF pressures produced by this degree of fluid loss would be expected to reduce or eliminate transmeningeal driving pressure, resulting at that point in a relative CSF volume homeostasis (in the supine position). Formal studies designed to determine an ideal volume of blood for EBP in the treatment of PDPH have generally failed to achieve better results with volumes greater than 10 mL, and there are few data to encourage the use of volumes greater than 20 mL [113]. It is notable that although the value of the EBP in the treatment of spontaneous intracranial hypotension is uncertain [55], much larger blood volumes (up to 100 mL) are generally recommended for this indication [114]. However, a recent case report highlights some potential complications from large-volume EBP [115], and practitioners are generally encouraged to use the smallest effective volume.

To allow for clot organization and regeneration of CSF (approximately 0.35 mL/min), it is common practice to have patients remain recumbent for a period of time following the EBP. Although the optimal duration of bed rest immediately following an EBP remains unknown, one small study suggested that maintaining the decubitus position for at least 1 and preferably 2 hours may result in a more complete resolution of symptoms [116]. Patients are usually advised to avoid lifting, Valsalva maneuvers (eg, straining with bowel movement), and air travel for 24 to 48 hours after EBP to minimize the risk of patch disruption.

Contraindications to the EBP are similar to those of any epidural needle placement: coagulopathy, systemic sepsis, fever, infection at the site, and patient refusal. Modifications of usual EBP technique have been suggested to accommodate the special needs of Jehovah's Witness patients [117]. Theoretical concerns have been expressed regarding the possibility of neoplastic seeding of the central nervous system in patients with cancer [118]. Although not free from concern and controversy, the EBP has been safely provided to patients with human immunodeficiency virus infection [119] and acute varicella

[120]. The EBP may also be indicated and performed, with decreased volumes of blood, in the pediatric population (0.2–0.3 mL/kg has been associated with successful EBP in adolescents) [121] and at extralumbar sites (eg, cervical) [122].

Minor side effects are common following the EBP. Patients should be warned to expect aching in the back, buttocks, or legs (seen in approximately 25% of patients) [109]. While usually short-lived, backache was noted to be persistent in 16% of patients following EBP, lasting 3 to 100 days (with a mean duration in this subgroup of 27.7 days) [123]. Despite these lingering symptoms, patient satisfaction with the EBP is high. Other frequent but benign after-effects of the EBP include transient neck ache [123], bradycardia [124], and modest temperature elevation [123].

Largely through extensive clinical experience, the EBP has been sufficiently proven to be safe. The risks are essentially the same as with other epidural procedures (infection, bleeding, nerve damage, and ADP). On occasion, the aforementioned temporary back and lower extremity radicular pain has been reported to be severe. With proper technique, infectious complications are vanishingly rare. Although controversial, a previous EBP does not appear to significantly influence the success of future epidural interventions [125]. Serious complications secondary to the EBP do occur, but have usually consisted of isolated case reports and have often been associated with significant deviations from standard practice [1].

Other epidural therapies
For various reasons, several alternatives to blood have been promoted as patch materials. The most commonly proposed materials (dextran-40, hydroxyethyl starch, gelatin, and fibrin glue) have been adapted for a perceived ability to provide prolonged epidural tamponade and/or result in sealing of a meningeal rent. In a rat model, experimental support for a "blood-like" effect was best shown for fibrin glue [104]. However, clinical use of these alternatives is limited to case reports and small series, and their use is uncommon in the United States [10]. Though not necessarily without merit, these options remain poorly defined, and reports of their use should still be considered preliminary.

PERSISTENT OR RECURRENT PDPH

Early reports of the EBP frequently cited success rates between 90% and 100%, but often did not include a strict definition of "success," had little or no follow-up, and failed to consider the influence of such confounding factors as needle size and tip design, severity of symptoms, or natural history of PDPH. The true efficacy of the EBP procedure is now known to be significantly lower than once thought. Persistent or recurrent headaches following the EBP, while not necessarily requiring consultation, warrant follow-up and thoughtful reevaluation.

The EBP is associated with nearly immediate symptomatic relief in more than 90% of cases, but appropriate follow-up reveals many patients experiencing incomplete relief, failure, and recurrence. In an uncontrolled, prospective, observational study of 504 consecutive patients treated with EBP following meningeal puncture with needles of various sizes, Safa-Tisseront and colleagues [110] reported some relief of symptoms in 93%. Yet on closer analysis, complete relief of symptoms was seen in only 75% of patients, with 18% experiencing incomplete relief. These investigators also found that the EBP was more likely to fail if the original meningeal puncture was made with needles larger than 20-gauge (Fig. 12). For needles larger than 20-gauge, the unqualified success rate of the EBP was only 62%, with 17% of patients reporting incomplete relief of symptoms and 21% experiencing failure. Not surprisingly, the majority of these large needles were Tuohy epidural needles.

Expectations of success with the EBP must be further tempered in obstetric patients (all young and female) following ADP with epidural needles. Under these circumstances, Williams and colleagues [126] noted complete relief of symptoms with EBP in only 34% of patients, partial relief in 54%, and no relief in 7% (results unknown in 5%). If performed, a second EBP resulted in complete relief in 50%, partial relief in 36%, and no relief in 14%. In a similar patient population, Banks and colleagues [109], despite initially observing complete or partial relief with EBP in 95% of patients, reported the return of moderate to severe symptoms in 31%, with a mean time to development of recurrent headache of 31.8 hours (range 12–96 hours). The rates of repeat EBP for the Williams and Banks studies were 27% and 19%, respectively. These studies clearly demonstrate the reduced efficacy of the EBP following meningeal punctures made with large needles, which not uncommonly make it necessary to consider repeating the procedure. Overall, success rates of a second EBP appear to be approximately equal to that of a first. The ideal timing and blood volume for repeat EBP is even more uncertain than for

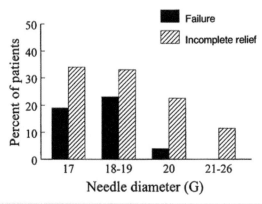

Fig. 12. Percentages of patients with incomplete relief of symptoms (including failures) and failure of the epidural blood patch versus the gauge of the needle performing meningeal puncture. (*From* Safa-Tisseront V, Thormann F, Malassine P, et al. Effectiveness of epidural blood patch in the management of post-dural puncture headache. Anesthesiology 2001;95:338; with permission.)

a primary procedure. A majority of United States anesthesiologists would wait at least 24 hours after recurrence of PDPH before performing a second EBP [10]. If more than one EBP is performed within a short period of time, practitioners should remain cognizant of the cumulative amount of blood used, as excessive volumes under these circumstances have been implicated in adverse outcomes [115].

Insufficient evidence exists to guide management following a second failed EBP. Given the frequency of PDPH and significant failure rate of the EBP, instances of sequential EBP failure are not unheard of, especially following large-gauge meningeal punctures. In an analysis of outcomes following ADP with 18-gauge Tuohy needles in an obstetric unit, Sadashivaiah [127] reported 3 of 48 patients (6.25%) requiring a third EBP to relieve the headache. Each failure of the EBP obviously necessitates an even more critical reconsideration of the diagnosis. Although experiences with managing repeated EBP failure have been published [128], such sporadic case reports are insufficient to guide others. However, one frequently cited and logical recommendation regarding repeat EBP, and particularly a third EBP, is to use some form of radiologic guidance to ensure accurate epidural blood placement. Other measures under these difficult circumstances may include any of the aforementioned "treatments," with open surgical repair usually constituting a last resort.

WHEN TO SEEK FURTHER CONSULTATION

Because the EBP has a relatively high rate of success and PDPH tends to improve even without specific treatment, many practitioners reasonably seek neurologic consultation in situations where symptoms have failed to resolve after an arbitrary duration (eg, 7–10 days) or number of EBPs (usually 2 or 3).

Consultation is always indicated in situations where serious non-PDPH is suspected or cannot reasonably be ruled out. As noted earlier, lateralizing neurologic signs, fever/chills, seizures, or change in mental status are not consistent with a diagnosis of PDPH or benign headache. Consultation is also appropriate for any headaches with atypical features. Proceeding with treatment measures directed toward PDPH under uncertain circumstances may hinder a correct diagnosis, cause critical delays in proper treatment, and can prove harmful. The EBP, for example, has occasionally been reported to produce detrimental increases in intracranial pressure.

As PDPH can be anticipated to resolve spontaneously, headaches that worsen over time and no longer have a positional nature should be strongly suspected to be secondary to SDH (especially if there are focal neurologic signs or decreases in mental status) [89]. Under these circumstances, a neurologic consultation should be obtained and diagnostic radiological studies performed.

Although headache and most associated symptoms, including auditory symptoms [32], resolve quickly following EBP, cranial nerve palsies generally resolve slowly (within 6 months), and may appropriately prompt a neurology consult for ongoing management and reassurance [25]. Although there are no accepted treatments for cranial nerve palsy associated with PDPH, it does not seem unreasonable to treat these conditions in a manner similar to idiopathic facial nerve (CN VII) palsy (Bell palsy). There is some evidence, for example, to suggest that corticosteroids administered early (within 72 hours of onset) may hasten resolution of symptoms from Bell palsy [129], and similar treatment has been suggested for cranial nerve palsy following meningeal puncture [26].

SUMMARY

More than a century after being first described, PDPH remains a significant clinical concern for several medical specialties. As with any complication, prevention is preferable to treatment. Identification and consideration of the risk factors for PDPH has resulted in an impressive reduction in the incidence of this iatrogenic problem.

Accidental meningeal puncture with epidural needles continues to be a major concern and challenge. The consequent PDPH symptoms tend to be more severe, of longer duration, and more difficult to treat than those seen with smaller gauge needles. While aggressive hydration and encouraging bed rest are the two most commonly used prophylactic measures in this setting, there is no evidence to support this practice. Several other prophylactic interventions after ADP appear promising, but each seems likely to be of limited value. Comparative studies may best help determine optimal management following ADP.

Many episodes of PDPH, especially those of mild to moderate severity, will resolve in a timely manner without specific treatment. Hydration, bed rest, and caffeine are of questionable value despite being among the most commonly advised treatment measures. However, in the absence of more definitive data, it is difficult to strongly discourage the use of these and numerous other benign and possibly helpful measures in the expectant management of PDPH of mild to moderate severity. Although alternatives have been proposed, EBP remains the definitive and sole proven treatment for PDPH, and should be encouraged and performed early (within 24 hours of diagnosis) if symptoms are severe.

Unfortunately, the published literature concerning PDPH has generally been of poor quality [55,79,130]. Many questions remain regarding the optimal means of preventing and treating this troublesome complication. Even much of what is "known" to this point has not been confirmed in follow-up studies. It is anticipated that these issues will be resolved in the future through well-designed clinical investigations.

References

[1] Harrington BE. Postdural puncture headache and the development of the epidural blood patch. Reg Anesth Pain Med 2004;29:136–63.
[2] Bier A. [Versuche ueber cocainsirung des rueckenmarkes]. Deutsche Zeitschrift Chirurgie 1899;51:361–8 [in German].

[3] Vandam LD, Dripps RD. Long-tern follow-up of patients who received 10,098 spinal anesthestics. Syndrome of decreased intracranial pressure (headache and ocular and auditory difficulties). J Am Med Assoc 1956;161(7):586–91.

[4] Hart JR, Whitacre RJ. Pencil-point needle in prevention of postspinal headache. J Am Med Assoc 1951;147:657–8.

[5] Tourtellotte WW, Haerer AF, Heller GL, et al. Post-lumbar puncture headaches. Springfield (IL): Charles C. Thomas; 1964.

[6] Moore DC. Headache. Complications of regional anesthesia. Springfield (IL): Charles C. Thomas; 1955;177–96.

[7] Gormley JB. Treatment of postspinal headache. Anesthesiology 1960;21:565–6.

[8] DiGiovanni AJ, Dunbar BS. Epidural injections of autologous blood for postlumbar-puncture headache. Anesth Analg 1970;49:268–71.

[9] Crawford JS. Experiences with epidural blood patch. Anaesthesia 1980;35:513–5.

[10] Harrington BE, Schmitt AM. Meningeal (postdural) puncture headache, unintentional dural puncture, and the epidural blood patch. A national survey of United States practice. Reg Anesth Pain Med 2009;34:430–7.

[11] Choi PT, Galinski SE, Takeuchi L, et al. PDPH is a common complication of neuraxial blockade in parturients: a meta-analysis of obstetrical studies. Can J Anaesth 2003;50: 460–9.

[12] Paech M, Banks S, Gurrin L. An audit of accidental dural puncture during epidural insertion of a Tuohy needle in obstetric patients. Int J Obstet Anesth 2001;10:162–7.

[13] Vercauteren MP, Hoffmann VH, Mertens E, et al. Seven-year review of requests for epidural blood patches for headache after dural puncture: referral patterns and the effectiveness of blood patches. Eur J Anaesthesiol 1999;16:298–303.

[14] Davies JM, Posner KL, Lee LA, et al. Liability associated with obstetric anesthesia. A closed claims analysis. Anesthesiology 2009;110:131–9.

[15] Lee LA, Posner KL, Domino KB, et al. Injuries associated with regional anesthesia in the 1980s and 1990s: a closed claims analysis. Anesthesiology 2004;101:143–52.

[16] Fitzgibbon DR, Posner KL, Domino KB, et al. Chronic pain management: American society of anesthesiologists closed claims project. Anesthesiology 2004;100:98–105.

[17] Brull R, McCartney CJL, Chan VWS, et al. Disclosure of risks associated with regional anesthesia: a survey of academic regional anesthesiologists. Reg Anesth Pain Med 2007;32: 7–11.

[18] Levine DN, Rapalino O. The pathophysiology of lumbar puncture headache. J Neurol Sci 2001;192:1–8.

[19] Kunkle EC, Ray BS, Wolff HG. Experimental studies on headache. Analysis of the headache associated with changes in intracranial pressure. Arch Neurol Psychiatr 1943;49: 323–58.

[20] Bernards CM. Sophistry in medicine: lessons from the epidural space. Reg Anesth Pain Med 2005;30:56–66.

[21] Harrington BE. Reply to Dr Colclough. Reg Anesth Pain Med 2005;30:318.

[22] Neal JM, Bernards C. Reply to Dr Colclough. Reg Anesth Pain Med 2005;30:318.

[23] Larrier D, Lee A. Anatomy of headache and facial pain. Otolaryngol Clin North Am 2003;36:1041–53.

[24] Day CJ, Shutt LE. Auditory, ocular, and facial complications of central neural block. A review of possible mechanisms. Reg Anesth 1996;21:197–201.

[25] Nishio I, Williams BA, Williams JP. Diplopia: a complication of dural puncture. Anesthesiology 2004;100:158–64.

[26] Fang JY, Lin JW, Li Q, et al. Trigeminal nerve and facial nerve palsy after combined spinal-epidural anesthesia for cesarean section. J Clin Anesth 2010;22:56–8.

[27] Lybecker H, Djernes M, Schmidt JF. Postdural puncture headache (PDPH): onset, duration, severity, and associated symptoms. An analysis of 75 consecutive patients with PDPH. Acta Anaesthesiol Scand 1995;39:605–12.

[28] Aida S, Taga K, Yamakura T, et al. Headache after attempted epidural block: the role of intrathecal air. Anesthesiology 1998;88:76–81.

[29] Reamy BV. Post-epidural headache: how late can it occur? J Am Board Fam Med 2009;22: 202–5.

[30] International Headache Society. International classification of headache disorders, 2nd edition. Cephalalgia 2004;24(Suppl 1):79.

[31] Chan TM, Ahmed E, Yentis SM, et al. Postpartum headaches: summary report of the National Obstetric Anaesthetic Database (NOAD) 1999. Int J Obstet Anesth 2003;12: 107–12.

[32] Sprung J, Bourke BA, Contreras MG, et al. Perioperative hearing impairment. Anesthesiology 2003;98:241–57.

[33] Lybecker H, Moller JT, May O, et al. Incidence and prediction of postdural puncture headache: a prospective study of 1021 spinal anesthesias. Anesth Analg 1990;70: 389–94.

[34] Wu CL, Rowlingson AJ, Cohen SR, et al. Gender and post-dural puncture headache. Anesthesiology 2006;105:613–8.

[35] Vallejo MC. Anesthetic management of the morbidly obese parturient. Curr Opin Anaesthesiol 2007;20:175–80.

[36] Kuntz KM, Kokmen E, Stevens JC, et al. Post-lumbar puncture headaches: experience in 501 consecutive procedures. Neurology 1992;42:1884–7.

[37] Faure E, Moreno R, Thisted R. Incidence of postdural puncture headache in morbidly obese parturients. Reg Anesth 1994;19:361–3.

[38] Angle P, Thompson D, Halpern S, et al. Second stage pushing correlates with headache after unintentional dural puncture in parturients. Can J Anaesth 1999;46: 861–6.

[39] Hannerz J. Postlumbar puncture headache and its relation to chronic tension-type headache. Headache 1997;37:659–62.

[40] Bader AM. The high risk obstetric patient: neurologic and neuromuscular disease in the obstetric patient. Anesthesiol Clin North America 1998;16:459–76.

[41] Echevarria M, Caba F, Rodriguez R. The influence of the menstrual cycle in postdural puncture headache. Reg Anesth Pain Med 1998;23:485–90.

[42] Amorim JA, Valenca MM. Postdural puncture headache is a risk factor for new postdural puncture headache. Cephalalgia 2007;28:5–8.

[43] Blanche R, Eisenach JC, Tuttle R, et al. Previous wet tap does not reduce success rate of labor epidural analgesia. Anesth Analg 1994;79:291–4.

[44] Halpern S, Preston R. Postdural puncture headache and spinal needle design. Metaanalysis. Anesthesiology 1994;81:1376–83.

[45] Kovanen J, Sulkava R. Duration of postural headache after lumbar puncture: effect of needle size. Headache 1986;26:224–6.

[46] Lambert DH, Hurley RJ, Hertwig L, et al. Role of needle gauge and tip configuration in the production of lumbar puncture headache. Reg Anesth 1997;22:66–72.

[47] Reina MA, de Leon-Casasola OA, Lopez A, et al. An in vitro study of dural lesions produced by 25-gauge Quincke and Whitacre needles evaluated by scanning electron microscopy. Reg Anesth Pain Med 2000;25:393–402.

[48] Richman J, Joe E, Cohen S, et al. Bevel direction and postdural puncture headache: a meta-analysis. Neurologist 2006;12:224–8.

[49] Reina MA, Dittmann M, Garcia AL, et al. New perspectives in the microscopic structure of human dura mater in the dorsolumbar region. Reg Anesth 1997;22:161–6.

[50] Seeberger MD, Kaufmann M, Staender S, et al. Repeated dural punctures increase the incidence of postdural puncture headache. Anesth Analg 1996;82:302–5.

[51] Singh S, Chaudry SY, Phelps AL, et al. A 5-year audit of accidental dural punctures, postdural puncture headaches, and failed regional anesthetics at a tertiary-care medical center. Scientific World Journal 2009;9:715–22.

[52] Goldszmidt E, Kern R, Chaput A, et al. The incidence and etiology of postpartum headaches: a prospective cohort study. Can J Anaesth 2005;52:971–7.

[53] Aya AG, Manguin R, Robert C, et al. Increased risk of unintentional dural puncture in nighttime obstetric epidural anaesthesia. Can J Anaesth 1999;46:665–9.

[54] Paech MJ, Whybrow T. The prevention and treatment of post dural puncture headache. ASEAN J Anaesthesiol 2007;8:86–95.

[55] Warwick WI, Neal JM. Beyond spinal headache: prophylaxis and treatment of low-pressure headache syndromes. Reg Anesth Pain Med 2007;32:455–61.

[56] Perlas A. Evidence for the use of ultrasound in neuraxial blocks. Reg Anesth Pain Med 2010;35(Suppl 1):S43–6.

[57] Yucel A, Ozyalcin S, Talu GK, et al. Intravenous administration of caffeine sodium benzoate for postdural puncture headache. Reg Anesth Pain Med 1999;24:51–4.

[58] Esmaoglu A, Akpinar H, Ugur F. Oral multidose caffeine-paracetamol combination is not effective for the prophylaxis of postdural puncture headache. J Clin Anesth 2005;17:58–61.

[59] Halker RB, Demaerschalk BM, Wellik KE, et al. Caffeine for the prevention and treatment of postdural puncture headache: debunking the myth. Neurologist 2007;13:323–7.

[60] Bussone G, Tullo V, d'Onofrio F, et al. Frovatriptan for the prevention of postdural puncture headache. Cephalalgia 2007;27:809–13.

[61] Sudlow C, Warlow C. Posture and fluids for preventing postdural puncture headache. Cochrane Database Syst Rev 2002;2:CD001790.

[62] Baraz R, Collis R. The management of accidental dural puncture during labor epidural analgesia: a survey of UK practice. Anaesthesia 2005;60:673–9.

[63] Strupp M, Brandt T, Muller A. Incidence of post-lumbar puncture syndrome reduced by reinserting the stylet: a randomized prospective study of 600 patients. J Neurol 1998;245:589–92.

[64] Moore JM. Continuous spinal anesthesia. Am J Ther 2009;16:289–94.

[65] Schier R, Guerra D, Aguilar J, et al. Epidural space identification: a meta-analysis of complications after air versus liquid as the medium for loss of resistance. Anesth Analg 2009;109:2012–21.

[66] Segal S, Arendt KW. A retrospective effectiveness study of loss of resistance to air or saline for identification of the epidural space. Anesth Analg 2010;110:558–63.

[67] Norris MC, Leighton BL, DeSimone CA. Needle bevel direction and headache after inadvertent dural puncture. Anesthesiology 1989;70:729–31.

[68] Duffy B. Don't turn the needle! Anaesth Intensive Care 1993;21:328–30.

[69] Simmons SW, Cyna AM, Dennis AT, et al. Combined spinal-epidural versus epidural analgesia in labour. Cochrane Database Syst Rev 2009;1:CD003401.

[70] Kuczkowski KM, Benumof JL. Decrease in the incidence of post-dural puncture headache: maintaining CSF volume. Acta Anaesthesiol Scand 2003;47:98–100.

[71] Charsley MM, Abram SE. The injection of intrathecal normal saline reduces the severity of postdural puncture headache. Reg Anesth Pain Med 2001;26:301–5.

[72] Ayad S, Bemian Y, Narouze S, et al. Subarachnoid catheter placement after wet tap for analgesia in labor: influence on the risk of headache in obstetric patients. Reg Anesth Pain Med 2003;28:512–5.

[73] Turkoz A, Kocum A, Eker HE, et al. Intrathecal catheterization after unintentional dural puncture during orthopedic surgery. J Anesth 2010;24(1):43–8.

[74] Newman M, Cyna A. Immediate management of inadvertent dural puncture during insertion of a labour epidural: a survey of Australian obstetric anaesthetists. Anaesth Intensive Care 2008;36:96–101.

[75] Stride PC, Cooper GM. Dural taps revisited: a 20-year survey from Birmingham Maternity Hospital. Anaesthesia 1993;48:247–55.

[76] Trivedi NS, Eddi D, Shevde K. Headache prevention following accidental dural puncture in obstetric patients. J Clin Anesth 1993;5:42–5.

[77] Al-metwalli RR. Epidural morphine injections for prevention of post dural puncture headache. Anaesthesia 2008;63:847–50.

[78] Scavone BM, Wong CA, Sullivan JT, et al. Efficacy of a prophylactic epidural blood patch in preventing post dural puncture headache in parturients after inadvertent dural puncture. Anesthesiology 2004;101:1422–7.

[79] Boonmak P, Boonmak S. Epidural blood patching for preventing and treating post-dural puncture headache. Cochrane Database Syst Rev 2010;1:CD001791.

[80] Leivers D. Total spinal anesthesia following early prophylactic epidural blood patch. Anesthesiology 1990;73:1287–9.

[81] Tobias MD, Pilla MA, Rogers C, et al. Lidocaine inhibits blood coagulation: implications for epidural blood patch. Anesth Analg 1996;82:766–9.

[82] Gutsche BB. Lumbar epidural analgesia in obstetrics: taps and patches. In: Reynolds F, editor. Epidural and spinal blockade in obstetrics. London: Balliere Tindall; 1990. p. 75–106.

[83] Naulty JS, Hertwig L, Hunt CO, et al. Influence of local anesthetic solution on postdural puncture headache. Anesthesiology 1990;72:450–4.

[84] Santanen U, Rautoma P, Luurila H, et al. Comparison of 27-gauge (0.41 mm) Whitacre and Quincke spinal needles with respect to post-dural puncture headache and non-dural puncture headache. Acta Anaesthesiol Scand 2004;48:474–9.

[85] Stella CL, Jodicke CD, How HY, et al. Postpartum headache: is your work-up complete? Am J Obstet Gynecol 2007;196:318,e1–318,e7.

[86] Somri M, Teszler CB, Vaida SJ, et al. Postdural puncture headache: an imaging-guided management protocol. Anesth Analg 2003;96:1809–12.

[87] Sharma R, Panda A. Ondansetron-induced headache in a parturient mimicking postdural puncture headache. Can J Anesth 2010;57:187–8.

[88] van de Beek D, Drake JM, Tunkel AR. Nosocomial bacterial meningitis. N Engl J Med 2010;362:146–54.

[89] Zeidan A, Farhat O, Maaliki H, et al. Does postdural puncture headache left untreated lead to subdural hematoma? Case report and review of the literature. Int J Obstet Anesth 2006;15:50–8.

[90] Bleeker CP, Hendriks IM, Booij LH. Postpartum post-dural puncture headache: is your differential diagnosis complete? Br J Anaesth 2004;93:461–4.

[91] Matthys LA, Coppage KH, Lambers DS, et al. Delayed postpartum preeclampsia: an experience of 151 cases. Am J Obstet Gynecol 2004;190:1464–6.

[92] Lockhart EM, Baysinger CL. Intracranial venous thrombosis in the parturient. Anesthesiology 2007;107:652–8.

[93] Vanden Eede H, Hoffmann VL, Vercauteren MP. Post-delivery postural headache: not always a classical post-dural puncture headache. Acta Anaesthesiol Scand 2007;51: 763–5.

[94] van Kooten F, Oedit R, Bakker SL, et al. Epidural blood patch in post dural puncture headache: a randomized, observer-blind, controlled clinical trial. J Neurol Neurosurg Psychiatry 2008;79:553–8.

[95] Sharma A, Cheam E. Acupuncture in the management of post-partum headache following neuraxial analgesia. Int J Obstet Anesth 2009;18:417–9.

[96] Choi A, Laurito CE, Cummingham FE. Pharmacologic management of postdural puncture headache. Ann Pharmacother 1996;30:831–9.

[97] Camann WR, Murray RS, Mushlin PS, et al. Effects of oral caffeine on postdural puncture headache. A double-blind, placebo-controlled trial. Anesth Analg 1990;70: 181–4.

[98] Carter BL, Pasupuleti R. Use of intravenous cosyntropin in the treatment of postdural puncture headache. Anesthesiology 2000;92:272–4.

[99] Connelly NR, Parker RK, Rahimi A, et al. Sumatriptan in patients with postdural puncture headache. Headache 2000;40:316–9.

[100] Rucklidge MW, Yentis SM, Paech MJ, et al. Synacthen depot for the treatment of postdural puncture headache. Anaesthesia 2004;59:138–41.

[101] Ashraf N, Sadeghi A, Azarbakht Z, et al. Hydrocortisone in post-dural puncture headache. Middle East J Anesthesiol 2007;19:415–22.

[102] Hakim S, Khan RM, Maroof M, et al. Methylergonovine maleate (methergine) relieves postdural puncture headache in obstetric patients. Acta Obstet Gynecol Scand 2005;84:100.

[103] Lin YT, Sheen MJ, Huang ST, et al. Gabapentin relieves post-dural puncture headache—a report of two cases. Acta Anaesthesiol Taiwan 2007;45:47–50.

[104] Kroin JS, Nagalla SK, Buvanendran A, et al. The mechanisms of intracranial pressure modulation by epidural blood and other injectates in a postdural puncture rat model. Anesth Analg 2002;95:423–9.

[105] Bart AJ, Wheeler AS. Comparison of epidural saline placement and epidural blood placement in the treatment of post-lumbar-puncture headache. Anesthesiology 1978;48:221–3.

[106] Liu SK, Chen KB, Wu RS, et al. Management of postdural puncture headache by epidural saline delivered with a patient-controlled pump—a case report. Acta Anaesthesiol Taiwan 2006;44:227–30.

[107] Vakharia SB, Thomas PS, Rosenbaum AE, et al. Magnetic resonance imaging of cerebrospinal fluid leak and tamponade effect of blood patch in postdural puncture headache. Anesth Analg 1997;84:585–90.

[108] Serpell MG, Haldane GJ, Jamieson DR, et al. Prevention of headache after lumbar puncture: questionnaire survey of neurologists and neurosurgeons in United Kingdom. Br Med J 1998;316:1709–10.

[109] Banks S, Paech M, Gurrin L. An audit of epidural blood patch after accidental dural puncture with a Tuohy needle in obstetric patients. Int J Obstet Anesth 2001;10:172–6.

[110] Safa-Tisseront V, Thormann F, Malassine P, et al. Effectiveness of epidural blood patch in the management of post-dural puncture headache. Anesthesiology 2001;95:334–9.

[111] Sandesc D, Lupei MI, Sirbu C, et al. Conventional treatment or epidural blood patch for the treatment of different etiologies of post dural puncture headache. Acta Anaesthesiol Belg 2005;56:265–9.

[112] Vilming ST, Kloster R, Sandvik L. When should an epidural blood patch be performed in postlumbar puncture headache? A theoretical approach based on a cohort of 79 patients. Cephalalgia 2005;25:523–7.

[113] Chen LK, Huang CH, Jean WH, et al. Effective epidural blood patch volumes for postdural puncture headache in Taiwanese women. J Formos Med Assoc 2007;106:134–40.

[114] Schievink WI. Spontaneous spinal cerebrospinal fluid leaks and intracranial hypotension. J Am Med Assoc 2006;295:2286–96.

[115] Riley CA, Spiegel JE. Complications following large-volume epidural blood patches for postdural puncture headaches. Lumbar subdural hematoma and arachnoiditis: initial cause or final effect? J Clin Anesth 2009;21:355–9.

[116] Martin R, Jourdain S, Clairoux M, et al. Duration of decubitus position after epidural blood patch. Can J Anaesth 1994;41:23–5.

[117] Jagannathan N, Tetzlaff JE. Epidural blood patch in a Jehovah's Witness patient with postdural puncture cephalgia. Can J Anaesth 2005;52:113.

[118] Bucklin BA, Tinker JH, Smith CV. Clinical dilemma: a patient with postdural puncture headache and acute leukemia. Anesth Analg 1999;88:166–7.

[119] Tom DJ, Gulevich SJ, Shapiro HM, et al. Epidural blood patch in the HIV-positive patient. Anesthesiology 1992;76:943–7.

[120] Martin DP, Bergman BD, Berger IH. Epidural blood patch and acute varicella. Anesth Analg 2004;99:1760–2.

[121] Janssens E, Aerssens P, Alliet P, et al. Post-dural puncture headaches in children: a literature review. Eur J Pediatr 2003;162:117–21.

[122] Waldman SD, Feldstein GS, Allen ML. Cervical epidural blood patch: a safe effective treatment for cervical post-dural puncture headache. Anesthesiol Rev 1987;14:23–4.

[123] Abouleish E, de la Vega S, Blendinger I, et al. Long-term follow-up of epidural blood patch. Anesth Analg 1975;54:459–63.

[124] Andrews PJD, Ackerman WE, Juneja M, et al. Transient bradycardia associated with extradural blood patch after inadvertent dural puncture in parturients. Br J Anaesth 1992;69:401–3.

[125] Hebl JR, Horlocker TT, Chantigian RC, et al. Epidural anesthesia and analgesia are not impaired after dural puncture with or without epidural blood patch. Anesth Analg 1999;89:390–4.

[126] Williams EJ, Beaulieu P, Fawcett WJ, et al. Efficacy of epidural blood patch in the obstetric population. Int J Obstet Anesth 1999;8:105–9.

[127] Sadashivaiah J. 18-G Tuohy needle can reduce the incidence of severe post dural puncture headache. Anaesthesia 2009;64:1379–80.

[128] Ho KY, Gan TJ. Management of persistent post-dural puncture headache after repeated epidural blood patch. Acta Anaesthesiol Scand 2007;51:633–6.

[129] Sullivan FM, Swan IR, Donnan PT, et al. Early treatment with prednisone or acyclovir in Bell's palsy. N Engl J Med 2007;357:1598–607.

[130] Choi PT, Galinski SE, Lucas S, et al. Examining the evidence in anesthesia literature: a survey and evaluation of obstetrical post-dural puncture headache reports. Can J Anaesth 2002;49:49–56.

Advances in Anesthesia 28 (2010) 147–159

ADVANCES IN ANESTHESIA

Current Concepts in the Management of Systemic Local Anesthetic Toxicity

Kinnari P. Khatri, MD[a], Leelach Rothschild, MD[a],
Sarah Oswald, MD[a], Guy Weinberg, MD[a,b,*]

[a]Department of Anesthesiology, University of Illinois Hospital, 1740 West Taylor Street, Suite 3200W, MC 515, Chicago, IL 60612, USA
[b]Jesse Brown VA Medical Center, 820 South Damen Chicago, IL 609612, USA

Local anesthetics are amphipathic compounds; they are both lipophilic and hydrophilic. The lipophilic component of the molecule allows local anesthetics to cross plasma and intracellular membranes, whereas the hydrophilic portion gives them the ability to interact with charged targets such as structural or catalytic proteins [1] and ion channels. When given at appropriate sites and doses, local anesthetics are safe. However, local anesthetic systemic toxicity (LAST) can occur from either accidental intravascular injection or when excessive amount of local anesthetic finds its way to the intravascular space. Patient factors can also reduce the threshold to LAST such that even normally safe serum concentrations of local anesthetic can lead to symptoms of clinical instability. Therefore, LAST is the end result of the interaction and contribution of patient-specific factors, the peak plasma concentration, and physicochemical properties of the specific local anesthetic [2]. Intrinsic anesthetic potency and the potential for causing acute cardiac and neurotoxicity parallel the lipid solubility of the drug.

The history of local anesthetics begins with the conquest of Peru by Pizarro in the early part of the 16th century and the introduction of the coca plant to Europe [2]. In 1850, Austrian von Scherzer first brought enough quantity of the coca plant to allow the isolation of cocaine by Niemann [3]. In the late 1880s Sigmund Freud suggested to his colleague Carl Koller the idea of using cocaine for its LA properties. In 1884 Koller performed the first eye surgery with the use of topical cocaine.

Shortly after the use of cocaine for topical anesthesia, physicians began to inject cocaine near peripheral nerves and into the spinal and epidural spaces [4]. In 1855 Alexander Wood first presented the idea of a nerve block by direct application of cocaine [2] and it was not long before the toxic effects of cocaine

*Corresponding author. Department of Anesthesiology, University of Illinois at Chicago, UIC Medical Center, 1740 West Taylor Street, Suite 3200W, MC 515, Chicago, IL 60612. E-mail address: guyw@uic.edu.

0737-6146/10/$ – see front matter
doi:10.1016/j.aan.2010.07.007

were identified. Cocaine not only led to addiction among medical staff but resulted in deaths among patients and medical staff alike. Before the introduction of cocaine as a local anesthetic, cocaine toxicity was reported in 1868 by Moreno y Maiz when he described cocaine-induced seizures in rats [4]. By 1887 J.B. Mattison had reported 30 cases of cocaine toxicity that involved a spectrum of symptoms from convulsions to death [3].

In 1919 Eggleston and Hatcher published a comprehensive summary of the prevention and treatment of LAST. They concluded that different local anesthetics were additive in their toxicity and that adding epinephrine to subcutaneous injection of local anesthetics apparently reduced the incidence of LAST [4]. In 1925 Tatum, Atkins and Collins identified that seizures from LAST could be controlled with barbiturate injection. By 1928 the medical community in the United States recognized a growing risk of mortality directly attributable to local anesthetics, which led to the formation of a specific ad hoc Council of the American Medical Association. The recommendations of the Council to treat toxicity from local anesthetics included cardiac massage and artificial respiration. The Council concluded that intracardiac adrenaline and digitalis were not useful to treat the toxicity [3].

As the frequency of central nervous system (CNS) and cardiovascular (CV) systemic toxicity from local anesthetics grew in number the medical community was prompted to search for new and less toxic local anesthetics [3]. Giesel isolated tropocaine in 1891 from a Javanese species of coca. Tropocaine proved to have similar degrees of toxicity to cocaine. However, structural modifications of tropocaine led to the preparation of newer local anesthetics such as eucaine, Holocaine, and orthoform [3]. In 1900 and 1905 Eihorn synthesized benzocaine and procaine, respectively. Procaine had relatively few side effects and quickly grew out of favor because of its low potency, slow onset, short duration of action, and limited ability to penetrate tissue [3]. Chloroprocaine was created by a chlorine substitution to the aromatic ring of procaine. Unfortunately, its use declined after 1980 because of reports of prolonged sensory and motor block following subarachnoid administration of an intended epidural dose. The last ester type local anesthetic to be developed was tetracaine in 1930. Tetracaine can be used to achieve 1.5 to 2.5 hours of spinal anesthesia as an isobaric, hypobaric, or hyperbaric solution [3]. It is also effective as a topical airway anesthetic. Lidocaine was created in 1944 and was first used clinically in 1948. It quickly became one of the most widely used local anesthetics because of its potency, rapid onset, and effectiveness for infiltration. The safety profile of lidocaine for neuraxial anesthesia was questioned in the late 1980s when numerous reports appeared of transient neurologic symptoms following uneventful spinal anesthesia and instances of cauda equina syndrome from high concentrations of lidocaine being administered through a continuous spinal catheter. All newer local anesthetics after the invention of lidocaine encompass the amide structure. Mepivacaine and prilocaine are both related to lidocaine and were introduced for clinical use in 1957 and 1960, respectively [3]. Prilocaine is limited for clinical use by its potential to cause methemoglobinemia.

The evolution of modern regional anesthesia begins with the invention of bupivacaine in 1957. Shortly after its synthesis bupivacaine was initially discarded for clinical use because it was found to be 4 times more toxic than its homolog mepivacaine [3] and was not introduced into clinical practice until 1965. Bupivacaine belongs to the family of n-alkyl-substituted pipecholyl xylidines having a butyryl substitution and an asymmetric carbon atom that represents a chiral center [5]. Bupivacaine is a long-acting amide local anesthetic that can be used for neuraxial block, peripheral nerve block, and infiltration. It can be used for a differential blockade because lower concentrations mainly provide sensory blockade, whereas motor blockade is only seen at higher concentrations [3].

Hollmen reported the first clinical descriptions of bupivacaine toxicity in 1966. A total of 133 patients were studied for toxic reactions during epidural and caudal anesthesia for abdominal and urological surgery [3]. Five out of 6 patients had mild to severe CNS toxicity manifesting as tremor or convulsions. One case involved hypotension and bradycardia after a caudal block.

In 1969 Beck and Martin reviewed 19,907 cases of paracervical blockade with bupivacaine in women during labor [6]. They found 23 cases of infant death and evidence of newborn acidosis associated with paracervical blockade with bupivacaine. It was not until 1983 that bupivacaine was abandoned for use in paracervical blockade [3].

In the early 1970s there were several human volunteer studies of bupivacaine toxicity. Most of these involved continuous infusion of bupivacaine until symptoms appeared [3]. The sample sizes for these studies were extremely small, consisting of only 3 to 6 patients. The main observed symptoms were CNS in nature (lightheadedness, muscle twitching, dizziness, lip numbness, tinnitus, and slurred speech).

The first case of severe cardiovascular toxicity was reported in 1977 by Edde and Deutsch, 10 years after the introduction of bupivacaine to clinical use. They described ventricular fibrillation in a patient undergoing an interscalene block with 100 mg of bupivacaine [2]. Albright's editorial in 1979 detailed bupivacaine-induced CV compromise such as ventricular arrhythmias, CV collapse and death. He implied a causal relationship between severe CV toxicity and the use of bupivacaine and etidocaine [7].

In the 1980s the pharmaceutical industry began to search for a less toxic, but potent and long-acting local anesthetic with reduced toxicity [3]. This led to the use of the potentially less toxic S-(−)-enantiomer of bupivacaine, levobupivacaine, and the new local anesthetic, ropivacaine. Ropivacaine was introduced into clinical practice in 1996 after evaluation in clinical trials starting in 1990. It is able to produce differential blockade and may have a better safety profile.

The latest focus on methods to reduce local anesthetic toxicity involves the delivery of local anesthetics mixed with substances capable of slowing release. Two approaches involve liposomes and microspheres. Boogaerts and colleagues [8] published the first study of epidural administration of liposomal bupivacaine in 1994.

MECHANISMS OF LAST

Bupivacaine is arguably the prototypical lipophilic amide local anesthetic with the highest potential for causing severe, even fatal clinical toxicity. Although all local anesthetics can produce LAST, the phenotype and mechanisms of bupivacaine toxicity have been the most widely studied. Therefore, the following descriptions of action behind CNS and CVS toxicity can presumably be generalized to most local anesthetics at sufficiently high concentrations.

CNS

Clinical central nervous system toxicity caused by bupivacaine consists of 2 phases. The first phase or the excitatory phase manifests as shivering, muscle twitching, and tremors progressing to tonic-clinic seizures [9]. The second or the inhibitory phase involves generalized depression leading to hypoventilation and respiratory arrest. The CNS symptoms usually occur before signs of cardiovascular toxicity. The specific mechanism underlying CNS toxicity involves neuronal desynchronization, possibly because of disturbances with the γ-aminobutyric acid neurotransmitter [10].

CVS

Cardiotoxicity from bupivacaine involves a 2-stage pattern similar to CNS toxicity. First, the central activation of the sympathetic nervous system produces tachycardia and hypertension, which can mask the direct cardiac depressant effects of bupivacaine. Malignant arrhythmias and contractile dysfunction shortly follow the initial sympathetic activation. The end result can be complete cardiovascular collapse.

Bupivacaine blocks cardiac sodium channels in a time- and voltage-dependent manner. The sodium channel block is intensified as heart rate is increased or membrane potential is more depolarized [11]. Bupivacaine has a preference for inactivated sodium channels over those in the resting or open configuration. At low concentrations, bupivacaine blocks sodium channels in a slow-in slow-out manner and at high concentrations the channel is blocked in a fast-in slow-out manner. Non–protein-bound free bupivacaine concentrations of 0.5 to 5 μg/mL slow conduction of cardiac action potentials, which leads to a prolonged PR interval and a widened QRS complex. The persistence of sodium channel blockade into diastole further slows cardiac conduction and can predispose the heart to re-entrant arrhythmias and/or unifocal, multifocal beats or ventricular tachycardias.

Local anesthetics also inhibit cardiac contractility in a nonstereoselective manner, which might result from various effects on mitochondrial energy metabolism, intracellular calcium regulation [12–14] inhibition of cAMP [15] or interference with other metabotropic signaling pathways. Bupivacaine reduces both the mitochondrial transmembrane potential and lipid-based respiration in mitochondria [16]. The former reduces efficiency of oxidative phosphorylation; the latter impairs the transport of lipid fuel necessary for the 70% of myocardial energy that is normally derived from fatty acid oxidation in the mitochondrial matrix. The observation that bupivacaine inhibits carnitine-acylcarnitine translocase was an important step in the discovery of lipid emulsion (see later discussion). This specific inhibition of carnitine fatty acyl transfer into the mitochondrial matrix might explain the relatively low dose of bupivacaine that leads to cardiovascular collapse [16]. Bupivacaine also impairs cardiac relaxation (lusitropy), an effect that may be caused by impairment of calcium handling in the sarcoplasmic reticulum [17].

EVOLUTION OF LIPID EMULSION (BENCH TO BEDSIDE) AS TREATMENT OF LOCAL ANESTHETIC TOXICITY

Several animal studies and case reports have demonstrated the effectiveness of intravenous lipid emulsion (ILE) infusion during resuscitation from symptomatic overdose of local anesthetic toxicity, and ILE has recently gained acceptance as a recommended treatment for LAST (Fig. 1). The investigation of ILE therapy for LAST resulted from unexpected clinical and laboratory observations. The first involved a patient with a history of isovaleric acidemia undergoing suction lipectomy. The surgeon used a tumescent solution containing 300 mL of 0.0075% bupivacaine and epinephrine 1:1,000,000 [18]. Minutes after the use of the tumescent solution the patient had ventricular dysrhythmias with hemodynamic instability. This patient was later discovered to have carnitine deficiency, and the investigators theorized that this could explain the patient's increased susceptibility to the toxic effects of bupivacaine [18].

During normal aerobic conditions carnitine is necessary for transport of fatty acids into the mitochondrial matrix. These fatty acids are the predominant energy source for the heart. Weinberg and colleagues [16] went on to show that bupivacaine inhibits carnitine metabolism in cardiac mitochondria. They found evidence that bupivacaine inhibited mitochondrial state III respiration when acylcarnitines are the available substrates. Therefore, because of the heart's respiratory dependence on fatty acids for energy and bupivacaine's inhibition of the enzyme carnitine-acylcarnitine translocase, the investigators postulated that this contributed to the relatively low ratio of the toxic dose of bupivacaine needed for cardiovascular collapse in relation to that producing seizures.

Because cytoplasmic accumulation of fatty acyl molecules was known to be arrhythmogenic, the investigators postulated that pretreatment with an infusion of lipids might aggravate bupivacaine-induced arrhythmias; they observed exactly the opposite effect in rats pretreated with lipid. Lipid infusion increased the dose of bupivacaine required to induce asystole in rats [19]. There was a 48% increase in the LD_{50} for bupivacaine when the rats were resuscitated with lipid infusion. Paradoxically, isolated hearts using lipid substrates are more sensitive to bupivacaine toxicity than when burning only carbohydrates [20].

The next set of experiments involved a dog model, a species closer in size to humans. Cardiovascular collapse occurred in all dogs after 10 mg/kg of bupivacaine injected intravascularly [21]. Cardiac massage alone failed to

AMERICAN SOCIETY OF
REGIONAL ANESTHESIA AND PAIN MEDICINE

Practice Advisory on Treatment of Local Anesthetic Systemic Toxicity

For Patients Experiencing Signs or Symptoms of Local Anesthetic Systemic Toxicity (LAST)

- **Get Help**
- **Initial Focus**
  - o *Airway management:* ventilate with 100% oxygen
  - o *Seizure suppression:* benzodiazepines are preferred
  - o *Basic and Advanced Cardiac Life Support (BLS/ACLS)* may require prolonged effort
- **Infuse 20% Lipid Emulsion (values in parenthesis are for a 70 kg patient)**
  - o *Bolus 1.5 mL/kg* (lean body mass) intravenously over 1 min (~100 mL)
  - o *Continuous infusion at 0.25 mL/kg/min* (~18 mL/min; adjust by roller clamp)
  - o Repeat bolus once or twice for persistent cardiovascular collapse
  - o Double the infusion rate to 0.5 mL/kg per minute if blood pressure remains low
  - o *Continue infusion* for at least 10 mins after attaining circulatory stability
  - o Recommended upper limit: approximately 10 mL/kg lipid emulsion over the first 30 mins
- **Avoid** vasopressin, calcium channel blockers, β-blockers, or local anesthetic
- **Alert** the nearest facility having cardiopulmonary bypass capability
- **Avoid propofol** in patients having signs of cardiovascular instability
- **Post LAST events** at www.lipidrescue.org and report use of lipid to www.lipidregistry.org

© 2010 American Society of Regional Anesthesia and Pain Medicine

ASRA hereby grants practitioners the right to reproduce this document as a tool for the care of patients who receive potentially toxic doses of LAs. Publication of these recommendations requires permission from ASRA.

The ASRA Practice Advisory on Local Anesthetic Toxicity is published in the society's official publication *Regional Anesthesia and Pain Medicine*, and can be downloaded from the journal Web site at www.rapm.org.

Neal JM, Weinberg GL, Bernards CM, et al. ASRA practice advisory on local anesthetic systemic toxicity. *Reg Anesth Pain Med* 2010;35:152-161.

Fig. 1. American Society of Regional Anesthesia practice advisory on the treatment of local anesthetic systemic toxicity. (*From* Neal JM, Weinberg GL, Bernards CM, et al. ASRA practice advisory on local anesthetic systemic toxicity. Reg Anesth Pain Med 2010;35:152–161; with permission. © 2010 American Society of Regional Anesthesia and Pain Medicine.)

resuscitate any of the dogs. An infusion of lipid emulsion plus internal cardiac massage led to full recovery whether the treatment was initiated immediately or 10 minutes after complete cardiovascular collapse. All 6 of the dogs in the experimental group recovered normal hemodynamic parameters but none of dogs in the control group survived.

CLINICAL USE OF ILE

In 2006 Rosenblatt and colleagues [22] published the first case report of successful lipid-based resuscitation of a patient with cardiac arrest secondary to LAST. The patient was given 40 mL of a 1:1 mixture of 0.5% bupivacaine plus 1.5%

mepivacaine for an interscalene brachial plexus block followed quickly by loss of consciousness and seizures. Within minutes of the seizure the patient's electrocardiograph (ECG) showed asystole. After 20 minutes of advanced cardiac life support, 100 mL of 20% lipid emulsion was administered via peripheral intravenous access and the patient rapidly recovered normal vital signs and normal sinus rhythm. Within 2.5 hours the patient was awake, alert and responsive, and extubated without any neurologic sequelae.

MECHANISMS OF ILE
Lipid Sink Mechanism
Lipid emulsion is a 20% formulation of fat emulsion and consists of 20% soybean oil, 1.2% egg yolk phospholipids, 2.25% glycerin, water, and sodium hydroxide. Egg yolk phospholipid exists in a 1% concentration with oil particles of about 0.5 μm in diameter and acts as the emulsifying agent. The emulsified fat droplets, when infused into an aqueous medium, such as blood, form a lipid compartment into which lipophilic substances, such as local anesthetics, are theoretically partitioned. As local anesthetics are drawn into the lipid sink a corresponding concentration gradient develops between tissue and blood causing the local anesthetics to move away from the heart or brain (areas of high concentration) to the lipid sink. In an experimental rat model, Weinberg and colleagues [19] demonstrated that radiolabeled bupivacaine added in vitro to lipid-treated rat plasma preferentially moves to the lipid phase. This concentration gradient reduces the total local anesthetic drug concentration in contact with tissue. The bupivacaine lipid/aqueous partition coefficient of 11.9 found in this model suggests that the lipid phase retains highly lipophilic drugs, such as bupivacaine. The solubility of long-acting local anesthetics in lipid emulsion and the high binding capacity of these emulsions likely explain the clinical efficacy when lipid emulsion is rapidly infused as in the treatment of LAST.

Alternative Mechanisms
ILE might also affect ATP synthesis in the myocyte by increasing intracellular fatty acid content and thereby overcoming the reduced ATP production secondary to local anesthetic block of fatty acid oxidation. Eledjam and colleagues [23] demonstrated that ATP repletion reverses bupivacaine toxicity in isolated myocardial strips. Van de Velde and colleagues [24] demonstrated in a dog model that infusion of 20% lipid emulsion improves contractility because of improved fatty acid oxidation. Furthermore, fatty acids have also been shown to increase calcium levels in cardiac myocytes. Lipid emulsion infusion may therefore directly increase intramyocyte calcium levels and lead to a direct positive inotropic effect [25]. Lipid emulsion was initially observed as acting faster in in vivo settings than was anticipated based on a simple lipid sink mechanism [26]. This suggested to the experimentalists that additional, potentially direct cardiotonic effects might be in play. Subsequently, Stehr and colleagues [27] demonstrated in isolated rat heart models that lipid emulsion reverses bupivacaine-induced contractile depression at concentrations that are

too low to provide a lipid sink phenomenon, suggesting an alternative, possibly metabolic explanation for the beneficial effect. Although the precise contribution of these mechanisms of benefit in ILE treatment of LAST remains unclear, it is likely that the key component is the local anesthetic binding property of the emulsion [28].

Potential Complications of ILE

Adverse effects of ILE have been reported largely in the setting of its use as a nutritional supplement, particularly in the neonatal intensive care unit. Some reported complications include pulmonary dysfunction, allergic reactions, increased liver function tests, hypercoagulability, thrombocytopenia, and hyperthermia [29]. The only published complication of ILE during resuscitation was reported by Marwick and colleagues [30] who described a single increased amylase level in a patient who had received 500 mL of lipid emulsion. Despite the increased amylase level, no clinical development of pancreatitis occurred, and no change in treatment was necessary. Therefore, the reported and potential complications of ILE probably do not outweigh its potential benefit, particularly in its use during the rescue of a patient with cardiovascular instability secondary to LAST.

ILE IN ACLS

ILE is a novel method for treating LAST that shows promise as an effective antidote for lipophilic drug poisoning, including local anesthetics (Fig. 2). Cardiovascular collapse is the most life-endangering complication of local anesthetic absorption or intravascular injection during regional anesthesia. Reports in the past several years have focused on the merits of ILE in the setting of standard resuscitation protocols.

Weinberg [31] published the first recommendation for the use of ILE in a letter to the editor in 2004 then a revised version in 2006 on an educational Web site (www.lipidrescue.org). These recommendations served as the basis for all subsequent recommendations for ILE. For instance, the Association of Anaesthetists of Great Britain and Ireland (AAGBI) published a set of guidelines for the management of LAST in 2007 that outline specific dosing information and recommend that lipid emulsion should be available in locations where potentially toxic doses of local anesthetics are administered [32]. The AAGBI's guidelines added credence to the use of ILE in the setting of LAST. One year later, in 2008, the American Society of Critical Care Anesthesiologists and the American Society of Anesthesiologists Committee on Critical Care Medicine as well as the Resuscitation Council (UK) incorporated the use of lipid emulsion in their published protocols for the treatment of LAST [33,34]. More recently, the American Society of Regional Anesthesia and Pain Medicine published practice guidelines for management of LAST that included specific recommendations for its prevention, diagnosis, and treatment [35]. The treatment guidelines included the use of ILE as an adjunct to airway management and good

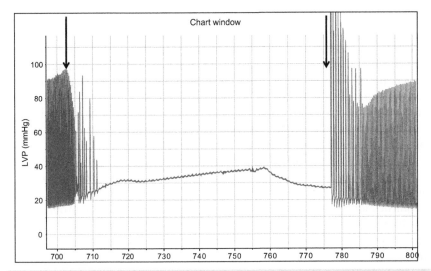

Fig. 2. Lipid emulsion therapy in an isolated heart experiment. Real-time trace of left ventricular pressure. Arrow B indicates the beginning of a 15-second infusion of 500 lM racemic bupivacaine. Arrow L indicates the beginning of infusion of 1% lipid emulsion. The interval between the arrows corresponds to mechanical asystole.

CPR, stating, "….lipid emulsion therapy can be instrumental in facilitating resuscitation, most probably by acting as a lipid sink that draws down the content of lipid-soluble local anesthetics from within cardiac tissue, thereby improving cardiac conduction, contractility, and coronary perfusion."

Lipid emulsion's success depends on prompt and effective airway management to prevent hypoxia and acidosis, which are known to potentiate LAST [36]. However, the question remains whether ILE should replace or supplement standard pharmacologic therapy. Recent reports highlight the detrimental effect that standard pharmacologic therapies might have in the setting of lipid emulsion administration. In a rat model, Hiller and colleagues [37] found that epinephrine doses equal to or greater than 10 µg/kg increased lactate concentration, worsened acidosis, and resulted in worse recovery at 15 minutes compared with lipid-treated animals. Prior studies by Weinberg and colleagues [38] in rat models of bupivacaine-induced asystole, showed that lipid is superior to epinephrine, vasopressin [39] or the combination of both vasopressors for measured hemodynamic variables at 10 minutes. Therefore, epinephrine might aggravate local anesthetic toxicity by severe systemic vasoconstriction and increased lactate production. These observations resulted in the 2010 American Society of Regional Anesthesia (ASRA) practice advisory recommending use of low-dose epinephrine, and avoiding vasopressin completely in the context of LAST.

Lipid emulsion might also be effective in preventing progression of clinically significant LAST. Clinicians are now perhaps more likely to administer lipid emulsion earlier in the progression of adverse reactions from local anesthetic toxicity, with the hope of preventing severe, refractory cardiovascular collapse following progression of LAST. For instance, Foxall and colleagues [40] reported using lipid emulsion to treat CNS toxicity and ventricular ectopy to prevent progression to cardiac arrest in a 75-year-old woman who experienced seizures following a posterior lumbar plexus block with levobupivacaine; this was the first reported use of lipid emulsion in a periarrest situation. Additional reports demonstrate the ability of lipid emulsion to effectively treat CNS symptoms and prevent further progression of LAST [41–43].

Although lipid emulsion is now a recommended treatment of local anesthetic toxicity, it still remains to be determined whether its use can be translated with similar efficacy to other lipophilic but nonlocal anesthetic drug toxicities. Local anesthetic-induced CNS disturbances and cardiovascular compromise are usually witnessed events in the perioperative environment. Generally, these events are addressed and treated with rapid institution of ABCs (airway, breathing, circulation) of basic life support. Adequate oxygenation is essential for lipid emulsion's efficacy in treating LAST. In settings such as emergency rooms, when the offending drug is unknown, the practitioner must decide whether lipid emulsion would contribute to standard resuscitation techniques. The physician must first consider whether a lipophilic toxin was ingested, and then decide whether in addition to following standard ACLS guidelines the patient will potentially benefit from administration of lipid emulsion.

AREAS OF FUTURE RESEARCH AND APPLICATION FOR OTHER DRUG TOXICITIES

Several animal models as well as case reports have sparked intense interest in lipid emulsion's potential lifesaving effects on resuscitation from poisonings of tricyclic antidepressants, beta blockers, and other lipophilic medications. Many of these medications share physicochemical properties with local anesthetics; it is believed that lipid emulsion exerts the same lipid sink effect with these lipophilic drugs, thereby decreasing the amount of active drug in the target tissue [44].

Animal Studies

Yoav and colleagues [45] used a rat model to show decreased mortality when clomipramine was given in a lipid infusion compared with a saline control. Following this observation, Bania and Chu [46] demonstrated the protective effects of pretreatment with lipid emulsion before toxic doses of amitriptyline were administered. Harvey and Cave [47] used a rabbit model to show a quicker recovery from clomipramine-induced hypotension with lipid emulsion rescue compared with controls treated with saline or sodium bicarbonate. Both rat [48] and canine [49] models of verapamil toxicity also supported the use of lipid emulsion in stabilizing and even resuscitating animals exposed to toxic doses of verapamil. Many other similar animal studies also point to lipid emulsion as having protective or even lifesaving effects when used in the setting of lipophilic drug toxicities.

Case Reports

The first report of lipid emulsion's successful use in a human as an antidote for a lipophilic, nonlocal anesthetic toxicity was described by Sirianni and colleagues [50]. This case involved a 17-year-old girl who had ingested enormous amounts of bupropion and lamotrigine, both known to potentially cause sodium channel blockade when taken in large quantities. Ten hours after the overdose, the patient experienced complete cardiovascular collapse with ensuing ventricular fibrillation and pulseless electrical activity. After more than 70 minutes of standard resuscitation, a single bolus of lipid emulsion was given as a last attempt to restore stable cardiac output. Approximately 1 minute later a normal pulse was observed and within 15 minutes, she returned to sinus rhythm and vasopressor therapy was decreased. This patient was subsequently discharged with minimal neurologic deficits. Another case report involves a 61-year-old man who presented to the emergency department with a Glascow Coma Scale (GCS) of 3 after overdosing on quetiapine and sertraline [51]. The patient was given a bolus of 20% lipid emulsion 4 hours after the overdose. Within seconds the patient's level of consciousness increased to a GCS of 9, and airway reflexes were restored within 15 minutes. The patient no longer needed intubation and was subsequently discharged to a psychiatric unit less than a day later, with GCS of 15.

SUMMARY

Recommendations about the use of lipid emulsion are complex and still evolving but several governing bodies have compiled guidelines on their Web sites to help standardize the treatment of LAST with lipid emulsion. ASRA has published a practice advisory on the treatment of local anesthetic systemic toxicity (Fig. 1) [35]. Two educational Web sites, www.lipidrescue.org and www.lipidregistry.org, provide additional information on ILE and a forum for posting and discussing cases of toxicity in which ILE was used.

References

[1] Butterworth JF 4th, Strichartz GR. Molecular mechanisms of local anesthesia: a review. Anesthesiology 1990;72:711–34.

[2] Feldman HS. Anesthetic toxicity. New York: Raven Press Ltd; 1994. p. 107–27.

[3] Ruetsch YA, Boni T, Borgeat A. From cocaine to ropivacaine: the history of local anesthetics drugs. Curr Top Med Chem 2001;1:175–82.

[4] Brown DL. Complications of regional anesthesia. New York: Springer; 2007. p. 61–70.

[5] Casati A, Putzu M. Bupivacaine, levobupivacaine and ropivacaine: are they clinically different? Best Pract Res Clin Anesthesiol 2004;19:247–68.

[6] Beck L, Martin K. [Hazards of paracervical block in obstetrics. A survey of 107 hospitals for women with a total of 32, 652 cases]. Geburtshilfe Frauenheilkd 1969;29(11):961–7 [in German].

[7] Albright GA. Cardiac arrest following regional anesthesia with etidocaine and bupivacaine. Anesthesiology 1979;51:285–7.

[8] Boogaerts JG, Lafont ND, Declercq AG, et al. Epidural administration of liposome associated bupivacaine for the management of postsurgical pain: a first study. J Clin Anesth 1994;6:315–20.

[9] Groban L. Central nervous system and cardiac effects from long acting amide local anesthetic toxicity in the intact animal model. Reg Anesth Pain Med 2003;1(8):3–11.

[10] Veering BT. Complications and local anesthetic toxicity in regional anesthesia. Curr Opin Anaesthesiol 2003;16:455–9.

[11] Clarkson CW, Hondeghem LM. Mechanism for bupivacaine depression of cardiac conduction: fast block of sodium channels during the action potential with slow recovery from block during diastole. Anesthesiology 1985;62:396–405.

[12] Sztark F, Ouhabi R, Dabadie P, et al. Effects of the local anesthetic bupivacaine on mitochondrial energy metabolism: change from uncoupling to decoupling depending on the respiration state. Biochem Mol Biol Int 1997;43:997–1003.

[13] Sztark F, Nouette –Gaulain K, Malgat M, et al. Absence of stereospecific effects of bupivacaine isomers on heart mitochondrial bioenergetics. Anesthesiology 1998;88:1340–9.

[14] Groban L, Deal DD, Vernon JC, et al. Does local anesthetic stereoselectivity or structure predict myocardial depression in anesthetized canines? Reg Anesth Pain Med 2002;27:460–8.

[15] Butterworth JF, Brownlow RC, Leith JP, et al. Bupivacaine inhibits cyclic-3′,53′-adenosine monophosphate production. Anesthesiology 1993;79(7):88–95.

[16] Weinberg GL, Palmer JW, VadeBoncouer TR, et al. Bupivacaine inhibits acylcarnitine exchange in cardiac mitochondria. Anesthesiology 2000;92(5):523–8.

[17] David JS, Ferreti C, Amour J, et al. Effects of bupivacaine, levobupivacaine and ropivacaine on myocardial relaxation. Can J Anaesth 2007;54:208–17.

[18] Weinberg GL, Laurito CE, Geldner P, et al. Malignant ventricular dysrhythmias in a patient with isovaleric acidemia receiving general and local anesthesia for suction lipectomy. J Clin Anesth 1997;9(8):668–70.

[19] Weinberg G, VadeBoncouer T, Ramaraju GA, et al. Pretreatment or resuscitation with a lipid infusion shifts the dose–response to bupivacaine-induced asystole in rats. Anesthesiology 1998;88:1071–5.

[20] Edelman LB, Ripper R, Kelly K, et al. Metabolic context affects hemodynamic response to bupivacaine in the isolated rat heart. Chem Biol Interact 2008;172(1):48–53.

[21] Weinberg G, Ripper R, Feinstein DL, et al. Lipid emulsion infusion rescues dogs from bupivacaine-induced cardiac toxicity. Reg Anesth Pain Med 2003;28:198–202.

[22] Rosenblatt MA, Abel M, Fischer GW, et al. Successful use of a 20% lipid emulsion to resuscitate a patient after a presumed bupivacaine-related cardiac arrest. Anesthesiology 2006;105:217–8.

[23] Eledjam JJ, de La Coussaye JE, Brugada J, et al. In vitro study on mechanisms of bupivacaine-induced depression of myocardial contractility. Anesth Analg 1989;69:732–5.

[24] Van de Velde M, Wouters PF, Rold N, et al. Long-chain triglycerides improve recovery from myocardial stunning in conscious dogs. Cardiovasc Res 1996;32:1008–15.

[25] Huang J, Xian H, Bacaner M. Long chain fatty acids activate calcium channels in ventricular myocytes. Proc Natl Acad Sci U S A 1992;89:6452–6.

[26] Weinberg G. Lipid rescue resuscitation from local anaesthetic cardiac toxicity. Toxicol Rev 2006;25(3):139–45.

[27] Stehr SN, Ziegeler JC, Pea A, et al. The effects of lipid infusion on myocardial function and bioenergetics in L-bupivacaine toxicity in the isolated rat heart. Anesth Analg 2007;104:186–92.

[28] Mazoit JX, Le Guen R, Beloeil H, et al. Binding of long-lasting local anesthetics to lipid emulsions. Anesthesiology 2009;110(2):380–6.

[29] Cave G, Harvey M. Intravenous ILE as antidote beyond local anesthetic toxicity: a systematic review. Acad Emerg Med 2009;16:815–24.

[30] Marwick PC, Levin AI, Coetzee AR. Recurrence of bupivacaine toxicity after lipid rescue from bupivacaine-induced cardiac arrest. Anesth Analg 2009;108:1344–6.

[31] Weinberg G. Reply to Drs. Goor, Groban, and Butterworth–Lipid rescue: caveats and recommendations for the "silver bullet". Reg Anesth Pain Med 2004;29(1):74–5.

[32] Association of Anaesthetists of Great Britain and Ireland. Guidelines for the management of severe localanaesthetic toxicity. Available at: http://aagbi.org/publications/guidelines/docs/la_toxicity_2010.pdf. Accessed August 21, 2010.

[33] Resuscitation Council of the United Kingdom. Cardiac arrest or cardiovascular collapse caused by local anaesthetic. Available at: http://www.resus.org.uk/pages/caLocalA.htm. Accessed August 21, 2010.

[34] Available at: http://www.asahq.org/clinical/Anesthesiology-CentricACLS.pdf. Accessed August 21, 2010.

[35] Neal JM, Bernards CM, Butterworth JF, et al. ASRA practice advisory on local anesthetic systemic toxicity. Reg Anesth Pain Med 2010;35(2):152–61.

[36] Harvey M, Cave G, Kazemi A. Intralipid infusion diminishes return of spontaneous circulation after hypoxic cardiac arrest in rabbits. Anesth Analg 2009;108(4):1163–8.

[37] Hiller D, Di Gregorio G, Ripper R, et al. Epinephrine impairs lipid resuscitation from bupivacaine overdose: a threshold effect. Anesthesiology 2009;111(3):1–8.

[38] Weinberg G, Di Gregorio G, Ripper R, et al. Resuscitation with lipid versus epinephrine in a rat model of bupivacaine overdose. Anesthesiology 2008;108:907–13.

[39] Di Gregorio G, Schwartz D, Ripper R, et al. ILE is superior to vasopressin in a rodent model of resuscitation from toxin-induced cardiac arrest. Crit Care Med 2009;37:993–9.

[40] Foxall G, McCahon R, Lamb J, et al. Levobupivacaine-induced seizures and cardiovascular collapse treated with lipid emulsion. Anaesthesia 2007;62:516–8.

[41] McCutchen T, Gerancher JC. Early lipid emulsion therapy may have prevented bupivacaine-associated cardiac arrest. Reg Anesth Pain Med 2008;33:178–80.

[42] Ludot H, Tharin JY, Belouadah M, et al. Successful resuscitation after ropivicaine and lidocaine-induced ventricular arrhythmia following posterior lumbar plexus block in a child. Anesth Analg 2008;106:1572–4.

[43] Litz RJ, Popp M, Stehr SN, et al. Successful resuscitation of a patient with ropivicaine-induced asystole after axillary plexus block using lipid infusion. Anaesthesia 2006;61:800–1.

[44] Leskiw U, Weinberg GL. Lipid resuscitation for local anesthetic toxicity, is it really lifesaving? Curr Opin Anaesthesiol 2009;22:667–71.

[45] Yoav G, Odelia G, Shaltiel C. A lipid emulsion reduced mortality from clomipramine overdose in rats. Vet Hum Toxicol 2002;44:30.

[46] Bania T, Chu J. Hemodynamic effect of lipid emulsion in amitriptyline toxicity [abstract]. Acad Emerg Med 2006;13(S1):117.

[47] Harvey M, Cave G. Lipid emulsion outperforms sodium bicarbonate in a rabbit model of clomipramine toxicity. Ann Emerg Med 2007;49:178–85.

[48] Tebbutt S, Havey M, Nicholson T, et al. Lipid emulsion prolongs survival in a rat model of verapamil toxicity. Acad Emerg Med 2006;13:134–9.

[49] Bania TC. Hemodynamic effects of intravenous fat emulsion in an animal model of severe verapamil toxicity resuscitated with atropine, calcium and normal saline. Acad Emerg Med 2007;14:105–11.

[50] Sirianni AJ, Osterhoudt KC, Callelo DP, et al. Use of lipid emulsion in the resuscitation of a patient with prolonged cardiovascular collapse after overdose of bupropion and lamotrigine. Ann Emerg Med 2008;51:412–5.

[51] Finn SDH, Uncles DR, Willers J, et al. Early treatment of quetiapine and sertraline overdose with lipid emulsion. Anaesthesia 2009;64:191–4.

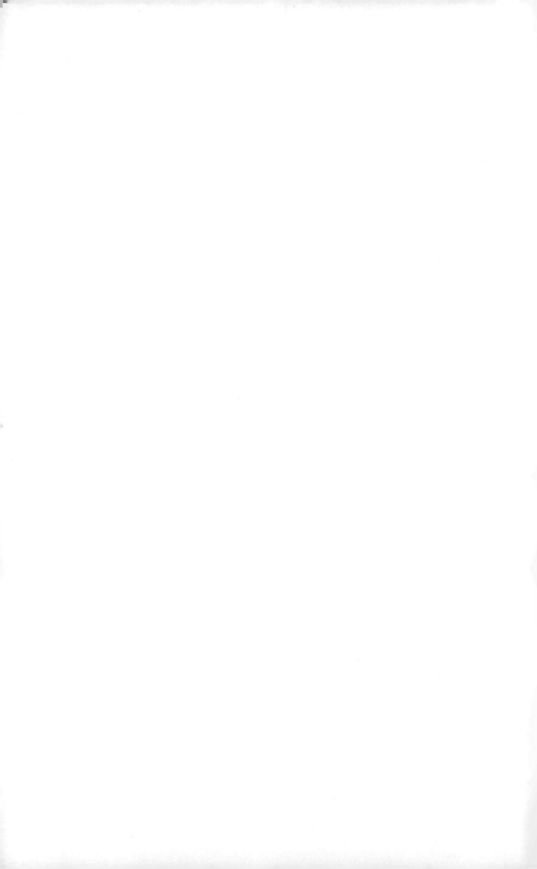

Advances in Anesthesia 28 (2010) 161–186

ADVANCES IN ANESTHESIA

Biomarkers: Understanding, Progress, and Implications in the Perioperative Period

Basem Abdelmalak, MD[a,b,*], Juan P. Cata, MD[a,b]

[a]Department of General Anesthesiology, E31, The Cleveland Clinic, 9500 Euclid Avenue, Cleveland, OH 44195, USA
[b]Department of Outcomes Research, The Cleveland Clinic, 9500 Euclid Avenue, Cleveland, OH 44195, USA

Patients with coronary artery disease undergoing major noncardiac surgery have a considerable risk of perioperative cardiac morbidity and mortality and compromised long-term outcome [1,2]. Several preoperative risk stratification scores, as well as strategies based on physical examination and history, have been developed to predict the risk of cardiac complications following various surgical procedures performed in different patient populations [3,4].

Some of these scores have limitations, and generating them may include cardiac stress testing, with its associated risks and costs [4]. Moreover, although there are many risk stratification tools concerning cardiac outcomes, few exist for important noncardiac complications, such as infectious, neurologic, and renal complications, or for noncardiac causes of mortality.

Biomarkers have attracted the attention of clinicians and investigators as a means of stratifying risk in different patient populations, including surgical patients. They generally entail simple, minimally invasive tests (blood draws) that have potentially high yield in assessing risk stratification [5,6]. Therefore, it is important to understand the biology, pathophysiology, and usefulness of biomarkers during the perioperative period, because these indicators may have predictive value for postoperative outcomes, especially when these biomarkers are added to existing risk stratification techniques. For instance, C-reactive protein (CRP) and N-terminal pro-brain natriuretic peptide (NT-proBNP) improved the average sensitivity of predicting perioperative major cardiovascular outcomes from 59% to 77% when added to a clinical risk

Support: Supported by internal funds. None of the authors has a personal financial interest in the topics discussed in this article.

*Corresponding author. Department of General Anesthesiology, E31, The Cleveland Clinic, 9500 Euclid Avenue, Cleveland, OH 44195. E-mail address: abdelmb@ccf.org.

0737-6146/10/$ – see front matter
doi:10.1016/j.aan.2010.08.001

prediction system [7]. The ultimate goal is to use these biomarkers to develop and evaluate therapies intended to improve surgical outcomes.

This article reviews and evaluates current knowledge and available evidence regarding the usefulness of some of the commonly studied infectious, inflammatory, neurologic, cardiac, and renal biomarkers in the perioperative period (Table 1).

CRP

Surgery induces an intense inflammatory response [8]. The release of inflammatory markers has been documented following cardiac surgery [9], and major noncardiac surgeries such as joint replacement, major vascular surgery, and colorectal surgery [10]. The perioperative inflammatory response is believed to contribute to poor perioperative outcomes. For example, 17% of postoperative deaths are attributed to cardiovascular causes [11]. Inflammation has been implicated in the pathophysiology of myocardial infarction; it is associated with the development of arterial plaque, starting with lipid deposition to plaque rupture and the resulting complications. If the underlying mechanism of

Table 1
Clinical perioperative biomarkers

Type	Name	Abbreviation	Source	Measured in
Cardiac	Cardiac troponin I	cTnI	Cardiac myocytes	Blood
	Cardiac troponin T	cTnT	Cardiac myocytes	Blood
	Brain natriuretic peptide	BNP	Cardiac myocytes	Blood
	Amino-terminal pro-Brain natriuretic peptide	NT-proBNP	Cardiac myocytes	Blood
Renal	Cystatin C	Cystatin C	Most nucleated cells	Blood and urine
	Neutrophil gelatinase-associated lipocalin	NGAL	Proximal tubular epithelial cells; also present in neutrophils	Blood and urine
	N-Acetyl-β-glucosaminidase	NAG	Proximal tubular epithelial cells	Blood and urine
	Kidney injury molecule-1	KIM-1	Proximal tubular epithelial cells	Blood and urine
Neurologic	S100β protein	S100β	Glial cells	Blood and CSF
	Neuron-specific enolase	NSE	Neurons	Blood and CSF
Systemic	C-reactive protein	CRP	Liver	Blood
	Procalcitonin	PCT	Thyroid (normal production) Extrathyroid (acute-phase reactant)	Blood

Abbreviation: CSF, cerebrospinal fluid.

perioperative myocardial infarction (PMI) is plaque rupture, then a negative stress test (which indicates that there is no flow-limiting stenosis) may fail to detect a nonobstructing plaque that may potentially rupture and cause cardiac ischemia or infarction [12]. In such circumstances, inflammatory markers such as CRP may more accurately predict perioperative cardiac morbidity and mortality [13]. There are many available markers of inflammation such as tumor necrosis factor (TNF) and the interleukins (IL) IL-2, IL-4. IL-6, IL-8, IL-10, and IL-14; however, this article focuses on CRP.

CRP, an acute-phase reactant produced in the liver, is a well-known marker of systemic inflammation; it greatly increases in response to acute injury. Its stable concentration over a long period of time is governed chiefly by the rate of hepatic production rather than by factors connected with its clearance [14]. CRP assays, being cost-effective, reliable, and fairly sensitive [15–17], seem to meet all criteria for the ideal biomarker. Indeed, the sensitivity of the high sensitivity CRP (hsCRP) assay seems to exceed even that of the original CRP assay.

In nonsurgical settings, CRP functions as a marker of atherosclerosis; when increased, it is considered a biochemical cardiovascular risk factor [18–20].

Cardiac Surgery

In cardiac surgery, postoperative serum concentrations of CRP are associated with the incidence of postoperative arrhythmias [9], and are predictive of septic complications, the need for catecholamine therapy, prolonged respiratory support, and prolonged intensive care unit (ICU) stay [21]. Moreover, Milazzo and colleagues [22] identified preoperative elevated concentrations of CRP as a predictor of recurrent ischemia up to six years postoperatively.

Noncardiac Surgery

The predictive power of CRP seems to be stronger than that of the clinical risk index [7]. Preoperative high levels are associated with short- and long-term morbidity and mortality after noncardiac [7]. Postoperative high levels of this marker are associated with complications after colorectal and bariatric surgeries [23–25].

So far, evidence provides no consensus on what value constitutes an abnormally increased hsCRP or even the range of detectable hsCRP in the general population. Because different studies have not used identical assays, a wide range exists in the values that are believed to constitute an increased level. Assays for hsCRP are new, only appearing commercially in the last decade. Most of the available clinical studies have accepted as normal or increased the values that have been designated as normal or increased by various laboratories, depending on the assay each laboratory used. However, more recent studies with the newer hsCRP assays have redefined a normal CRP level in a healthy individual as approximately ≤ 3 mg/L. Other clinicians might recognize an even lower cutoff (≤ 1 mg/L) as normal. Although the present assays are highly sensitive, these current values may change with future advances in technology and in the criteria governing specific assays [13,26–29].

Interventions that moderate the inflammatory response may reduce adverse outcomes [30]. Clinical studies show that, in some circumstances, a simple antiinflammatory intervention such as corticosteroid administration is associated not only with lower perioperative CRP levels but also with improved clinical outcomes [31,32]. In a randomized trial of 88 patients undergoing laparoscopic cholecystectomy, 8 mg of dexamethasone given 90 minutes before incision correlated with significantly lower CRP levels, significantly reduced postoperative fatigue, less nausea and vomiting, and a faster return to recreational activities [33]. Therefore, interventions targeted to decrease CRP levels, or to prevent their perioperative increase, may be warranted [34].

In conclusion, CRP has been shown to be a valuable marker in predicting poor postoperative outcomes in both cardiac and noncardiac surgery. It may also be promising in the study of various antiinflammatory strategies intended to prevent such poor outcomes, and thereby improve recovery. However, additional investigation is needed to identify what should be accepted as normal or abnormal concentrations in the perioperative period.

BRAIN OR B-TYPE NATRIURETIC PEPTIDE AND NT-ProBNP

Congestive heart failure (CHF) has been shown to be a predictor of PMI following vascular surgery [3,35–37]. It increases the odds of dying from a PMI 12-fold if diagnosed within 12 months of a vascular surgery [1]. Diagnosis of CHF is a clinical challenge. Traditionally, the diagnostic approach begins with a thorough history and physical examination, complemented by chest radiographic examination and echocardiography. However, the history and physical examination can be misleading [38], and chest radiographic examination has its own limitations [39]. Echocardiography can also be misleading, in that 30% to 70% of patients with CHF present with a normal (>50%) or only mildly depressed left ventricular ejection fraction. Diastolic dysfunction may underlie CHF in many of these patients [40]. Most patients with asymptomatic left ventricular dysfunction remain undiagnosed [38]. Brain natriuretic peptide (BNP) and NT-proBNP have emerged as promising biomarkers, as simple and reliable tests that may be useful in establishing the diagnosis of CHF and correlating with its severity [38,41].

BNP is a 32-amino acid polypeptide secreted by cardiomyocytes in response to excessive ventricular or atrial stretching, or during ischemia. NT-proBNP is a 76-amino acid N-terminal fragment that is biologically inactive and is coreleased in the same conditions as BNP [42,43]. Biologically, they are distinguished by a significantly different half-life: NT-ProBNP has a longer half-life, 1 to 2 hours, in contrast with 20 minutes for BNP.

In nonsurgical settings, clinical studies have shown that plasma BNP is a powerful predictor of adverse cardiovascular events in patients with heart failure, acute coronary syndromes, primary pulmonary hypertension, and valvular disease [44–46].

Cardiac Surgery

In cardiothoracic surgery patients, 2 recent clinical studies showed the importance of BNP and NT-proBNP. High levels BNP and NT-proBNP have been associated with the development of atrial fibrillation in patients undergoing cardiac or thoracic oncology surgery [47,48]. Moreover, NT-proBNP may be useful in the assessment of potential donor hearts and in the follow-up of patients undergoing lung transplantation [49,50]. A recent study indicates that plasma BNP levels do not correlate with left ventricular function after cardiac surgery but do correlate with the E/E' ratio, which is an echocardiographic indicator of filling pressures and diastolic function [51].

Noncardiac Surgery

In noncardiac surgery, many investigators have confirmed that either preoperative BNP [52–56] or NT-proBNP [57–60] are helpful in predicting outcomes (Fig. 1). A clear example comes from Breidhardt and colleagues [61], who showed that preoperative increase of BNP predicts major perioperative cardiovascular complications in patients undergoing orthopedic surgery, and that the combination of BNP and the American Society of Anesthesiologists score is superior to BNP alone in predicting in-hospital cardiac events.

In light of these studies, both BNP and NT-proBNP are promising markers for postoperative cardiac outcomes. The current evidence does not support a universal cutoff point for BNP or NT-proBNP levels beyond which poor outcomes are anticipated, because existing studies have used different assays and various statistical methods to obtain their cutoffs; moreover, some did not indicate how they obtained their cutoff [62]. The specified cutoff points have varied between 40 and 189 pg/mL for BNP [52–56] and between 280 and 533 pg/mL for NT-proBNP [57–60]. Additional investigations are needed in order for consensus to be reached on what constitutes increased and predictive levels of both markers. Interventions should be sought that reduce concentrations of these 2 markers, and trials designed to assess the effects of these interventions on surgical outcomes.

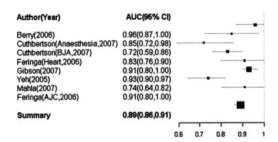

Author(Year)	AUC(95% CI)
Berry(2006)	0.96(0.87,1.00)
Cuthbertson(Anaesthesia,2007)	0.85(0.72,0.98)
Cuthbertson(BJA,2007)	0.72(0.59,0.86)
Feringa(Heart,2006)	0.83(0.76,0.90)
Gibson(2007)	0.91(0.80,1.00)
Yeh(2005)	0.93(0.90,0.97)
Mahla(2007)	0.74(0.64,0.82)
Feringa(AJC,2006)	0.91(0.80,1.00)
Summary	**0.89(0.86,0.91)**

Fig. 1. The area under the curve (95% confidence interval) for each study and overall, evaluating the usefulness of BNP and NT-proBNP in noncardiac surgery. (*From* Karamchandani K, Abdelmalak B, Sun Z, et al. Pre-op BNP as a predictor for post-op cardiac morbidity after noncardiac surgery – a meta-analysis. Anesthesiology 2008:A470; with permission.)

CARDIAC TROPONINS

Troponins are proteins of the contractile system of the cardiac cells that act together through the tropomyosin complex to regulate muscle contraction [63]. Cardiac troponins have become the biomarker of choice for the diagnosis of acute myocardial ischemia and infarction [64]. Cardiac troponin T (cTnT) levels are detectable 3 to 12 hours after myocardial injury, and the concentration is in direct proportion to the extent of myocardial injury [65–67].

Cardiac troponins have also been used in the perioperative period to evaluate myocardial ischemia and infarction. Early studies considered them the best tool for diagnosing PMI in patients having noncardiac and cardiac surgery. Several investigators have shown that increased preoperative and postoperative levels of cTnI are associated with poor postoperative clinical outcomes [68]. However, at present, no single cutoff value has been recommended for use in the diagnosis of PMI. Moreover, cTnI may increase even before aortic cross-clamping and cardiac manipulation [69]. Martin and colleagues [70] suggested that cTnI levels lower than 0.15 µg/L were not associated with myocardial ischemia in the perioperative period of cardiac surgery. In contrast, cTnI levels higher than 0.15 µg/L were a strong indicator of ischemic damage.

Thielmann and colleagues [71] showed that preoperative cTnI levels higher than 1.15 ng/mL were associated with longer ICU stay and with higher in-hospital mortality. Moreover, levels of 0.15 ng/mL or higher were associated with higher morbidity and mortality 6 months after surgery [72]. In a study conducted by Lehrke and colleagues [73], cTnT measurement 48 hours after surgery was a strong predictor of severe cardiac failure and high postoperative mortality. A cTnT value exceeding 0.46 µg/L 48 hours after surgery carried a 6.7-fold risk of cardiac death.

Cardiac troponins have also been used to identify clinical outcomes in patients undergoing major vascular surgery [74]. Early studies by Lee and colleagues [75] and Meltzer and colleagues [76] suggested an association between increased levels of cTn and postoperative outcomes. More recently, Landesberg and colleagues [77] showed that levels of cTnI greater than 0.6 ng/mL and cTnT greater than 0.03 ng/mL were independently associated with a respectively 2.15-fold and 1.89-fold increase in mortality. The investigators of the Coronary Artery Revascularization Prophylaxis (CARP) trial used cTnI to define PMI. They found that cTnI levels of 0.1 µg/L or higher occurred in 27% of patients undergoing elective vascular surgery and that these levels were a strong predictor of long-term risk of death among patients with diabetes [78]. Preoperative concentrations of cTnI were predictive of postoperative cardiac outcomes in major noncardiac surgery patients and their predictive power was mildly improved by adding preoperative BNP concentration into the model (Fig. 2).

In agreement with these last 2 studies, Filipovic and colleagues [79] found an association between cTnI levels and all-cause mortality 1 year after major noncardiac surgery, but a subsequent study by the same group of investigators could not show this association [80]. Controversies surround the validity of

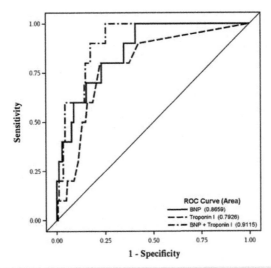

Fig. 2. The predictive value of preoperative BNP, troponin I, individually and combined for postoperative cardiac outcomes in patients having major noncardiac surgery. (*From* Abdelmalak B, You J, Tang W, et al. Combining pre-operative BNP and cTnI in predicting cardiac outcomes from major non-cardiac surgery. Anesthesiology 2009:A1229; with permission.)

cTnT in patients with impaired renal function. However, Feringa and colleagues [81] showed that, after adjustment for estimate of the glomerular filtration rate, minor increases in troponin T from 0.03 to 0.09 ng/mL were strongly associated with late mortality and major adverse cardiac events after major vascular surgery.

In summary, cTn assays are important diagnostic tools in the perioperative period. The most recently developed assays are much more sensitive than the older generations; however, what their absolute cutoff values should be as markers for myocardial infarction remains unclear, because very low levels of cTn may represent increased permeability of myocytes resulting from inflammation.

PROCALCITONIN

Procalcitonin (PCT) is a 116-amino acid peptide produced by the c-cells in the thyroid. Its concentration in the serum of healthy individuals is low (<0.1 ng/mL); however, it may be considered an acute-phase reactant because of its production and release during inflammatory stress [63,82]. Traditionally identified as a marker for infectious conditions, PCT at increased levels has been shown more recently to be associated with noninfectious processes such as trauma, surgery, cardiogenic shock, burns, heat stroke, acute respiratory distress syndrome, and rejection after transplantation [83–87]. In these conditions it is produced outside the thyroid by the liver and circulating mononuclear cells.

Cardiac Surgery

Procalcitonin has been investigated in the context of cardiac surgery. It is not clear whether the type of cardiac surgery influences the surge of PCT after surgery. Prat and colleagues [88] could not identify differences in PCT levels between patients undergoing coronary artery bypass graft (CABG) and open heart valvular surgery. In contrast, Sponholz and colleagues [89] and Franke and colleagues [90] reported that valvular surgery induces larger increments of PCT levels than on-pump CABG, and this in turn induces larger increases than off-pump CABG.

Procalcitonin seems to be predictive of poor outcomes after cardiac surgery. An early study by Loebe and colleagues [91] showed that an increased PCT level, higher than 1 ng/mL, after cardiac surgery was predictive of poor postoperative outcomes. Two recent studies showed that procalcitonin significantly increased in patients who underwent cardiac surgery and subsequently developed infectious and noninfectious complications, compared with patients who did not experience complications [88,92]. Procalcitonin proved more accurate than CRP in predicting those complications [92]. In heart transplantation, PCT is also a reliable marker in the diagnosis and monitoring of postoperative infections [93,94]. Moreover, PCT levels were not affected by the use of immunosuppressants [94,95].

Noncardiac Surgery

Schneider and colleagues [96] retrospectively analyzed the association of PCT concentration with postoperative mortality, morbidity, and length of stay in 220 patients who were admitted after surgery to an ICU. The researchers found a significant and logarithmic association between PCT concentration and outcome. Moreover, PCT was an independent predictor of mortality and duration of hospital stay after surgery in the survivors. In patients undergoing oncologic surgery, PCT seems to be a more useful marker than CRP for monitoring the postoperative course and diagnosing severe bacterial infections [97,98]. Procalcitonin is also superior to high sensitivity CRP (hsCRP) as an independent predictor of graft failure in renal transplantation [99]. However, Mommertz and colleagues [100] found no association between perioperative neurologic deficit and PCT in patients who had carotid endarterectomy.

In summary, PCT is being intensively investigated as a biomarker. Although there is a paucity of large randomized controlled trials, current evidence suggests that PCT may be useful in predicting complications after cardiac surgery. Additional studies are needed to establish the role of PCT in patients undergoing noncardiac surgery.

BIOMARKERS OF KIDNEY DYSFUNCTION

Acute kidney injury (AKI) remains a common postoperative complication. The incidence of dialysis-dependent acute renal failure after cardiac surgery is approximately 1%, and approximately half of these patients die from this complication [101–103]. Early detection of AKI in the perioperative period may permit early renoprotective interventions, which may in turn translate into more favorable postoperative outcomes; thus, simple and specific biomarkers would be useful to monitor AKI.

Cystatin C

Cystatin C is a 13-kDa endogenous cysteine proteinase inhibitor that is synthesized at a constant rate and released into the plasma by all nucleated cells in the body. It is freely filtered at the glomerulus, not secreted or reabsorbed, and nearly completely catabolized by proximal renal tubular cells. Cystatin C can be measured in plasma and urine [104]. Cystatin C has a lower variability of measurements, a shorter half-life, and a lower distribution volume than creatinine [105]. Because of these properties, it has been suggested that it may be more sensitive than creatinine to early and mild changes in kidney function [106–108]. However, factors such as age, gender, and body mass index may still affect the serum levels of this protein [104,109,110]. A recent study by Villa and colleagues [111] showed that cystatin C correlated better with glomerular filtration rate than creatinine in patients in ICUs with mild kidney dysfunction. Moreover, a meta-analysis conducted by Dharnidharka and colleagues [106] indicated that the serum cystatin C concentration was a more sensitive indicator of renal dysfunction than serum creatinine.

Cardiac surgery

Several investigators have studied the clinical value of cystatin C in identifying patients with, or at risk for, renal dysfunction after cardiac surgery [112,113]. In a cohort study of 110 elderly patients having cardiac surgery requiring cardiopulmonary bypass, serum cystatin C could not detect mild renal injury earlier than plasma creatinine [114]. Similar results were reported by Liangos and colleagues [115], who found that cystatin C levels 2 hours after cardiopulmonary bypass could not predict AKI. However, these results are disputed by a recent study demonstrating that serum cystatin C predicted AKI about 2 days earlier than clinically significant increases in creatinine [116]. Increased levels of urinary cystatin C have also been associated with early detection of kidney dysfunction after cardiac surgery [117]. In a prospective study of 376 patients, Ledoux and colleagues [113] found that preoperative estimation of renal function from serum cystatin C was strongly associated with hospital morbidity and mortality.

Noncardiac surgery

In contrast with cardiac surgery, cystatin C seems to correlate better with kidney dysfunction in the setting of noncardiac surgery. Lebkowska and colleagues [118] showed that patients with delayed graft function after cadaveric renal transplantation showed significantly higher levels of cystatin C than those with normal graft function. Cystatin C correlated with perioperative levels of neutrophil gelatinase–associated lipocalin (NGAL) and creatinine. Moreover, cystatin C has also been used to detect early kidney dysfunction in living-related donor kidney transplantation. Gourishankar and colleagues [119] found that cystatin C correlated with all other markers of kidney function and detected acute changes in kidney function immediately after donor nephrectomy.

Cystatin C has been used clinically to monitor the perioperative effect of nephrotoxic agents such as cyclooxygenase inhibitors or the effect of a variety of perioperative interventions on kidney function. In a randomized, controlled, double-blinded trial, Puolakka and colleagues [120] found that cystatin C levels were not affected by the administration of parecoxib in patients undergoing laparoscopic hysterectomy, and accordingly the researchers suggested that 80 mg of this analgesic was not associated with perioperative kidney dysfunction. Cystatin C has also been used to evaluate the effects of perioperative fluid optimization in patients undergoing surgery [121]. Boldt and colleagues [122] assessed the effect of different kinds of colloid therapy (albumin vs hydroxyethylstarch) on patients undergoing cardiac surgery and found that differences in the increase of cystatin C after surgery did not reach statistical significance between the 2 groups being studied.

Cystatin C has also been used to investigate the effects of sevoflurane on kidney function. Laisalmi and colleagues [123] showed in a double-blinded controlled study that cystatin C levels did not differ in healthy women undergoing breast surgery who received ketorolac during high fresh gas flow of sevoflurane anesthesia. They concluded that, in healthy women, the use of ketorolac is not associated with kidney injury in patients having general anesthesia with sevoflurane.

In conclusion, the role of cystatin C in detecting renal impairment after cardiac surgery is not well established. However, in renal transplantation and other noncardiac surgeries, cystatin C may have more reliable predictive value.

Neutrophil Gelatinase-associated Lipocalin

NGAL, a 25-kDa protein that belongs to the superfamily of lipocalins, has been measured in plasma and urine. NGAL binds to 2 receptors, the megalin multi-scavenger complex and the 24p3 receptors. It has been suggested that NGAL also acts as an acute-phase reactant that is increased not only during the infective process but also during noninfective systemic diseases. The kidney can release NGAL in response to damage or stress, and thus serum or urinary NGAL can be used to detect AKI [124,125]. It has also been suggested that serum and urinary NGAL may be useful in distinguishing between septic and nonseptic AKI. Bagshaw and colleagues [126] found that septic kidney injury was associated with higher initial and peak values of urinary and serum NGAL than nonseptic kidney dysfunction. Several investigators have also studied the predictive value of NGAL in the perioperative setting, as discussed later [127–130].

Cardiac surgery

Urinary and serum levels of NGAL were increased in patients with postoperative kidney injury after cardiac surgery [131,132]. In addition, a study by Che and colleagues [133] found that urinary NGAL was highly predictive of kidney dysfunction. Its predictive value was higher than that of other markers such as cystatin C, urinary interleukin 18, serum creatinine and N-acetyl-β-D-glucosaminidase. These results were partially replicated by McIlroy and colleagues [134], who observed that urinary NGAL detected AKI only in patients with a preoperative estimated glomerular filtration rates of 90 to 120 mL/min.

Noncardiac surgery
Serum NGAL has been tested in liver transplantation. Intraoperative increases of NGAL were significantly associated with postoperative acute kidney dysfunction. Moreover, the difference between intraoperative and preoperative levels was also predictive of renal dysfunction. This delta value is particularly important because proper intraoperative interventions targeted to reduce or prevent increases of NGAL may mitigate or prevent postoperative kidney injury [135].

Several researchers have investigated the predictive value of NGAL in patients undergoing renal transplantation. They found that NGAL performs better than serum creatinine in detecting graft dysfunction [136–138].

In conclusion, NGAL seems to have a reasonable predictive value for postoperative renal failure. However, additional studies are needed before it can be recommended for routine use.

N-Acetyl-β-Glucosaminidase

N-Acetyl-β-glucosaminidase (NAG), a proximal tubular epithelial cell glycosidase of 130 kDa, is normally excreted in low amounts in urine [139]. Early clinical studies showed that NAG is increased after kidney injury and can predict acute renal dysfunction in critically ill patients [140–142].

Cardiac surgery
In a small pilot study, Backlund and colleagues [143] showed that the urinary NAG/creatinine ratio increased during aortic operations. The researchers observed that the NAG/creatinine ratio increased soon after the induction of anesthesia and before the aortic cross-clamp. It was argued that early intraoperative increases in NAG might be related to hypotension or administration of nephrotoxic drugs such as antibiotics [144]. Also, increased NAG levels were found in patients with low intraoperative hematocrit who received blood transfusion during cardiac surgery [145]. In an early clinical study of 36 patients, a positive correlation was found between serum creatinine levels and urinary excretion of NAG after cardiac surgery [146]. However, Gormley and colleagues [147] found that, although NAG concentration increased in patients undergoing cardiac surgery, it did not adequately predict postoperative AKI [115,148].

Noncardiac surgery
NAG has been extensively used to assess volatile anesthesia-induced nephropathy. For instance, an early study investigated the comparative effects of 2 hours of hypotensive anesthesia with sevoflurane or isoflurane under 5 L/min total gas flow in patients having no preoperative renal dysfunction. Patients who received sevoflurane showed a transient increase of the NAG index; the researchers

therefore concluded that sevoflurane in hypotensive patients caused a temporary, reversible disturbance of renal tubular function [149]. Kanbak and colleagues [150] investigated the effect of sevoflurane on kidney dysfunction in patients undergoing liver transplantation and showed that NAG increased during the intraoperative period, with a peak level occurring during the anhepatic phase. The researchers concluded that increased NAG concentrations did not correlate with blood urea nitrogen and creatinine levels. In a double-blinded, placebo-controlled study, NAG was used as a biomarker to detect renal injury in patients who received ketorolac for mastectomy surgery performed under sevoflurane-based anesthesia. The investigators could not show significant differences in NAG levels in patients who received or did not receive ketorolac [151].

NAG has also been used to assess the effect of perioperative renoprotective interventions. For instance, a prospective randomized, double-blind study investigated the effects of N-acetylcysteine infusion in patients undergoing abdominal aortic repair. The researchers found that N-acetylcysteine does not decrease renal injury as assessed by an increase in the urinary NAG/creatinine ratio [144]. NAG was also measured in a randomized controlled trial that ascertained whether the administration of N-acetylcysteine prevented AKI in 30 patients undergoing knee arthroplasty. Similar to the study discussed earlier, NAG increased in the perioperative period and the infusion of N-acetylcysteine did not prevent AKI [152]. NAG was one of the biomarkers used by Izumi and colleagues [153] to assess the efficacy of human atrial natriuretic peptide in patients with renal dysfunction undergoing cardiac surgery. The researchers found that the administration of human atrial natriuretic peptide prevented the increase of NAG associated with surgery and improved creatinine clearance.

In summary, NAG has been one of the most extensively studied biomarkers of AKI in the perioperative context. A postoperative increase of NAG is an indicator of AKI, but its long-term predictive value for renal failure is controversial.

Kidney Injury Molecule-1

During kidney injury, the kidney injury molecule-1 (KIM-1) glycoprotein is shed from cells into the urine. Ninety percent of KIM-1 expression in the human kidney occurs in the proximal tubule system, which might explain why KIM-1 seems to be specific to ischemic acute tubular necrosis (ATN) [154]. In patients with established acute renal failure, urinary KIM-1 levels are useful in assessing its severity, and have a prognostic value [155]. Han and colleagues [156] showed that patients with acute ischemic ATN had significantly higher levels of KIM-1 than patients with other forms of kidney dysfunction.

Cardiac surgery

In patients undergoing cardiac surgery, KIM-1 was increased before an increase in serum creatinine was detected [130]. Moreover, KIM-1 was a better biomarker than urinary NAG, NGAL, and IL-18 for predicting AKI in a cohort of 103 patients who underwent cardiac surgery [115].

Noncardiac surgery
The expression of KIM-1 has been assessed in cadaveric-donor and living-donor kidneys. The levels of expression of KIM-1 were significantly higher in cadaveric-donor kidneys than in living-donor kidneys [157]. In 2007, van Timmeren and colleagues [158] reported that high KIM-1 excretion was a predictor of graft loss. This predictive value was independent of donor age, creatinine clearance, and proteinuria, and was associated with hazard ratios of a magnitude similar to those of proteinuria. However, a later study by Hall and colleagues [136] found that KIM-1 was not a predictor of graft dysfunction in 98 patients who underwent cadaveric-donor kidney transplant. In summary, KIM-1 is an attractive biomarker of AKI but, because of the small number of clinical trials, its real predictive value in the perioperative context is unclear.

BIOMARKERS FOR NEUROLOGIC INJURY
The ideal biochemical serum marker of central nervous system injury would be highly specific and sensitive for the brain and/or spinal cord, would be released only after damage of central nervous tissue, and would rapidly cross the blood-brain barrier into the blood stream. Thus early detection of the marker would allow clinicians to initiate neuroprotective measures before irreversible damage occurs.

S100b Protein
The S100b protein is a low molecular weight glial protein of approximately 10 kDa that belongs to a multigenic family of calcium-mediated proteins (S100 proteins) [159]. S100b is currently labeled as a marker of generalized blood-brain barrier dysfunction that is released into the cerebrospinal fluid (CSF) after neuronal injury [160]. S100b has a half-life of 25 minutes [161]. Increased S100b is observed after infarction and after traumatic and toxic injury of the central nervous system [162–165]. However, S100b measurements differ depending on the assay used for its detection. Thus, researchers have suggested the need for international standardization among methods to measure S100b, to facilitate effective assessment of the predictive validity of this biomarker in clinical practice [166].

Cardiac surgery
Several clinical studies have shown that the S100b protein increased in patients undergoing cardiac surgery using cardiopulmonary bypass [167–169]. Serum S100b levels seem to be influenced by the age and gender of patients, by the use of cardiotomy suction or cell saver, and on-pump versus off-pump cardiac surgery, all of which might explain the varying and, in some instances, contradictory results of different trials [170,171]. Also, genetic factors may influence serum concentrations of S100b. Kofke and colleagues [172] showed that S100b levels were higher in ApoE4 carriers than in ApoE2 and ApoE3. Kilminster and colleagues [173] showed that S100b protein release during and after cardiopulmonary bypass

correlated positively with both age of patient and duration of extracorporeal perfusion. However, the relationship between S100b levels and neurologic/neuropsychological outcomes remains controversial [174]. In a small cohort study, serum levels of S100b protein higher than 0.3 μg/L were more commonly observed in patients who had postoperative sleep disturbances after cardiac surgery [175]. The timing of S100b sampling may be important if this biomarker is used to predict outcomes. Georgiadis and colleagues [176] showed that S100b levels 24 hours after the operation had a sensitivity and specificity of approximately 90% in identifying patients with postoperative cerebral lesions.

Noncardiac surgery
Serum levels of S100b have also been studied in the perioperative period of noncardiac surgery [177,178]. In patients with chronic cervical myelopathy who underwent uncomplicated spine surgery, S100b did not predict functional outcomes; however, in patients with a complicated postoperative course, S100b had prognostic significance [179]. The same group of researchers investigated the predictive value of S100b in patients with intradural spine lesions. The postoperative time course of serum S100b did not correlate with functional outcomes [180]. Cerebrospinal levels of S100b were measured by Winnerkvist and colleagues [178] to identify patients at risk of neurologic complications in the perioperative period of surgery for thoracoabdominal aneurysm. The researchers found that patients who developed neurologic complications had significantly higher levels of S100b; however, the concentrations of this biomarker began to increase after the onset of clinical symptoms. In a small study in patients undergoing major vascular surgery, the serum concentration of S100b increased during the perioperative period, but the cerebrospinal levels remained low in some patients. The researchers argued that, in the absence of central nervous injury, surgical trauma itself may be responsible for the observed serum S100b increments [181,182].

Several studies have investigated the predictive value of S100b in the context of carotid endarterectomy (CEA), but the results remain controversial. In a cohort of 43 patients, intraoperative serum concentrations of S100b increased during catorid endarterectomy; however, these increased concentrations failed to predict cognitive outcome [183]. S100b did not significantly increase in patients undergoing CEA under local anesthesia [184]. Wijeyaratne and colleagues [185] also found no significant differences in S100b levels between patients who underwent CEA under either general or local anesthesia.

In conclusion, S100b has been extensively studied in the perioperative context and seems to be a sensitive marker of brain barrier dysfunction, but the lack of a large clinical trial and the uncertainty about the correct timing for sampling make its recommendation as a long-term predictor of neurologic outcomes improbable.

Neuron-specific Enolase
Neuron-specific enolase (NSE), located in neurons and neuroendocrine cells, is a neuronal form of the cytoplasmic glycolytic enzyme enolase. It has

a molecular weight of 78 kDa and a dimeric structure composed of two γ subunits [186,187].

Cardiac surgery

In patients undergoing cardiac surgery, Ramlawi and colleagues [170] were able to show a significant association between postoperative neurocognitive dysfunction and NSE. However, no relationship between NSE concentrations and perioperative diffusion-weighted imaging lesions on magnetic resonance scanning was found in patients who had aortic valve replacement [169]. In a small cohort of patients, those who had the ApoE4 allele showed significantly higher postoperative levels of NSE than those with ApoE2 and ApoE3 [172]. Carriers of ApoE4 had an increased likelihood of developing Alzheimer disease [188]. Therefore, it is possible that genetic susceptibility explains increased levels of some biomarkers and postoperative cognitive dysfunction after cardiac surgery.

Noncardiac surgery

Lases and colleagues [182] investigated the predictive value of NSE in patients undergoing aortic aneurysm repair. The researchers concluded that neither NSE nor S100b added useful clinical information to that gleaned from the motor-evoked potential monitoring during surgery. In patients undergoing orthotopic liver transplantation, postreperfusion levels of NSE correlated highly with decreased regional cerebral oxygen saturation levels; however, the investigators did not assess neurologic outcomes [189].

NSE has been the focus of research in patients undergoing carotid endarterectomy (CEA). It increases during and after CEA, but its serum levels seem to depend on the anesthetic technique used during surgery [185]. In a study by Sahlein and colleagues [183], NSE failed to predict cognitive dysfunction in patients undergoing CEA. NSE was also used to assess neurologic damage in a randomized controlled trial that compared CEA with carotid artery stenting (CAS). The researchers found that NSE levels were significantly higher in the CAS group of patients than in those who underwent CEA [190].

In summary, NSE increases after the perioperative neurologic insult of cardiac or noncardiac surgery; however, its long-term predictive value remains uncertain.

SUMMARY

Biomarkers have attracted the attention of clinicians and investigators as a means of stratifying risk in surgical patients because of their simple, minimally invasive nature and their potentially high yield in improving risk stratification. Existing biomarkers, and those currently being developed and studied, may lead to improved clinical practices, with earlier detection of organ injury prompting more timely intervention to improve surgical outcomes. This article reviews and evaluates current knowledge and available evidence regarding the usefulness of commonly studied infectious, inflammatory, neurologic, cardiac, and renal biomarkers in the perioperative period.

The inflammatory marker CRP has been shown to be a valuable marker in predicting poor postoperative outcomes in both cardiac and noncardiac surgery. It is also promising in the study of various antiinflammatory strategies intended to prevent such poor outcomes and thereby improve recovery.

However, additional investigation is needed to identify what should be accepted as normal or abnormal concentrations in the perioperative period.

Among cardiac markers; both BNP and NT-proBNP are promising markers for postoperative cardiac outcomes. However, additional investigations are needed for consensus to be reached on what constitutes an unsafe level of both markers, and we encourage investigations of measures to decrease concentrations of these 2 markers, and to assess the effects of these interventions on surgical outcomes. Also, cTn assays are important diagnostic tools in the perioperative period of cardiac and noncardiac surgery. The most recently developed assays are much sensitive than older versions, but definition of specific values that serve as markers for myocardial infarction remain unclear.

The infectious marker PCT is a biomarker being intensively investigated. Current evidence suggests that PCT may be useful in predicting complications after cardiac surgery, but additional studies are needed to establish the value of measuring PCT in patients undergoing noncardiac surgery.

Among renal function/outcomes markers, the role of cystatin C in detecting renal impairment after cardiac surgery is not well established. However, in renal transplantation, cystatin C may have more predictive value. NGAL seems to have a reasonable predictive value for postoperative renal failure. However, additional studies are needed before it can be recommended for routine use. NAG has been one of the most extensively studied biomarkers of perioperative AKI. A postoperative increase of NAG is an indicator of AKI, but its long-term predictive value for renal failure is not established. KIM-1 is an attractive biomarker of AKI but, because of the small number of clinical trials to date, its predictive value in the perioperative period is still unclear.

The neurologic marker S100b has been extensively studied in the perioperative period and is a sensitive marker of brain barrier dysfunction. Lack of evidence from any large clinical trials, and uncertainty about proper sampling protocols, make its recommendation as a long-term predictor of neurologic outcomes improbable at this time. NSE increases with perioperative neurologic insult following cardiac or noncardiac surgery, but any long-term predictive value is unproven.

References

[1] Sprung J, Abdelmalak B, Gottlieb A, et al. Analysis of risk factors for myocardial infarction and cardiac mortality after major vascular surgery. Anesthesiology 2000;93:129–40.

[2] Mangano DT, Browner WS, Hollenberg M, et al. Long-term cardiac prognosis following noncardiac surgery. The Study of Perioperative Ischemia Research Group. JAMA 1992;268:233–9.

[3] Lee TH, Marcantonio ER, Mangione CM, et al. Derivation and prospective validation of a simple index for prediction of cardiac risk of major noncardiac surgery. Circulation 1999;100:1043–9.

[4] Fleisher LA, Beckman JA, Brown KA, et al. ACC/AHA 2007 Guidelines on Perioperative Cardiovascular Evaluation and Care for Noncardiac Surgery: Executive Summary: A Report of the American College of Cardiology/American Heart Association Task Force on Practice Guidelines (Writing Committee to Revise the 2002 Guidelines on Perioperative Cardiovascular Evaluation for Noncardiac Surgery): developed in collaboration with the American Society of Echocardiography, American Society of Nuclear Cardiology, Heart Rhythm Society, Society of Cardiovascular Anesthesiologists, Society for Cardiovascular Angiography and Interventions, Society for Vascular Medicine and Biology, and Society for Vascular Surgery. Circulation 2007;116:1971–96.

[5] Kuller LH, Tracy RP, Shaten J, et al. Relation of C-reactive protein and coronary heart disease in the MRFIT nested case-control study. Multiple Risk Factor Intervention Trial. Am J Epidemiol 1996;144:537–47.

[6] Ridker PM, Buring JE, Shih J, et al. Prospective study of C-reactive protein and the risk of future cardiovascular events among apparently healthy women. Circulation 1998;98:731–3.

[7] Choi JH, Cho DK, Song YB, et al. Preoperative NT-proBNP and CRP predict perioperative major cardiovascular events in non-cardiac surgery. Heart 2010;96:56–62.

[8] Rassias AJ, Procopio MA. Stress response and optimization of perioperative care. Dis Mon 2003;49:522–54.

[9] Laffey JG, Boylan JF, Cheng DC. The systemic inflammatory response to cardiac surgery: implications for the anesthesiologist. Anesthesiology 2002;97:215–52.

[10] Desborough JP. The stress response to trauma and surgery. Br J Anaesth 2000;85:109–17.

[11] Monk TG, Saini V, Weldon BC, et al. Anesthetic management and one-year mortality after noncardiac surgery. Anesth Analg 2005;100:4–10.

[12] Brennan ML, Penn MS, Van Lente F, et al. Prognostic value of myeloperoxidase in patients with chest pain. N Engl J Med 2003;349:1595–604.

[13] Rossi E, Biasucci LM, Citterio F, et al. Risk of myocardial infarction and angina in patients with severe peripheral vascular disease: predictive role of C-reactive protein. Circulation 2002;105:800–3.

[14] Pepys MB, Baltz ML. Acute phase proteins with special reference to C-reactive protein and related proteins (pentaxins) and serum amyloid A protein. Adv Immunol 1983;34:141–212.

[15] Ledue TB, Weiner DL, Sipe JD, et al. Analytical evaluation of particle-enhanced immunonephelometric assays for C-reactive protein, serum amyloid A and mannose-binding protein in human serum. Ann Clin Biochem 1998;35(Pt 6):745–53.

[16] Tracy RP. Inflammation in cardiovascular disease: cart, horse, or both? Circulation 1998;97:2000–2.

[17] Wilkins J, Gallimore JR, Moore EG, et al. Rapid automated high sensitivity enzyme immunoassay of C-reactive protein. Clin Chem 1998;44:1358–61.

[18] Rifai N, Joubran R, Yu H, et al. Inflammatory markers in men with angiographically documented coronary heart disease. Clin Chem 1999;45:1967–73.

[19] Ridker PM, Cushman M, Stampfer MJ, et al. Inflammation, aspirin, and the risk of cardiovascular disease in apparently healthy men. N Engl J Med 1997;336:973–9.

[20] Kuller LH, Tracy RP, Shaten J, et al. Relation of C-reactive protein and coronary heart disease in the MRFIT nested case-control study. Multiple Risk Factor Intervention Trial. Am J Epidemiol 1996;144:537–47.

[21] Boeken U, Feindt P, Zimmermann N, et al. Increased preoperative C-reactive protein (CRP)-values without signs of an infection and complicated course after cardiopulmonary bypass (CPB)-operations. Eur J Cardiothorac Surg 1998;13:541–5.

[22] Milazzo D, Biasucci LM, Luciani N, et al. Elevated levels of C-reactive protein before coronary artery bypass grafting predict recurrence of ischemic events. Am J Cardiol 1999;84:459–61, A9.

[23] Woeste G, Muller C, Bechstein WO, et al. Increased serum levels of C-reactive protein precede anastomotic leakage in colorectal surgery. World J Surg 2010;34:140–6.

[24] Mackay GJ, Molloy RG, O'Dwyer PJ. C-reactive protein as a predictor of postoperative infective complications following elective colorectal resection. Colorectal Dis 2010 Feb 15. [E-pub ahead of print].

[25] Woodard GA, Peraza J, Bravo S, et al. One year improvements in cardiovascular risk factors: a comparative trial of laparoscopic Roux-en-Y gastric bypass vs. adjustable gastric banding. Obes Surg 2010;20:578–82.

[26] Ackland GL, Scollay JM, Parks RW, et al. Pre-operative high sensitivity C-reactive protein and postoperative outcome in patients undergoing elective orthopaedic surgery. Anaesthesia 2007;62:888–94.

[27] Amar D, Zhang H, Park B, et al. Inflammation and outcome after general thoracic surgery. Eur J Cardiothorac Surg 2007;32:431–4.

[28] Owens CD, Ridker PM, Belkin M, et al. Elevated C-reactive protein levels are associated with postoperative events in patients undergoing lower extremity vein bypass surgery. J Vasc Surg 2007;45:2–9 [discussion: 9].

[29] Nagaoka S, Yoshida T, Akiyoshi J, et al. C-reactive protein levels predict survival in hepatocellular carcinoma. Liver Int 2007;27:1091–7.

[30] Ridker PM, Morrow DA. C-reactive protein, inflammation, and coronary risk. Cardiol Clin 2003;21:315–25.

[31] Nagelschmidt M, Fu ZX, Saad S, et al. Perioperative high dose methylprednisolone improves patients outcome after abdominal surgery. Eur J Surg 1999;165:971–8.

[32] Komori KIM, Matsumoto T, Kume M, et al. Cytokine patterns and the effects of a preoperative steroid treatment in the patients with abdominal aortic aneurysms. Int Angiol 1999;18: 193–7.

[33] Bisgaard T, Klarskov B, Kehlet H, et al. Preoperative dexamethasone improves surgical outcome after laparoscopic cholecystectomy: a randomized double-blind placebo-controlled trial. Ann Surg 2003;238:651–60.

[34] Abdelmalak B, Maheshwari A, Mascha E, et al. Design and organization of the Dexamethasone, Light Anesthesia and Tight Glucose Control (DeLiT) Trial: a factorial trial evaluating the effects of corticosteroids, glucose control, and depth-of-anesthesia on perioperative inflammation and morbidity from major non-cardiac surgery. BMC Anesthesiol 2010;10:11.

[35] Reilly D, McNeely M, Doerner D, et al. Self-reported exercise tolerance and the risk of serious perioperative complications. Arch Intern Med 1999;159:2185–92.

[36] Aziz I, Lee J, Kopchok G, et al. Cardiac risk stratification in patients undergoing endoluminal graft repair of abdominal aortic aneurysm: a single-institution experience with 365 patients. J Vasc Surg 2003;38:56–60.

[37] Liu L, Leung J. Predicting adverse postoperative outcomes in patients aged 80 years or older. J Am Geriatr Soc 2000;48:405–12.

[38] Mair J, Friedl W, Thomas S, et al. Natriuretic peptides in assessment of left-ventricular dysfunction. Scand J Clin Lab Invest Suppl 1999;230:132–42.

[39] Chakko S, Woska D, Martinez H, et al. Clinical, radiographic, and hemodynamic correlations in chronic congestive heart failure: conflicting results may lead to inappropriate care. Am J Med 1991;90:353–9.

[40] Tarantini L, Faggiano P, Cioffi G, et al. [Diastolic heart failure: a disease in search of his own identity]. Monaldi Arch Chest Dis 2003;60:79–84 [in Italian].

[41] Qi W, Mathisen P, Kjekshus J, et al. Natriuretic peptides in patients with aortic stenosis. Am Heart J 2001;142:725–32.

[42] Levin ER, Gardner DG, Samson WK. Natriuretic peptides. N Engl J Med 1998;339: 321–8.

[43] Goetze JP, Christoffersen C, Perko M, et al. Increased cardiac BNP expression associated with myocardial ischemia. FASEB J 2003;17:1105–7.

[44] Bettencourt P, Azevedo A, Pimenta J, et al. N-terminal-pro-brain natriuretic peptide predicts outcome after hospital discharge in heart failure patients. Circulation 2004;110:2168–74.

[45] de Lemos JA, Morrow DA, Bentley JH, et al. The prognostic value of B-type natriuretic peptide in patients with acute coronary syndromes. N Engl J Med 2001;345:1014–21.

[46] Tsunoda Y, Sakahira K, Nakano S, et al. Antagonism of acupuncture analgesia by naloxone in unconscious man. Bull Tokyo Med Dent Univ 1980;27:89–94.

[47] Wazni OM, Martin DO, Marrouche NF, et al. Plasma B-type natriuretic peptide levels predict postoperative atrial fibrillation in patients undergoing cardiac surgery. Circulation 2004;110:124–7.

[48] Cardinale D, Colombo A, Sandri MT, et al. Increased perioperative N-terminal pro-B-type natriuretic peptide levels predict atrial fibrillation after thoracic surgery for lung cancer. Circulation 2007;115:1339–44.

[49] Dronavalli VB, Ranasinghe AM, Venkateswaran RJ, et al. N-terminal pro-brain-type natriuretic peptide: a biochemical surrogate of cardiac function in the potential heart donor. Eur J Cardiothorac Surg 2010;38:181–6.

[50] Leon I, Vicente R, Moreno I, et al. Plasma levels of N terminal pro-brain natriuretic peptide as a prognostic value in primary graft dysfunction and a predictor of mortality in the immediate postoperative period of lung transplantation. Transplant Proc 2009;41:2216–7.

[51] Salustri A, Cerquetani E, Piccoli M, et al. Relationship between B-type natriuretic peptide levels and echocardiographic indices of left ventricular filling pressures in post-cardiac surgery patients. Cardiovasc Ultrasound 2009;7:49.

[52] Cuthbertson BH, Card G, Croal BL, et al. The utility of B-type natriuretic peptide in predicting postoperative cardiac events and mortality in patients undergoing major emergency non-cardiac surgery. Anaesthesia 2007;62:875–81.

[53] Cuthbertson BH, Amiri AR, Croal BL, et al. Utility of B-type natriuretic peptide in predicting perioperative cardiac events in patients undergoing major non-cardiac surgery. Br J Anaesth 2007;99:170–6.

[54] Berry C, Kingsmore D, Gibson S, et al. Predictive value of plasma brain natriuretic peptide for cardiac outcome after vascular surgery. Heart 2006;92:401–2.

[55] Gibson SC, Payne CJ, Byrne DS, et al. B-type natriuretic peptide predicts cardiac morbidity and mortality after major surgery. Br J Surg 2007;94:903–9.

[56] Dernellis J, Panaretou M. Assessment of cardiac risk before non-cardiac surgery: brain natriuretic peptide in 1590 patients. Heart 2006;92:1645–50.

[57] Mahla E, Baumann A, Rehak P, et al. N-terminal pro-brain natriuretic peptide identifies patients at high risk for adverse cardiac outcome after vascular surgery. Anesthesiology 2007;106:1088–95.

[58] Feringa HH, Bax JJ, Elhendy A, et al. Association of plasma N-terminal pro-B-type natriuretic peptide with postoperative cardiac events in patients undergoing surgery for abdominal aortic aneurysm or leg bypass. Am J Cardiol 2006;98:111–5.

[59] Feringa HH, Schouten O, Dunkelgrun M, et al. Plasma N-terminal pro-B-type natriuretic peptide as long-term prognostic marker after major vascular surgery. Heart 2007;93:226–31.

[60] Yeh HM, Lau HP, Lin JM, et al. Preoperative plasma N-terminal pro-brain natriuretic peptide as a marker of cardiac risk in patients undergoing elective non-cardiac surgery. Br J Surg 2005;92:1041–5.

[61] Breidthardt T, Kindler CH, Schindler C, et al. B-type natriuretic peptide in patients undergoing orthopaedic surgery: a prospective cohort study. Eur J Anaesthesiol 2010;27: 690–5.

[62] Karamchandani K, Abdelamalak B, Sun Z, et al. Pre-Op BNP as a predictor for post-op cardiac morbidity after non-cardiac surgery – a meta-analysis [abstract]. Annual Meeting of the American Society of Anesthesiologists. Orlando (FL), October 17–22, 2008.

[63] Guyton AC, Hall JE. Textbook of medical physiology. 11th edition. Philadelphia: Elsevier Saunders; 2006.

[64] Mangano DT. Beyond CK-MB. Biochemical markers for perioperative myocardial infarction. Anesthesiology 1994;81:1317–20.

[65] Berridge BR, Pettit S, Walker DB, et al. A translational approach to detecting drug-induced cardiac injury with cardiac troponins: consensus and recommendations from the Cardiac Troponins Biomarker Working Group of the Health and Environmental Sciences Institute. Am Heart J 2009;158:21–9.

[66] Thygesen K, Alpert JS, White HD, et al. Universal definition of myocardial infarction. Circulation 2007;116:2634–53.

[67] Ammann P, Fehr T, Minder EI, et al. Elevation of troponin I in sepsis and septic shock. Intensive Care Med 2001;27:965–9.

[68] Abdelmalak B, Jing You MS, Tang WHW, et al. Combining pre-operative BNP and cTnI in predicting cardiac outcomes from major non-cardiac surgery [abstract]. Annual Meeting of the American Society of Anesthesiologists. New Orleans (LA), October 16–21, 2009.

[69] McDonough JL, Labugger R, Pickett W, et al. Cardiac troponin I is modified in the myocardium of bypass patients. Circulation 2001;103:58–64.

[70] Martin CB, Shaw AD, Gal J, et al. The comparison and validity of troponin I assay systems in diagnosing myocardial ischemic injury after surgical coronary revascularization. J Cardiothorac Vasc Anesth 2005;19:288–93.

[71] Thielmann M, Massoudy P, Neuhauser M, et al. Risk stratification with cardiac troponin I in patients undergoing elective coronary artery bypass surgery. Eur J Cardiothorac Surg 2005;27:861–9.

[72] Paparella D, Scrascia G, Paramythiotis A, et al. Preoperative cardiac troponin I to assess midterm risks of coronary bypass grafting operations in patients with recent myocardial infarction. Ann Thorac Surg 2010;89:696–702.

[73] Lehrke S, Steen H, Sievers HH, et al. Cardiac troponin T for prediction of short- and long-term morbidity and mortality after elective open heart surgery. Clin Chem 2004;50:1560–7.

[74] Barbagallo M, Casati A, Spadini E, et al. Early increases in cardiac troponin levels after major vascular surgery is associated with an increased frequency of delayed cardiac complications. J Clin Anesth 2006;18:280–5.

[75] Lee TH, Thomas EJ, Ludwig LE, et al. Troponin T as a marker for myocardial ischemia in patients undergoing major noncardiac surgery. Am J Cardiol 1996;77:1031–6.

[76] Metzler H, Gries M, Rehak P, et al. Perioperative myocardial cell injury: the role of troponins. Br J Anaesth 1997;78:386–90.

[77] Landesberg G, Shatz V, Akopnik I, et al. Association of cardiac troponin, CK-MB, and postoperative myocardial ischemia with long-term survival after major vascular surgery. J Am Coll Cardiol 2003;42:1547–54.

[78] McFalls EO, Ward HB, Moritz TE, et al. Predictors and outcomes of a perioperative myocardial infarction following elective vascular surgery in patients with documented coronary artery disease: results of the CARP trial. Eur Heart J 2008;29:394–401.

[79] Filipovic M, Jeger R, Probst C, et al. Heart rate variability and cardiac troponin I are incremental and independent predictors of one-year all-cause mortality after major noncardiac surgery in patients at risk of coronary artery disease. J Am Coll Cardiol 2003;42:1767–76.

[80] Filipovic M, Jeger RV, Girard T, et al. Predictors of long-term mortality and cardiac events in patients with known or suspected coronary artery disease who survive major non-cardiac surgery. Anaesthesia 2005;60:5–11.

[81] Feringa HH, Bax JJ, de Jonge R, et al. Impact of glomerular filtration rate on minor troponin T elevations for risk assessment in patients undergoing operation for abdominal aortic aneurysm or lower extremity arterial obstruction. Am J Cardiol 2006;98:1515–8.

[82] Schuetz P, Christ-Crain M, Muller B. Biomarkers to improve diagnostic and prognostic accuracy in systemic infections. Curr Opin Crit Care 2007;13:578–85.

[83] Maier M, Wutzler S, Lehnert M, et al. Serum procalcitonin levels in patients with multiple injuries including visceral trauma. J Trauma 2009;66:243–9.

[84] Meisner M, Tschaikowsky K, Hutzler A, et al. Postoperative plasma concentrations of pro-calcitonin after different types of surgery. Intensive Care Med 1998;24:680–4.

[85] Wanner GA, Keel M, Steckholzer U, et al. Relationship between procalcitonin plasma levels and severity of injury, sepsis, organ failure, and mortality in injured patients. Crit Care Med 2000;28:950–7.

[86] Mimoz O, Benoist JF, Edouard AR, et al. Procalcitonin and C-reactive protein during the early posttraumatic systemic inflammatory response syndrome. Intensive Care Med 1998;24:185–8.

[87] Reith HB, Mittelkotter U, Debus ES, et al. Procalcitonin in early detection of postoperative complications. Dig Surg 1998;15:260–5.

[88] Prat C, Ricart P, Ruyra X, et al. Serum concentrations of procalcitonin after cardiac surgery. J Card Surg 2008;23:627–32.

[89] Sponholz C, Sakr Y, Reinhart K, et al. Diagnostic value and prognostic implications of serum procalcitonin after cardiac surgery: a systematic review of the literature. Crit Care 2006;10:R145.

[90] Franke A, Lante W, Fackeldey V, et al. Pro-inflammatory cytokines after different kinds of cardio-thoracic surgical procedures: is what we see what we know? Eur J Cardiothorac Surg 2005;28:569–75.

[91] Loebe M, Locziewski S, Brunkhorst FM, et al. Procalcitonin in patients undergoing cardio-pulmonary bypass in open heart surgery–first results of the Procalcitonin in Heart Surgery study (ProHearts). Intensive Care Med 2000;26(Suppl 2):S193–8.

[92] Jebali MA, Hausfater P, Abbes Z, et al. Assessment of the accuracy of procalcitonin to diag-nose postoperative infection after cardiac surgery. Anesthesiology 2007;107:232–8.

[93] Madershahian N, Wittwer T, Strauch J, et al. Kinetic of procalcitonin in the early postop-erative course following heart transplantation. J Card Surg 2008;23:468–73.

[94] Staehler M, Hammer C, Meiser B, et al. Procalcitonin: a new marker for differential diag-nosis of acute rejection and bacterial infection in heart transplantation. Transplant Proc 1997;29:584–5.

[95] Eberhard OK, Langefeld I, Kuse ER, et al. Procalcitonin in the early phase after renal trans-plantation–will it add to diagnostic accuracy? Clin Transplant 1998;12:206–11.

[96] Schneider CP, Yilmaz Y, Kleespies A, et al. Accuracy of procalcitonin for outcome predic-tion in unselected postoperative critically ill patients. Shock 2009;31:568–73.

[97] Montagnana M, Minicozzi AM, Salvagno GL, et al. Postoperative variation of C-reactive protein and procalcitonin in patients with gastrointestinal cancer. Clin Lab 2009;55:87–92.

[98] Gorisek B, Miksic NG, Krajnc P, et al. The role of procalcitonin in gynaecological surgery. J Int Med Res 2009;37:918–26.

[99] van Ree RM, de Vries AP, Oterdoom LH, et al. Plasma procalcitonin is an independent predictor of graft failure late after renal transplantation. Transplantation 2009;88:279–87.

[100] Mommertz G, Langer S, Koeppel T, et al. The role of procalcitonin as predictor for neurological deficits after carotid endarterectomy. J Cardiovasc Surg (Torino) 2009;50:665–8.

[101] Mangano CM, Diamondstone LS, Ramsay JG, et al. Renal dysfunction after myocardial revascularization: risk factors, adverse outcomes, and hospital resource utilization. The Multicenter Study of Perioperative Ischemia Research Group. Ann Intern Med 1998;128:194–203.

[102] Chertow GM, Levy EM, Hammermeister KE, et al. Independent association between acute renal failure and mortality following cardiac surgery. Am J Med 1998;104:343–8.

[103] Conlon PJ, Stafford-Smith M, White WD, et al. Acute renal failure following cardiac surgery. Nephrol Dial Transplant 1999;14:1158–62.

[104] Taglieri N, Koenig W, Kaski JC. Cystatin C and cardiovascular risk. Clin Chem 2009;55:1932–43.

[105] Herget-Rosenthal S, Bokenkamp A, Hofmann W. How to estimate GFR-serum creatinine, serum cystatin C or equations? Clin Biochem 2007;40:153–61.

[106] Dharnidharka VR, Kwon C, Stevens G. Serum cystatin C is superior to serum creatinine as a marker of kidney function: a meta-analysis. Am J Kidney Dis 2002;40:221–6.

[107] Tamsen A, Hartvig P, Fagerlund C, et al. Patient controlled analgesic therapy, part 2: individual analgesic demand and analgesic plasma concentrations of pethidine in postoperative pain. Clin Pharmacokinet 1982;7:164–75.

[108] Herget-Rosenthal S, Marggraf G, Husing J, et al. Early detection of acute renal failure by serum cystatin C. Kidney Int 2004;66:1115–22.

[109] Vinge E, Lindergard B, Nilsson-Ehle P, et al. Relationships among serum cystatin C, serum creatinine, lean tissue mass and glomerular filtration rate in healthy adults. Scand J Clin Lab Invest 1999;59:587–92.

[110] White CA, Akbari A, Doucette S, et al. Effect of clinical variables and immunosuppression on serum cystatin C and beta-trace protein in kidney transplant recipients. Am J Kidney Dis 2009;54:922–30.

[111] Villa P, Jimenez M, Soriano MC, et al. Serum cystatin C concentration as a marker of acute renal dysfunction in critically ill patients. Crit Care 2005;9:R139–43.

[112] Song D, Heise DA, White PF. Facial electromyography correlates with the level of sedation and pain in outpatients undergoing lithotripsy. Anesthesiology 1998;89:A928 [abstract].

[113] Ledoux D, Monchi M, Chapelle JP, et al. Cystatin C blood level as a risk factor for death after heart surgery. Eur Heart J 2007;28:1848–53.

[114] Ristikankare A, Poyhia R, Kuitunen A, et al. Serum cystatin C in elderly cardiac surgery patients. Ann Thorac Surg 2010;89:689–94.

[115] Liangos O, Tighiouart H, Perianayagam MC, et al. Comparative analysis of urinary biomarkers for early detection of acute kidney injury following cardiopulmonary bypass. Biomarkers 2009;14:423–31.

[116] Haase-Fielitz A, Bellomo R, Devarajan P, et al. Novel and conventional serum biomarkers predicting acute kidney injury in adult cardiac surgery–a prospective cohort study. Crit Care Med 2009;37:553–60.

[117] Koyner JL, Bennett MR, Worcester EM, et al. Urinary cystatin C as an early biomarker of acute kidney injury following adult cardiothoracic surgery. Kidney Int 2008;74:1059–69.

[118] Lebkowska U, Malyszko J, Lebkowska A, et al. Neutrophil gelatinase-associated lipocalin and cystatin C could predict renal outcome in patients undergoing kidney allograft transplantation: a prospective study. Transplant Proc 2009;41:154–7.

[119] Gourishankar S, Courtney M, Jhangri GS, et al. Serum cystatin C performs similarly to traditional markers of kidney function in the evaluation of donor kidney function prior to and following unilateral nephrectomy. Nephrol Dial Transplant 2008;23:3004–9.

[120] Puolakka PA, Rintala S, Yli-Hankala A, et al. The effect of parecoxib on kidney function at laparoscopic hysterectomy. Ren Fail 2009;31:284–9.

[121] Harten J, Crozier JE, McCreath B, et al. Effect of intraoperative fluid optimisation on renal function in patients undergoing emergency abdominal surgery: a randomised controlled pilot study (ISRCTN 11799696). Int J Surg 2008;6:197–204.

[122] Boldt J, Brosch C, Ducke M, et al. Influence of volume therapy with a modern hydroxyethylstarch preparation on kidney function in cardiac surgery patients with compromised renal function: a comparison with human albumin. Crit Care Med 2007;35:2740–6.

[123] Laisalmi M, Teppo AM, Koivusalo AM, et al. The effect of ketorolac and sevoflurane anesthesia on renal glomerular and tubular function. Anesth Analg 2001;93:1210–3.

[124] Mishra J, Mori K, Ma Q, et al. Neutrophil gelatinase-associated lipocalin: a novel early urinary biomarker for cisplatin nephrotoxicity. Am J Nephrol 2004;24:307–15.

[125] Bolignano D, Donato V, Coppolino G, et al. Neutrophil gelatinase-associated lipocalin (NGAL) as a marker of kidney damage. Am J Kidney Dis 2008;52:595–605.

[126] Bagshaw SM, Bennett M, Haase M, et al. Plasma and urine neutrophil gelatinase-associated lipocalin in septic versus non-septic acute kidney injury in critical illness. Intensive Care Med 2010;36:452–61.

[127] Bennett M, Dent CL, Ma Q, et al. Urine NGAL predicts severity of acute kidney injury after cardiac surgery: a prospective study. Clin J Am Soc Nephrol 2008;3:665–73.

[128] Dent CL, Ma Q, Dastrala S, et al. Plasma neutrophil gelatinase-associated lipocalin predicts acute kidney injury, morbidity and mortality after pediatric cardiac surgery: a prospective uncontrolled cohort study. Crit Care 2007;11:R127.

[129] Mishra J, Dent C, Tarabishi R, et al. Neutrophil gelatinase-associated lipocalin (NGAL) as a biomarker for acute renal injury after cardiac surgery. Lancet 2005;365:1231–8.

[130] Han WK, Wagener G, Zhu Y, et al. Urinary biomarkers in the early detection of acute kidney injury after cardiac surgery. Clin J Am Soc Nephrol 2009;4:873–82.

[131] Tuladhar SM, Puntmann VO, Soni M, et al. Rapid detection of acute kidney injury by plasma and urinary neutrophil gelatinase-associated lipocalin after cardiopulmonary bypass. J Cardiovasc Pharmacol 2009;53:261–6.

[132] Xin C, Yulong X, Yu C, et al. Urine neutrophil gelatinase-associated lipocalin and interleukin-18 predict acute kidney injury after cardiac surgery. Ren Fail 2008;30:904–13.

[133] Che M, Xie B, Xue S, et al. Clinical usefulness of novel biomarkers for the detection of acute kidney injury following elective cardiac surgery. Nephron Clin Pract 2010;115:c66–72.

[134] McIlroy DR, Wagener G, Lee HT. Neutrophil gelatinase-associated lipocalin and acute kidney injury after cardiac surgery: the effect of baseline renal function on diagnostic performance. Clin J Am Soc Nephrol 2010;5:211–9.

[135] Niemann CU, Walia A, Waldman J, et al. Acute kidney injury during liver transplantation as determined by neutrophil gelatinase-associated lipocalin. Liver Transpl 2009;15: 1852–60.

[136] Hall IE, Yarlagadda SG, Coca SG, et al. IL-18 and urinary NGAL predict dialysis and graft recovery after kidney transplantation. J Am Soc Nephrol 2010;21:189–97.

[137] Malyszko J, Malyszko JS, Mysliwiec M. Serum neutrophil gelatinase-associated lipocalin correlates with kidney function in renal allograft recipients. Clin Transplant 2009;23: 681–6.

[138] Kusaka M, Kuroyanagi Y, Mori T, et al. Serum neutrophil gelatinase-associated lipocalin as a predictor of organ recovery from delayed graft function after kidney transplantation from donors after cardiac death. Cell Transplant 2008;17:129–34.

[139] Price RG. The role of NAG (N-acetyl-beta-D-glucosaminidase) in the diagnosis of kidney disease including the monitoring of nephrotoxicity. Clin Nephrol 1992;38(Suppl 1): S14–9.

[140] Hultberg B, Ravnskov U. The excretion of N-acetyl-beta-glucosaminidase in glomerulonephritis. Clin Nephrol 1981;15:33–8.

[141] Perez-Blanco FJ, Garbin-Fuentes I, Perez-Chica G, et al. Urinary activity of N-acetyl-beta-glucosaminidase and progression of retinopathy in non-insulin-dependent diabetes mellitus. Clin Nephrol 1997;48:388–9.

[142] Westhuyzen J, Endre ZH, Reece G, et al. Measurement of tubular enzymuria facilitates early detection of acute renal impairment in the intensive care unit. Nephrol Dial Transplant 2003;18:543–51.

[143] Backlund M, Kellokumpu I, Scheinin T, et al. Effect of temperature of insufflated CO_2 during and after prolonged laparoscopic surgery. Surg Endosc 1998;12:1126–30.

[144] Hynninen MS, Niemi TT, Poyhia R, et al. N-acetylcysteine for the prevention of kidney injury in abdominal aortic surgery: a randomized, double-blind, placebo-controlled trial. Anesth Analg 2006;102:1638–45.

[145] Huybregts RA, de Vroege R, Jansen EK, et al. The association of hemodilution and transfusion of red blood cells with biochemical markers of splanchnic and renal injury during cardiopulmonary bypass. Anesth Analg 2009;109:331–9.

[146] Jorres A, Kordonouri O, Schiessler A, et al. Urinary excretion of thromboxane and markers for renal injury in patients undergoing cardiopulmonary bypass. Artif Organs 1994;8: 565–9.

[147] Gormley SM, McBride WT, Armstrong MA, et al. Plasma and urinary cytokine homeostasis and renal dysfunction during cardiac surgery. Anesthesiology 2000;93:1210–6 [discussion: 5A].

[148] Hamada Y, Kanda T, Anzai T, et al. N-acetyl-beta-D-glucosaminidase is not a predictor, but an indicator of kidney injury in patients with cardiac surgery. J Med 1999;30:329–36.

[149] Hara T, Fukusaki M, Nakamura T, et al. Renal function in patients during and after hypotensive anesthesia with sevoflurane. J Clin Anesth 1998;10:539–45.

[150] Kanbak M, Karagoz AH, Erdem N, et al. Renal safety and extrahepatic defluorination of sevoflurane in hepatic transplantations. Transplant Proc 2007;39:1544–8.

[151] Laisalmi M, Eriksson H, Koivusalo AM, et al. Ketorolac is not nephrotoxic in connection with sevoflurane anesthesia in patients undergoing breast surgery. Anesth Analg 2001;92:1058–63.

[152] Laisalmi-Kokki M, Pesonen E, Kokki H, et al. Potentially detrimental effects of N-acetylcysteine on renal function in knee arthroplasty. Free Radic Res 2009;43:691–6.

[153] Izumi K, Eishi K, Yamachika S, et al. The efficacy of human atrial natriuretic peptide in patients with renal dysfunction undergoing cardiac surgery. Ann Thorac Cardiovasc Surg 2008;14:294–302.

[154] van Timmeren MM, van den Heuvel MC, Bailly V, et al. Tubular kidney injury molecule-1 (KIM-1) in human renal disease. J Pathol 2007;212:209–17.

[155] Liangos O, Perianayagam MC, Vaidya VS, et al. Urinary N-acetyl-beta-(D)-glucosaminidase activity and kidney injury molecule-1 level are associated with adverse outcomes in acute renal failure. J Am Soc Nephrol 2007;18:904–12.

[156] Han WK, Bailly V, Abichandani R, et al. Kidney injury molecule-1 (KIM-1): a novel biomarker for human renal proximal tubule injury. Kidney Int 2002;62:237–44.

[157] Schroppel B, Kruger B, Walsh L, et al. Tubular expression of KIM-1 does not predict delayed function after transplantation. J Am Soc Nephrol 2010;21:536–42.

[158] van Timmeren MM, Vaidya VS, van Ree RM, et al. High urinary excretion of kidney injury molecule-1 is an independent predictor of graft loss in renal transplant recipients. Transplantation 2007;84:1625–30.

[159] Karlberg P, Moore RE, Oliver TK Jr. Thermogenic and cardiovascular responses of the newborn baby to noradrenaline. Acta Paediatr Scand 1965;54:225–38.

[160] Marchi N, Rasmussen P, Kapural M, et al. Peripheral markers of brain damage and blood-brain barrier dysfunction. Restor Neurol Neurosci 2003;21:109–21.

[161] Jonsson H, Johnsson P, Alling C, et al. S100beta after coronary artery surgery: release pattern, source of contamination, and relation to neuropsychological outcome. Ann Thorac Surg 1999;68:2202–8.

[162] Persson L, Hardemark HG, Gustafsson J, et al. S-100 protein and neuron-specific enolase in cerebrospinal fluid and serum: markers of cell damage in human central nervous system. Stroke 1987;18:911–8.

[163] Abraha HD, Butterworth RJ, Bath PM, et al. Serum S-100 protein, relationship to clinical outcome in acute stroke. Ann Clin Biochem 1997;34(Pt 5):546–50.

[164] Cakir Z, Aslan S, Umudum Z, et al. S-100beta and neuron-specific enolase levels in carbon monoxide-related brain injury. Am J Emerg Med 2010;28:61–7.

[165] Schultke E, Sadanand V, Kelly ME, et al. Can admission S-100beta predict the extent of brain damage in head trauma patients? Can J Neurol Sci 2009;36:612–6.

[166] Einav S, Itshayek E, Kark JD, et al. Serum S100B levels after meningioma surgery: a comparison of two laboratory assays. BMC Clin Pathol 2008;8:9.

[167] Johnsson P, Lundqvist C, Lindgren A, et al. Cerebral complications after cardiac surgery assessed by S-100 and NSE levels in blood. J Cardiothorac Vasc Anesth 1995;9: 694–9.

[168] Blomquist S, Johnsson P, Luhrs C, et al. The appearance of S-100 protein in serum during and immediately after cardiopulmonary bypass surgery: a possible marker for cerebral injury. J Cardiothorac Vasc Anesth 1997;11:699–703.

[169] Stolz E, Gerriets T, Kluge A, et al. Diffusion-weighted magnetic resonance imaging and neurobiochemical markers after aortic valve replacement: implications for future neuroprotective trials? Stroke 2004;35:888–92.

[170] Ramlawi B, Rudolph JL, Mieno S, et al. Serologic markers of brain injury and cognitive function after cardiopulmonary bypass. Ann Surg 2006;244:593–601.

[171] Kobayashi J, Tashiro T, Ochi M, et al. Early outcome of a randomized comparison of off-pump and on-pump multiple arterial coronary revascularization. Circulation 2005;112:1338–43.

[172] Kofke WA, Konitzer P, Meng QC, et al. The effect of apolipoprotein E genotype on neuron specific enolase and S-100beta levels after cardiac surgery. Anesth Analg 2004;99:1323–5.

[173] Kilminster S, Treasure T, McMillan T, et al. Neuropsychological change and S-100 protein release in 130 unselected patients undergoing cardiac surgery. Stroke 1999;30:1869–74.

[174] Westaby S, Saatvedt K, White S, et al. Is there a relationship between serum S-100beta protein and neuropsychologic dysfunction after cardiopulmonary bypass? J Thorac Cardiovasc Surg 2000;119:132–7.

[175] Iskesen I, Kurdal AT, Yilmaz H, et al. Sleep disturbances after cardiac surgery with or without elevated S100B levels. Acta Cardiol 2009;64:741–6.

[176] Georgiadis D, Berger A, Kowatschev E, et al. Predictive value of S-100beta and neuron-specific enolase serum levels for adverse neurologic outcome after cardiac surgery. J Thorac Cardiovasc Surg 2000;119:138–47.

[177] Saranteas T, Tachmintzis A, Katsikeris N, et al. Perioperative thyroid hormone kinetics in patients undergoing major oral and maxillofacial operations. J Oral Maxillofac Surg 2007;65:408–14.

[178] Winnerkvist A, Anderson RE, Hansson LO, et al. Multilevel somatosensory evoked potentials and cerebrospinal proteins: indicators of spinal cord injury in thoracoabdominal aortic aneurysm surgery. Eur J Cardiothorac Surg 2007;31:637–42.

[179] Marquardt G, Setzer M, Szelenyi A, et al. Significance of serial S100b and NSE serum measurements in surgically treated patients with spondylotic cervical myelopathy. Acta Neurochir (Wien) 2009;151:1439–43.

[180] Marquardt G, Setzer M, Szelenyi A, et al. Prognostic relevance of serial S100b and NSE serum measurements in patients with spinal intradural lesions. Neurol Res 2009;31:265–9.

[181] Anderson RE, Winnerkvist A, Hansson LO, et al. Biochemical markers of cerebrospinal ischemia after repair of aneurysms of the descending and thoracoabdominal aorta. J Cardiothorac Vasc Anesth 2003;17:598–603.

[182] Lases EC, Schepens MA, Haas FJ, et al. Clinical prospective study of biochemical markers and evoked potentials for identifying adverse neurological outcome after thoracic and thoracoabdominal aortic aneurysm surgery. Br J Anaesth 2005;95:651–61.

[183] Sahlein DH, Heyer EJ, Rampersad A, et al. Failure of intraoperative jugular bulb S-100B and neuron-specific enolase sampling to predict cognitive injury after carotid endarterectomy. Neurosurgery 2003;53:1243–9 [discussion: 1249–50].

[184] Aleksic M, Heckenkamp J, Reichert V, et al. S-100B release during carotid endarterectomy under local anesthesia. Ann Vasc Surg 2007;21:571–5.

[185] Wijeyaratne SM, Collins MA, Barth JH, et al. Jugular venous neurone specific enolase (NSE) increases following carotid endarterectomy under general, but not local, anaesthesia. Eur J Vasc Endovasc Surg 2009;38:262–6.

[186] Schmechel D, Marangos PJ, Brightman M. Neurone-specific enolase is a molecular marker for peripheral and central neuroendocrine cells. Nature 1978;276:834–6.

[187] Pahlman S, Esscher T, Bergvall P, et al. Purification and characterization of human neuron-specific enolase: radioimmunoassay development. Tumour Biol 1984;5:127–39.

[188] Skoog I, Hesse C, Aevarsson O, et al. A population study of apoE genotype at the age of 85: relation to dementia, cerebrovascular disease, and mortality. J Neurol Neurosurg Psychiatry 1998;64:37–43.

[189] Plachky J, Hofer S, Volkmann M, et al. Regional cerebral oxygen saturation is a sensitive marker of cerebral hypoperfusion during orthotopic liver transplantation. Anesth Analg 2004;99:344–9.

[190] Capoccia L, Speziale F, Gazzetti M, et al. Comparative study on carotid revascularization (endarterectomy vs stenting) using markers of cellular brain injury, neuropsychometric tests, and diffusion-weighted magnetic resonance imaging. J Vasc Surg 2010;51: 584–91, e1–3 [discussion: 592].

Advances in Anesthesia 28 (2010) 187–210

ADVANCES IN ANESTHESIA

Single or Multiple Guidance Methods for Peripheral Nerve Blockade in Modern-Day Practice of Regional Anesthesia

Anupama Wadhwa, MBBS[a],*, Ralf E. Gebhard, MD[b], Detlef Obal, MD, DESA[a]

[a]Department of Anesthesiology & Perioperative Medicine, University of Louisville Hospital, 530 South Jackson Street, Louisville, KY 40202, USA
[b]Departments of Anesthesiology and Orthopedics and Rehabilitation, Miller School of Medicine, University of Miami, Room C302 JMH Central, 1611 NW 12th Avenue, Miami, FL 33136, USA

Regional anesthesia has traditionally been performed with the help of a single modality, which has depended on the availability of technology at the time of performance of these blocks. The transitions from paresthesia-guided to nerve stimulation to ultrasound-guided nerve blocks have helped advance regional anesthesia as a science rather than an art, and have taken it to a higher level of sophistication. However, the visual information obtained with the use of ultrasonography remains subject to interpretation by the user and, consequently, is limited by the ability to optimize the sonographic image, variations in formal training of applied ultrasound physics, and overall experience in ultrasonography. Even though ultrasound visualization by itself is presumably associated with minimal risks, the safety claimed by ultrasound enthusiasts may not necessarily result in the safest clinical practice.

There is current debate as to whether the use of nerve stimulation or ultrasonography is superior as a nerve localization instrument for regional anesthesia; there is also a proposal that the use of dual or multiple guidance modalities may further expand the opportunities to employ regional anesthesia versus use of a single method. Regional anesthesia reliably works if the correct amount of the correct local anesthetic is placed within the correct fascial plane in correct proximity to the nerve. Nerve stimulation is generally able to provide one or two of these objectively, that is, depositing a local anesthetic near the nerve to be blocked. Anesthesiologists traditionally have used larger doses of local anesthetics with this technique to ascertain block success, as it is not possible to stimulate the nerve again after even a small dose of local anesthetic has been deposited. Ultrasonography does not solve all of these problems but it

*Corresponding author. E-mail address: wadhwaanu@me.com.

0737-6146/10/$ – see front matter
doi:10.1016/j.aan.2010.08.002

does provide extra information, such as direct visualization of nerve structures that need to be blocked, the appropriate spread of the local anesthetic around the nerve and within the correct fascial plane, and visualization of the surrounding perineural structures that need to be avoided. These advantages may improve success and reduce complications; however, experts have suggested that such claims may be premature [1]. The success rate and expertise of practitioner groups varies, making it very difficult to compare the results of studies from different institutions and operators. Use of one approach should not preclude the use of another, and the debate on the best methods needs to be more outcome-oriented than target-oriented. The guidance modalities used in each case must depend on the availability of equipment, the hospital setting, the individual patient's needs, and the expertise of the practitioner. Current technologies aiding in block performance include feeling loss of tissue resistances with blunt needles, eliciting paresthesia, peripheral nerve stimulation (PNS), ultrasonography, and injection pressures [2,3]. However, addition of sophisticated modalities may not necessarily improve the success rate nor decrease the complication rate of peripheral nerve blocks, especially in the hands of experienced physicians.

In this review, the authors present the outcomes of randomized, controlled studies that compare single to dual guidance for regional anesthesia, concentrating on PNS in comparison with ultrasound guidance, or the combined use of the two technologies.

EVOLUTION OF REGIONAL ANESTHESIA

In 1885, William Halsted performed the first brachial plexus block under direct visualization by applying cocaine directly to nerves that had been surgically exposed. Going forward, but before the invention of nerve stimulation, the nerves or nerve roots were recognized by the presence of paresthesia. Almost 100 years ago a German physician, Kulenkampff [4], used transcutaneous insertion of a needle and located nerves using the paresthesia technique. Paresthesia is a phenomenon whereby mechanical stimulation of a nerve results in a sensory feeling described as "an electric shock" in the sensory distribution of the nerve being contacted. Moore [5] stated "no paresthesias—no anesthesia," which is still part of the controversy regarding the use of nerve stimulation. The knowledge of anatomy and its common variations are core to performing this technique, as is the ability to appreciate the fascial planes and tissue layers with the use of blunt needles. Patient understanding and cooperation greatly enhance success with this method. The success rate with these techniques is about 60% to 70% [6]. Moreover, paresthesia has been demonstrated to have poor sensitivity for needle to nerve contact [7].

Nerve stimulation became common in the late twentieth century and changed the face of regional anesthesia. In 1912, a peripheral nerve stimulator was introduced by Perthes, but the technique did not gain popularity until 1962, when a smaller and portable instrument was devised [8]. PNS provides an accurate approximation of the proximity of the stimulating needle tip to a nerve or plexus by using an electric current to elicit an objective functional motor response. One obvious advantage is that PNS causes minimal discomfort to patients, because the low stimulating currents (0.3–1.5 mA) readily stimulate the larger A-alpha motor fibers more than C pain fibers when short pulse duration (0.1 ms) is used [9]; this is in contrast to the paresthesia technique, which by its nature causes varying degrees of discomfort. A second advantage of PNS is that patient cooperation is not needed during the procedure, so a block can be performed in a lightly or moderately sedated patient, providing an extra degree of comfort. In addition, the incidence of nerve damage may be decreased with PNS as compared with paresthesia techniques [10–12], and the success rate with PNS may be equal to or greater than that from eliciting paresthesias [13]. Problems with this technique, however, are that a motor response may not be elicited if the tip of the needle is in contact with just the sensory portions of a given nerve [14], and a response to a stimulating current less than 0.5 mA does not guarantee extraneural placement [3,7,15,16].

HISTORY OF ULTRASONOGRAPHY AND ITS EVOLVING USE IN REGIONAL ANESTHESIA

Doppler and sonography became common for the placement of supraclavicular blocks as early as 1978 [17]. Ting and Sivagnanaratnam [18] first used ultrasound to confirm needle placement and observe local anesthetic spread during axillary nerve blocks in 1989. These investigators reported a 100% success rate with no complications during this pilot study, and that they were able to visualize the needle tip and axillary anatomy at all times. Subsequently, Kapral and colleagues [19] demonstrated that ultrasound-guided supraclavicular blocks resulted in safe and more effective anesthesia than axillary blocks for the brachial plexus distribution.

Marhofer and colleagues [20] demonstrated improved success of "3-in-1" lower extremity blocks performed under ultrasound guidance as compared with nerve stimulation. These investigators further showed a reduction in the volume of local anesthetic required to produce an effective block with ultrasound guidance than with nerve stimulation [21]. The use of ultrasound localization of nerves was further advanced when a group of researchers in Toronto demonstrated high-quality images of the brachial plexus with ultrasound [22]. This group also confirmed the findings by Urmey [23] that contact of a stimulating needle with the nerves does not necessarily initiate a motor response [14,22].

Within the past 6 years, Brian Sites and his colleagues [24–27] have developed and published core competencies training for ultrasound-guided regional anesthesia, and developed curricula focused on ultrasound physics and establishing appropriate learning metrics and behavior during ultrasonographic skill development. These guidelines for education and training in ultrasound-guided regional anesthesia have been adapted and published by the American and European Societies of Regional Anesthesia, and comprise formal guidelines and minimum expectations required of regional anesthesia practitioners, educators, and researchers in an attempt to create uniformity of practice in different parts of the world. The studies reviewed in this article lack this kind of consistency, but the authors hope that researchers in the future will follow these guidelines and that reviewers of their articles will have an easier time comparing studies from various countries.

UPPER EXTREMITY BLOCKS

Evidence for Interscalene and Supraclavicular Blocks

The upper extremity is especially well suited for ultrasound-guided regional anesthesia. High-frequency linear array transducers (10–15 Hz) provide very high-resolution images of the brachial plexus (Table 1) [28]. Supraclavicular blocks have regained popularity, because the dreaded complication of pneumothorax may be dramatically reduced with ultrasound-guided placement compared with the traditional landmark technique [17,19,29–32]. The interscalene and supraclavicular regions are rich in vessels and nerves, which helps allow clear identification of anatomic structures; conversely, it provides little room for error while performing regional blocks. Therefore, it seems likely that using ultrasound-guided regional anesthesia for the upper extremity may prevent severe complications (eg, vascular puncture and intravascular injection leading to local anesthetic systemic toxicity). However, differences between ultrasound-guided and PNS-guided blocks, as well as the combination of both techniques, are difficult to evaluate based on data available to date. Liu and colleagues [33] investigated ultrasound-guided and PNS-guided interscalene blocks in 219 patients, mainly to assess postoperative neurologic symptoms (PONS). These investigators found no difference in the failure rate, time to perform blocks, patient satisfaction, or postoperative neurologic outcome between techniques; however, they demonstrated fewer needle passes and quicker onset of motor block with ultrasound guidance [33]. This lack of difference in success (100% in both groups) could be attributed to the high volume of local anesthetic used in their study (55–65 mL mepivacaine 1.5% with sodium bicarbonate). In addition, this same group recently published a large prospective clinical registry of ultrasound-guided regional interscalene and supraclavicular blocks for shoulder surgery, demonstrating a 99.8% success rate of surgical anesthesia. The incidence of vascular puncture and permanent nerve injury was similarly low, at 0% (95% confidence interval [CI], 0%–0.3%), whereas the incidence of PONS was reported to be only 0.4% (95% CI, 0.1%–1%) [34].

By contrast, Kapral and colleagues [35] performed interscalene blocks using ultrasound in 160 patients, using a much lower volume of local anesthetic (20 mL of 0.75% ropivacaine). This study demonstrated both a quicker onset of sensory blockade and a stronger motor blockade in all nerves of the upper extremity, and detected anatomic variances in 11% of patients in the ultrasound group. In addition, they demonstrated an increased success rate in the ultrasound group (99%) versus the PNS group (90%). As elegantly described in the accompanying editorial [36], this could be caused by the methodological flaws of the study. For example, they used multiple injections for the ultra-sound-guided group to ensure complete circumferential spread, but only a single stimulation for the PNS group, especially targeting for a twitch for middle and lower trunks only. Kapral and colleagues also highlight the lesser-known anatomic variation of the brachial plexus that constitutes roots located within the anterior or middle scalene muscles.

A single study performed by Williams and colleagues [30] compared combined ultrasound and PNS with anatomically guided PNS in 80 patients. These investigators demonstrated a higher success rate in complete block (95% vs 85%) and surgical anesthesia in the ultrasound group. Less time was required to perform the block in the ultrasound group (5.0 ± 2.4 minutes vs 9.8 ± 7.5 minutes, $P = .0001$).

The addition of nerve stimulation to ultrasound may not offer any advantage in supraclavicular blocks because about 13% of patients have no twitch response even after needle nerve contact, but will have successful surgical anesthesia [3,37].

Authors' opinion
Interscalene and supraclavicular blocks should be performed under ultrasound guidance not only to avoid vascular or intrathecal puncture but also for a more circumferential spread of the local anesthetic, which is likely to increase the success rate. Ultrasonography would identify the abnormal location of one of the trunks within the scalene muscles. However, based on only one study in both interscalene (160 patients) and supraclavicular (80 patients) areas, it is difficult to comment as to whether using ultrasound and nerve stimulation guidance in combination will improve block quality, speed of onset, or duration of regional anesthesia.

Evidence for Infraclavicular Blocks

Compared with the supraclavicular area where the divisions of the brachial plexus are in close proximity to each other, the brachial plexus divides into cords below the clavicle. These cords surround the axillary artery laterally, medially, and posteriorly. Thus, methods for this block that use multiple-injection techniques are likely to achieve higher success rates than single-injection techniques. Eight randomized controlled studies have compared ultrasound-guided and PNS-guided infraclavicular blocks in adult patients [38–42]. Overall, 370 patients were included in these comparisons, with 37 to 103 patients per study. All studies reported a high success rate with either ultrasound guidance or with nerve stimulation guidance, without being able to demonstrate a clear difference between the 2 modes of nerve identification [38–41]. However, visualization of major anatomic structures by ultrasound appears to shorten the time to achieve a successful block [38,39]. Most studies failed to demonstrate a better quality of nerve blockade with one method over the other [38–40], but there was a trend toward a higher success rate in the ultrasound-guided groups [40]. Although limited by his small sample size, Gurkan and colleagues [41] demonstrated that

Table 1
Randomized control trials comparing ultrasonography, peripheral nerve stimulation, or both for nerve block of upper extremities

Study	Technique (No of patients)	Outcomes	Complications
Interscalene block			
Soeding et al [90]	US vs Landmark and paresthesia (40)	• Better sensory and motor block with US	Less paresthesia with US
Kapral et al [35]	US vs PNS (160)	• 99% success rate with US vs 91% with PNS	None studied
Liu et al [33]	US vs PNS (219)	• Prolonged duration of block with US • Fewer needle passes (1 vs 3) with US • Faster motor onset with US	Similar postoperative neurologic symptoms at 1 wk and 4–6 wk
Supraclavicular block			
Williams et al [30]	USPNS vs PNS (80)	• Shorter procedure time with US (5 vs 10 min) • 85% vs 78% surgical anesthesia in USPNS vs PNS group	No complications in either group
Infraclavicular block			
Dingemans et al [42]	US vs USPNS (72)	• Faster performance with US alone • Greater success with US alone	Three axillary artery punctures (2 in US vs 1 in USPNS) and 1 prolonged paresthesia (US)
Gurkan et al [41]	US vs USPNS (80)	• Faster performance with US	No complications noted
Dhir and Ganapathy [91]	Nonstimulating catheter vs Stimulating catheter vs USPNS (66)	• Greater primary and secondary success with US	
Sauter et al [40]	US vs PNS (80)	• Fewer needle passes with US • No difference in success rate	Blood aspiration less frequent in US, more paresthesia in US (8 vs 1)
Brull et al [38]	US vs dual-point PNS (103)	• Faster surgical readiness with US • Faster block performance with US	Paresthesia in 45% PNS vs 6% US
Taboada et al [39]	US vs PNS (35)	• Similar onset of sensory and motor block • Onset time shorter with US (3 vs 6 min) • No difference in success rate (89% vs 91%)	Vascular puncture; but no significant differences between both groups

Study	Comparison	Findings	Comments
De Tran et al [92]	US (Single injection vs 2 injections)	• No difference in success rate (97% with single injection vs 93% with double injection) • No difference in onset time, imaging time, total anesthesia-related time • Block-related pain was less with dual injection	Block-related pain less in 2-injection group; no other differences in complications
Axillary block			
Soeding et al [90]	US vs Landmark and paresthesia (40)	• US quicker and more complete sensory and motor block	Less paresthesia with US
Liu et al [93]	Three groups: US or PNS with double injections vs US with single injection (90)	• Shorter procedure time with US • 90% success rate in the 2-injection groups vs 70% in the single-injection group	Higher incidence of paresthesia, axillary vessel puncture, and subcutaneous hematoma in the 2-injection PNS group
Sites et al [94]	US vs Transarterial (TA) (56)	• 100% success with US vs 71% with TA • Faster procedure time (8 vs 11 min) with US	None noted
Casati et al [46]	US vs PNS (60) 4 separate injections for all 4 nerves	• Reduced needle passes (4 vs 8 with US) and shorter sensory block onset time (14 vs 18 min) with US • 100% success rate with both groups • No difference in motor block	Procedure-related pain 20% in US and 48% in PNS group
Chan et al [45]	US vs PNS vs USPNS (188)	• Shorter procedure time with US (9 vs 11 min) • Success rate 95% in US, 92% in USPNS, and 86% in PNS • Complete sensory block 81%–83% with US vs 62% with PNS	Less paresthesia with US
Yu et al [95]	US-guided 4-point vs PNS one puncture (80)	• Shorter procedure time with US (5 vs 14 min) • Shorter onset times for individual nerves • Higher success rate (100% with US vs 78% with PNS)	Fewer punctures of blood vessels in US group (0% vs 40%)

Abbreviations: PNS, peripheral nerve stimulation-guided; US, ultrasound-guided; USPNS, ultrasound-guided and peripheral nerve stimulation–guided combination.

the complication rate (eg, vascular puncture) was lower in the ultrasound-guided than in the PNS-guided group.

In contrast to the previous studies, Dingemans and colleagues [42] compared the combination of nerve stimulation and ultrasound guidance with ultrasound guidance alone for infraclavicular blocks. The trainee performing the block in all patients visualized the spread of the local anesthetic posterior to and to each side of the axillary artery in the ultrasound-only group with the minimum number of injections. The combined group received a single injection of local anesthetic after obtaining a distal motor response to nerve stimulation. Dingemans and colleagues concluded that infraclavicular nerve blocks were performed faster with a higher success rate in the ultrasound-only group. Patients with single injections in both groups had a similar success rate (86%), which reinforces the improved success with multiple injections.

Authors' opinion
The majority of studies suggest that approaches using ultrasound guidance alone allow quicker performance and faster onset or surgical readiness of regional anesthesia, with fewer needle passes than nerve stimulation with or without ultrasound in the infraclavicular region. Thus nerve stimulation does not provide any additional benefit to ultrasound guidance in the infraclavicular region; however, ultrasound guidance seems to have a definite benefit over nerve stimulation alone in all aspects of regional anesthesia success as defined by onset time, success rate, and surgical anesthesia.

Evidence for Axillary Blocks/Single Nerve Blocks

Axillary brachial plexus block is performed at the level of terminal nerves surrounding the axillary artery in a sheath. Radial and musculocutaneous nerves are often missed with single-injection techniques. Multiple-injection techniques have been shown to provide a higher success rate and a shorter onset time compared with single-injection techniques, even though they take longer to perform [43]. If each of the 4 major nerves is blocked with localization by nerve stimulation rather than paresthesia, the success rate is more than 90%. Ultrasound techniques also have high success rates because it is possible to make multiple injections with visual confirmation around the 4 major nerves.

Multiple studies have focused on the effect of ultrasound on success rate, complications, and performance time of axillary brachial blockade. Morros and colleagues [44] demonstrated similar success rates with nerve stimulation–guided and combined ultrasound-guided and nerve stimulation–guided axillary plexus block, but the complication rate (eg, vascular puncture 8% vs 28%) dropped significantly as did the onset time of sensory and motor blockade with ultrasound-guided blocks. However, more time (350 seconds vs 291 seconds) was required to perform the procedure when nerve stimulation was combined with ultrasound.

The largest study conducted in axillary ultrasound-guided regional anesthesia by Chan and colleagues [45] (188 patients) had 3 groups (ultrasound alone, ultrasound with PNS, and PNS alone). The results clearly demonstrated that ultrasound, with or without PNS, was superior to PNS alone in terms of blockade of the 3 major nerves—radial, median, and ulnar. However, there was no clinical difference in terms of surgical anesthesia between groups (95%, 92%, and 86% in ultrasound, ultrasound with PNS, and PNS groups, respectively). In addition, complications such as postoperative axillary bruising and pain were less frequent in the groups in which ultrasound was used during block placement.

By contrast, Casati and colleagues [46] found no difference in success rate (100% in both groups) or time to onset of motor block with axillary blocks performed with ultrasound or nerve stimulation guidance with 4 separate injections. On the other hand, onset of sensory block was faster with ultrasound guidance compared with electrical guidance (14 minutes vs 18 minutes). Patient satisfaction was higher in the ultrasound group as well. In fact, almost 53% of patients with multiple nerve stimulations reported the procedure as painful [47], whereas 98% of patients receiving their blocks with ultrasound guidance reported high satisfaction and acceptance of their procedures [48]. Thus, ultrasound guidance may have an advantage in the performance of axillary plexus block in terms of patient comfort. Bloc and colleagues [49] confirmed this finding in their recent study comparing comfort of the patient during axillary block placement with PNS and ultrasound guidance.

Authors' opinion
Overall patient comfort and satisfaction seem to be greater in patients receiving ultrasound-guided axillary blocks simply because nerve stimulation in this area is uncomfortable, requires more time, and use of ultrasound may be associated with a higher success rate. In terms of success rate, there is no evidence that dual guidance is superior to ultrasound alone in this region. Vascular puncture and bruising are likely to be reduced with use of ultrasound for axillary plexus block; thus, the authors recommend the routine use of ultrasound for this site.

LOWER EXTREMITY BLOCKS
Unlike the upper extremities, there are relatively few studies that compare ultrasound with nerve stimulation guidance for lower extremity blocks, and in those available the total number of study subjects is small, allowing for limited interpretation of the results (Tables 2 and 3). A recent evidence-based review summarized the benefits of ultrasound versus nerve stimulation for lower extremity nerve block [50]. The conclusion was that there is level Ib evidence to make a grade A recommendation that ultrasound guidance improves onset and success of sensory block, decreases local anesthetic requirements, and needs decreased time to perform the lower extremity peripheral nerve blocks.

Complications with regional anesthesia are relatively rare; thus, it is difficult to comment on outcomes and safety based on 200 total patients undergoing femoral, 3-in-1, or fascia iliaca blocks, and slightly more than 200 patients undergoing sciatic nerve block. Comments can be made, however, about the

Table 2
Randomized control trials comparing ultrasonography, peripheral nerve stimulation, or both for nerve blocks of lower extremities

Study	Technique (No of patients)	Outcomes	Complications
3-in-1 or Femoral Nerve Block			
Marhofer et al [20]	US vs PNS (40)	• 95% success with US vs 85% with PNS • Reduced onset time with US (16 vs 27 min)	Arterial punctures (3 in PNS vs 0 in US)
Marhofer et al [21]	US vs PNS (60)	• 95% success rate with US compared with PNS (80%) • Reduced LA (20 mL vs 30 mL) with US • 33%–57% reduction in LA with US compared with other studies using PNS	None reported
Casati et al [54]	US vs PNS (60)	• 42% reduction in MEAV of 0.5% ropivacaine with US-guided blocks	
Mariano et al [55]	US vs PNS (40) catheter placement	• 100% success with US vs 85% with PNS. Successful placement in 15% failed patients with US • Less time with US (11 vs 13 min) • More patient comfort	0% vs 20% intravascular punctures with US vs PNS
Subgluteal sciatic nerve block			
Danelli et al [56]	US vs PNS	• 37% lower $MEAV_{50}$ with US vs PNS	None

Popliteal sciatic nerve block

Danelli et al [61]	US vs PNS (44)	• Less procedure time (2 min with US vs 5 min with PNS) • Decreased onset of block time (12 vs 18 min) for common peroneal nerve	None
Mariano et al [62]	US vs PNS (40) catheter placement	• Less procedure time (median time 5 min with US vs 10 min with PNS) and less failure rate (100% success with US vs 80% success rate with PNS)	None
Perlas et al [63]	US vs PNS (67)	• Higher block success rate (90% vs 61%) and faster sensory and motor block onset (10–60 min)	None
van Geffen et al [64]	US vs PNS (40)	• 100% success with US and 83% with PNS	
Midfemoral sciatic nerve block			
Domingo-Triado et al [96]	USPNS vs PNS (61)	• 54% reduction in the volume of LA injected	None

Abbreviations: LA, local anesthetic; MEAV, minimum effective anesthetic volume; PNS, peripheral nerve stimulation–guided; US, ultrasound-guided; USPNS, ultrasound-guided and peripheral nerve stimulation–guided combination.

Study	Technique (No of patients)	Outcomes	Complications
Table 3 Retrospective analysis of interscalene, axillary, femoral, and popliteal nerve blocks			
Orebaugh et al [97]	USPNS vs PNS (248)	• More time to perform blocks with PNS (7 vs 2 min) • More needle insertions with PNS (median 6 vs 2)	Fewer vascular punctures with USPNS (12 vs 3)

success rate and block quality in these small studies, but even these results are subject to each institution's expertise in performing these blocks. Abnormal location of femoral nerve makes it difficult to identify with ultrasound [51] or nerve stimulation alone, and ultrasound may not be of additional value in femoral nerve blocks with normal anatomy in terms of block efficacy. However, when in question, dual guidance may help the anesthesiologist to identify the desired target. For instance, at times the femoral nerve may not be very visible on the ultrasound screen and fascial structures either lateral or posterolateral to the femoral artery may appear as femoral nerve [52]. Here the authors present studies related to femoral and sciatic catheters that have included ultrasound-guided blocks in one of their study groups.

Evidence for Femoral Nerve Blocks and Catheter Placement

There is only one study that provides an anatomic basis to an educated approach to dual-guidance techniques to block peripheral nerves. Although not a direct comparison between the 2 techniques, a study by Nader and colleagues [53] demonstrates the anatomic basis for recommending dual-guidance techniques for femoral nerve blocks. Their cadaver dissections revealed that the branch to the quadriceps muscle originates from the lateral part of the common femoral nerve in 95% and medially in 5% of the specimens, while the fascicular branch to the sartorius muscle arises from the medial side of the common femoral nerve. A quadriceps contraction was elicited in 1.2% and 96% of the specimens when the medial and lateral aspects of the femoral nerve were stimulated, respectively. By contrast, a sartorius muscle contraction was elicited in 94% and 0% when stimulating the medial and lateral part of the femoral nerve, respectively. The investigators concluded that using out-of-plane ultrasound imaging at the inguinal crease to direct the stimulating needle to the lateral half of the femoral nerve should be associated with a higher probability of encountering the motor branch to the quadriceps muscle.

One of the proven advantages of ultrasound-guided femoral nerve block over nerve stimulation–guided blocks is the reduction of anesthetic dose. Studies have shown up to a 42% reduction in the mean effective anesthetic volume of local anesthetic needed to block the femoral nerve (15 mL in ultrasound vs 28 mL in PNS) [21,54]. With logistic regression and probit transformation, the estimated effective dose (ED_{95}) for ultrasound was half of that for PNS (22 mL vs 41 mL) [21,54].

Adding nerve stimulation to ultrasound guidance (USPNS) does not seem to offer any advantages in terms of either a partial or complete block 40 minutes after local anesthetic injection (96% vs 88%; $P = .19$) [52]. There were more needle redirections in the USPNS group (4 vs 1, $P<.001$), with a higher percentage of patients requiring 2 or more needle attempts (44% vs 19%, $P<.01$), and the time to perform the block in USPNS group was longer (188 vs 148 seconds, $P = .01$). Thus, the addition of nerve stimulation to an ultrasound-guided femoral block did not improve efficacy as defined by the quality of the sensory and motor blocks, but did prolong the time to perform the procedure.

In a study by Mariano and colleagues [55], perineural catheters placed with ultrasound guidance (n = 20) took a median of 5.0 (range 3.9–10.0) minutes compared with 8.5 (4.8–30.0) minutes for the group using electrical stimulation (n = 20; $P=.012$). All ultrasound-guided catheters were placed within the parameters of the protocol (n = 20) versus only 85% of nerve stimulation–guided catheters (n = 20; $P = .086$). Patients in the ultrasound group found catheter placements to cause less discomfort than did those in the nerve stimulation group. There were no vascular punctures with ultrasound guidance, compared with 4 in the nerve stimulation group ($P = .039$).

Authors' opinion
One of the major roles of the use of ultrasound will be to reduce the amount of local anesthetic required to block the femoral nerve and to reduce the incidence of vascular puncture; however, addition of nerve stimulation to ultrasound does not seem to offer further advantage in terms of time required to perform femoral blocks or their success rate. Successful continuous catheter placement may be facilitated with ultrasound guidance. Based on the anatomic study, an in-plane technique directed toward the lateral, rather than the medial, aspect of the nerve may have a higher likelihood of success with the femoral block when single or dual guidance is used.

Evidence for Sciatic Nerve Blocks

A single study [56] has examined an ultrasound-guided method to block the sciatic nerve at the subgluteal level, using the "up and down" method. Subjects in the ultrasound-guided group were reported to have a 37% reduction in mepivacaine requirements compared with those in the nerve stimulation–guided group. The reason for the lack of studies for this anatomic approach is probably because the sheer bulk of the gluteus maximums muscle makes the sciatic nerve more difficult to visualize at this anatomic approach [57], and nerve stimulation using palpable anatomic landmarks reliably provides quick and easy access to the sciatic nerve [58,59]. Abbas and Brull [60] mention in a letter to the editor their routine use of ultrasound at this level; however, it remains to be seen whether addition of ultrasound offers any advantage to this block.

Authors' opinion
Given that only one study has been performed comparing the subgluteal sciatic nerve block with the 2 guidance techniques, it would be reasonable only to comment on the reduced local anesthetic requirement with ultrasound guidance.

Distal Sciatic Blocks at the Level of Midfemoral or Popliteal Region
Five randomized controlled trials (RCTs), including a total of 251 patients, have compared the use of ultrasound versus nerve stimulation guidance for sciatic nerve block at the popliteal level, which seems to be the preferred approach for many groups because of the ease of visualization of the nerve at this level. Danelli and colleagues [61] reported that although the onset times for sensory and motor blocks were comparable with the 2 methods, ultrasound guidance reduced needle redirections ($P = .01$), was associated with less procedural pain ($P = .002$), and required less time to perform ($P = .002$). The success rate was 100% for ultrasound-guided versus 82% for nerve stimulation–guided procedures ($P = .116$).

Mariano and colleagues [62] reported that perineural catheters placed with ultrasound guidance took a median of 5 (range 4–11) minutes compared with 10 (2–15) minutes for stimulation guidance ($P = .034$). Subjects in the ultrasound group experienced less pain during catheter placement, scoring a median discomfort of 0 (0.0–2.1) compared with 2.0 (0.0–5.0) for the stimulation group ($P = .005$) on a numeric rating scale of 0 to 10.

Perlas and colleagues [63] concluded that ultrasound guidance enhances the quality of single-injection popliteal sciatic nerve block compared with nerve stimulation–guided block using either a tibial or peroneal end point. Ultrasound guidance resulted in higher success rate (89% vs 60%), and faster onset and progression of sensorimotor block, without an increase in block procedure time or complications.

van Geffen and colleagues [64] concluded that the use of ultrasound localization for distal sciatic nerve block in the popliteal fossa reduced the required dose of local anesthetic (17 vs 37 mL, $P<.001$), reduced the number of needle passes required, and was associated with a higher success rate than nerve stimulation (100% vs 75%; $P = .017$), without changing block characteristics. A faster onset of both sensory and motor blockade with no change in block duration was also demonstrated.

Authors' opinion
The sciatic nerve may be visualized with a high degree of success at the popliteal level with ultrasonography because of its superficial location. This delineation allows for a higher success rate compared with nerve stimulation techniques, and to faster onset of nerve block. There also seems to be less procedural pain and reduced local anesthetic requirements when ultrasound is employed in this area. These advantages could be attributed to a variable division of the sciatic nerve above the popliteal crease [65,66], which may prevent a complete circumferential spread of local anesthetic around both

branches of sciatic nerve when using nerve stimulation alone. It may be advantageous to use dual guidance at this site.

Evidence for Neuraxial Blocks

Studies have shown a strong correlation between depth of the epidural space from the skin as measured by ultrasound and as measured by loss of resistance via an epidural needle [67–69]. Subsequently, Grau and colleagues [70–72] completed 3 RCTs in adult obstetric patients (Table 4). Overall, these studies suggest that when used to identify the epidural space, level, and depth from skin to epidural space preprocedure, ultrasound reduces the number of punctures and the number of levels attempted, and improves the quality of resultant analgesia. Even in a patient population with expectation of difficult placement, either because of abnormal anatomy or previous history of difficult placement, catheter placement with ultrasound assistance resulted in higher patient satisfaction [72].

These same investigators subsequently demonstrated positive impacts on both patient care and in regional anesthesia education for neuraxial techniques [73] (see comment on education in ultrasound-guided anesthesia later in this article).

Some additional studies performed in the pediatric population and case reports published on ultrasound guidance for drainage of spinal abscess and use of ultrasound to guide lumbar facet nerve block [74] are beyond the scope of this review.

Authors' opinion

Only 3 RCTs have been published on the use of ultrasound guidance in neuraxial blockade. Unfortunately, these studies are all from the same center with

Table 4
Comparison of use of ultrasonography for neuraxial blocks vs landmark technique

Study	Technique (No. of patients)	Outcomes	Complications
Grau et al [70]	US vs Landmark (300)	• Reduced number of puncture attempts and planes • Improved quality of analgesia • No difference in patient satisfaction	Higher incidence of headache and backache in the control group
Grau et al [71]	US vs Landmark (80)	• Reduced number of puncture attempts and planes • Improved quality of analgesia	
Grau et al [72]	US vs Landmark (72)	• Reduced number of puncture attempts and planes • Improved quality of analgesia	

the same first author, who is an expert in ultrasonography of the spine. Therefore, more studies on patient populations other than obstetrics are needed to determine whether catheter placement guided by sonography of the neuraxis increases the speed or reliability of epidural analgesia/anesthesia. Although regional anesthesia performed in the obstetric population requires extensive experience, it would be interesting to determine whether the described results are reproducible in the thoracic spine, and in elderly patients or those with more challenging anatomic conditions.

COMPARISON OF COMPLICATIONS BETWEEN GUIDANCE METHODS

Very few studies have actually shown a reduction of significant complications with ultrasound guidance as compared with nerve stimulation guidance. Renes and colleagues [75,76] demonstrated decreased occurrence of phrenic nerve block by using ultrasound in comparison with nerve stimulation for both supraclavicular blocks (0% ultrasound vs 53% PNS) and interscalene brachial plexus blocks (12% ultrasound vs 93% PNS). These investigators also reported objective evidence of impairment in the nerve stimulation group, including a significant reduction of forced expiratory volume in 1 second, forced vital capacity, and peak expiratory flow, along with evidence of paresis of the ipsilateral hemidiaphragm. A case report also described sparing of the phrenic nerve when an ultrasound-guided interscalene block was performed in a patient who had contralateral pneumonectomy [77].

A preliminary report from one of the largest studies on peripheral nerve blocks indicates that there is a reduction in the incidence of unintentional vascular puncture with the use of ultrasound because the practitioner can easily see the structures that need to be avoided (5% incidence with ultrasound vs 13% with PNS) [78]. Even though it seems intuitive that the needle tip may be visualized with ultrasound, occasional reports of seizures and cardiac arrest caused by local anesthetic toxicity have been reported even with the use of ultrasound [79,80]. Gnaho and colleagues [79] reported cardiac arrest while performing a sciatic block with a combined ultrasound and PNS technique. Barrington and colleagues [78] showed a similar incidence of local anesthetic systemic toxicity (0.98 per 1000 patients) with peripheral nerve blocks performed with either ultrasound or PNS techniques. By contrast, Auroy and colleagues [81] reported an incidence of between 0.75 and 2 incidents per 1000 patients in an earlier study performing peripheral nerve blocks with nerve stimulation. There was a trend toward lower local anesthetic toxicity in the ultrasound group (1.2 vs 0.8 per 1000 patients). Although the incidence of paresthesia was higher in the ultrasound group (20.5 vs 10.8 per 1000 patients), the late or long-term neurologic deficits were higher in the nerve stimulation group [78]. As noted previously, ultrasound-guided supraclavicular and interscalene blocks are associated with an extremely low incidence of vascular punctures and permanent nerve injury [34].

LIMITATIONS OF ULTRASOUND-GUIDED REGIONAL ANESTHESIA

Anesthesiologists using ultrasound in clinical practice need to appreciate and correctly interpret common ultrasound-generated, tissue-generated, and overlapping artifacts. Sono-anatomy of peripheral nerves is complex and continuing to be delineated. Accurate needle placement is facilitated by an "in-plane" approach, which can be challenging given narrow ultrasound beam widths. Higher-resolution images correlate with better image quality, which is a balance between spatial resolution (with higher frequencies) and depth of penetration (with lower frequencies); therefore, the authors expect that future ultrasound technology may be able to balance both these factors, and will increase the accuracy of nerve localization and perineural local anesthetic delivery.

Nerves may appear hypo- or hyperechoic on ultrasonography. In general, the hypoechoic areas correlate with the neural tissue and the hyperechoic structures correlate with the connective tissue. Because brachial plexus nerve roots may appear to be unifascicular or oligofascicular, they often produce hypoechoic shadows unlike the more peripheral nerves. The ratio of neural to non-neural tissue increases from 1:1 to 1:2 when comparing interscalene and supraclavicular regions with infraclavicular regions of the brachial plexus [82]. Different regions of the brachial plexus thus often manifest varying degrees of echogenicity, potentially confusing an ultrasound novice.

There are very few studies demonstrating the effectiveness of using ultrasound during placement of catheters at various sites [62,83]. An editorial by Mariano and colleagues [84] recently pointed out that a high or very high success rate with single-shot peripheral nerve blocks may not necessarily translate into a high success rate for perineural catheter placement, as the angle of the needle is very important for perineural catheter insertion, and it is difficult to visualize a catheter tip in relation to the target nerve as easily as it is to visualize needles with 2-dimensional ultrasound. Addition of stimulating catheters with the use of ultrasound may be an interesting area to study for improvement in the success rate of catheter placements.

Lastly, the cost of an ultrasound machine as compared with nerve stimulation equipment, and the effort and cost of training physicians in the core competencies of ultrasound-guided blocks, are among the major challenges faced by anesthesiologists attempting to incorporate ultrasound-guided regional anesthesia into their daily practice.

ADVANTAGES OF ULTRASOUND-GUIDED REGIONAL ANESTHESIA

High-resolution sonography provides visual information that is not obtainable by any other nerve localization method. The trained practitioner can image the vessels and nerves, including details up to 1 mm, depending on the frequency of the applied transducer and the quality of the ultrasound machine [85]. However, fascicles with small diameters (<1 mm) are not discerned with current high-frequency ultrasound technology and may only display about 33% of the total number of fascicles in a peripheral nerve [85]. If the needle tip is visualized, intraneural placement can be relatively easily discerned. PNS does not have the sensitivity to exclude direct needle tip to nerve contact or even intraneural placement, even with low stimulation currents [3]. In addition, studies show a reduction of the total dose of local anesthetic required to achieve surgical block when ultrasound was used compared with nerve stimulation alone. This dose sparing is in the range of 25% to 42% [54,86–89]. Thus, in summary, there may be an advantage of ultrasound in avoiding intravascular and intraneural injections, and a possible reduction of total amount of local anesthetic used.

RECOMMENDATIONS FOR DUAL GUIDANCE OF REGIONAL ANESTHESIA

Dual guidance of peripheral nerve blockade procedures with both nerve stimulation and ultrasound is definitely warranted under certain specific circumstances. Abnormal location of nerves makes it difficult to identify them reliably in all cases with ultrasound alone. Therefore, the combination of ultrasound and nerve stimulation is recommended in these cases. One important example of common abnormal nerve location involves the femoral nerve, as mentioned earlier. Additional indications are listed below and largely derive from situations involving difficulties with using either technique alone, because of either patient- or provider-imposed limitations. Based on the lack of concordance between the current output and the needle tip to nerve, it may be more useful and appropriate to use PNS (in conjunction with ultrasound) as a qualitative tool ("yes or no") to confirm the location of peripheral nerve rather than attempting to achieve a predefined minimum current output.

Recommended Indications for Dual Guidance Methods
- Nerves with common anatomic variability or abnormal anatomy: a combination helps to identify peripheral neural structures
- Deep blocks such as sciatic and lumbar plexus: poor ultrasound visualization
- Obesity/morbid obesity: poor ultrasound visualization
- Lymphedema, subcutaneous emphysema: poor ultrasound visualization
- Unsure of anatomy or structures
- Novice sonologist/regional anesthesiologist
- Need to perform an additional block after a failed or partial initial block
- Catheter techniques: initial localization with ultrasound followed by insertion of stimulating catheter may improve the perineural placement, as catheters may be difficult to visualize with ultrasound.

SUMMARY

Ultrasound guidance for peripheral nerve block performance is a relatively new technique. Consequently, available data in the literature are somewhat limited and interpretations are preliminary. Although nerve stimulation has been the standard of care for several decades and has been proved to be safe in experienced hands, the success rate varies in the hands of inexperienced care providers. However, does this justify the call for dual guidance, or is it more appropriate to provide additional training to produce higher predictability with one or the other modality?

Considering that dual guidance does not consistently produce better results with regional anesthesia, to add ultrasound to a very successful nerve stimulation–based practice will add cost for an experienced regional anesthesiologist, who may find little value in adding ultrasonography to routine practice. Although the literature comparing dual guidance with single guidance generally indicates better success rates with some blocks, it is important to realize that groups with high success rates and short procedural times reportedly using peripheral nerve stimulators alone also use multiple guidance techniques. Such techniques may be in the form of a strong anatomic background that includes a good knowledge of anatomic variations, good feel of the tissue and fascial planes with blunt needles, and paying attention to patients' reporting of paresthesia or pain on injection [59].

In essence, ultrasound guidance or nerve stimulation, alone or in combination, allow high success rates with peripheral nerve blocks. Whether purchase of new equipment and adjustment to a relatively new technique will be efficient for individual institutions depends on the nature of the practice, the number of challenging patients (difficult anatomies, high number of comorbidities), and the expertise of the personnel in one technology or another. The literature favors neither sole technique nor dual techniques strongly, other than for cases in which difficult anatomy reduces success with a "single" technique approach. Nevertheless, in cases of doubt combinations of various techniques (eg, ultrasound or nerve stimulation) will help to avoid serious–although rare–complications.

Future developments, including reduced costs and improvements in image quality available with ultrasound machines, as well as formal training in ultrasound-guided techniques, seem likely to turn the tide toward ultrasound-based techniques as an integral part of regional anesthesia practice.

References

[1] Hadzic A, Sala-Blanch X, Xu D. Ultrasound guidance may reduce but not eliminate complications of peripheral nerve blocks. Anesthesiology 2008;108(4):557–8.

[2] Gadsden JC, Lindenmuth DM, Hadzic A, et al. Lumbar plexus block using high-pressure injection leads to contralateral and epidural spread. Anesthesiology 2008;109(4):683–8.

[3] Robards C, Hadzic A, Somasundaram L, et al. Intraneural injection with low-current stimulation during popliteal sciatic nerve block. Anesth Analg 2009;109(2):673–7.

[4] Kulenkampff D. Zur Anaesthesierung des Plaxus brachialis. [On anesthesia of the brachial plexus]. Zentralblatt fuer Chirurgie 1911;38:13.

[5] Moore DC. "No paresthesias-no anesthesia," the nerve stimulator or neither? Reg Anesth 1997;22(4):388–90.

[6] Sia S, Bartoli M, Lepri A, et al. Multiple-injection axillary brachial plexus block: a comparison of two methods of nerve localization-nerve stimulation versus paresthesia. Anesth Analg 2000;91(3):647–51.

[7] Perlas A, Niazi A, McCartney C, et al. The sensitivity of motor response to nerve stimulation and paresthesia for nerve localization as evaluated by ultrasound. Reg Anesth Pain Med 2006;31(5):445–50.

[8] Greenblatt GM, Denson JS. Needle nerve stimulator locator: nerve blocks with a new instrument for locating nerves. Anesth Analg 1962;41:599–602.

[9] Pither CE. Insulation of needles. Anaesthesia 1988;43(11):991.

[10] Selander D. Paresthesias or no paresthesias? Nerve complications after neural blockades. Acta Anaesthesiol Belg 1988;39(3 Suppl 2):173–4.

[11] Selander D. Peripheral nerve damage and regional anaesthesia. Br J Anaesth 1995;75(1):116–7.

[12] Selander D, Edshage S, Wolff T. Paresthesiae or no paresthesiae? Nerve lesions after axillary blocks. Acta Anaesthesiol Scand 1979;23(1):27–33.

[13] Goldberg ME, Gregg C, Larijani GE, et al. A comparison of three methods of axillary approach to brachial plexus blockade for upper extremity surgery. Anesthesiology 1987;66(6):814–6.

[14] Urmey WF, Stanton J. Inability to consistently elicit a motor response following sensory paresthesia during interscalene block administration. Anesthesiology 2002;96(3):552–4.

[15] Urmey WF. Using the nerve stimulator for peripheral or plexus nerve blocks. Minerva Anestesiol 2006;72(6):467–71.

[16] Chan VW, Brull R, McCartney CJ, et al. An ultrasonographic and histological study of intraneural injection and electrical stimulation in pigs. Anesth Analg 2007;104(5):1281–4 [tables of contents].

[17] la Grange P, Foster PA, Pretorius LK. Application of the Doppler ultrasound bloodflow detector in supraclavicular brachial plexus block. Br J Anaesth 1978;50(9):965–7.

[18] Ting PL, Sivagnanaratnam V. Ultrasonographic study of the spread of local anaesthetic during axillary brachial plexus block. Br J Anaesth 1989;63(3):326–9.

[19] Kapral S, Krafft P, Eibenberger K, et al. Ultrasound-guided supraclavicular approach for regional anesthesia of the brachial plexus. Anesth Analg 1994;78(3):507–13.

[20] Marhofer P, Schrogendorfer K, Koinig H, et al. Ultrasonographic guidance improves sensory block and onset time of three-in-one blocks. Anesth Analg 1997;85(4):854–7.

[21] Marhofer P, Schrogendorfer K, Wallner T, et al. Ultrasonographic guidance reduces the amount of local anesthetic for 3-in-1 blocks. Reg Anesth Pain Med 1998;23(6):584–8.

[22] Perlas A, Chan VW, Simons M. Brachial plexus examination and localization using ultrasound and electrical stimulation: a volunteer study. Anesthesiology 2003;99(2):429–35.

[23] Urmey WF. Interscalene block: the truth about twitches. Reg Anesth Pain Med 2000;25(4):340–2.

[24] Sites BD, Chan VW, Neal JM, et al. The American Society of Regional Anesthesia and Pain Medicine and the European Society of Regional Anaesthesia and Pain Therapy joint committee recommendations for education and training in ultrasound-guided regional anesthesia. Reg Anesth Pain Med 2009;34(1):40–6.

[25] Sites BD, Gallagher JD, Cravero J, et al. The learning curve associated with a simulated ultrasound-guided interventional task by inexperienced anesthesia residents. Reg Anesth Pain Med 2004;29(6):544–8.

[26] Sites BD, Brull R, Chan VW, et al. Artifacts and pitfall errors associated with ultrasound-guided regional anesthesia. Part I: understanding the basic principles of ultrasound physics and machine operations. Reg Anesth Pain Med 2007;32(5):412–8.

[27] Sites BD, Neal JM, Chan V. Ultrasound in regional anesthesia: where should the "focus" be set? Reg Anesth Pain Med 2009;34(6):531–3.

[28] Sites BD, Brull R. Ultrasound guidance in peripheral regional anesthesia: philosophy, evidence-based medicine, and techniques. Curr Opin Anaesthesiol 2006;19(6):630–9.

[29] Chan VW, Perlas A, Rawson R, et al. Ultrasound-guided supraclavicular brachial plexus block. Anesth Analg 2003;97(5):1514–7.

[30] Williams SR, Chouinard P, Arcand G, et al. Ultrasound guidance speeds execution and improves the quality of supraclavicular block. Anesth Analg 2003;97(5):1518–23.

[31] Perlas A, Lobo G, Lo N, et al. Ultrasound-guided supraclavicular block: outcome of 510 consecutive cases. Reg Anesth Pain Med 2009;34(2):171–6.

[32] Tsui BC, Doyle K, Chu K, et al. Case series: ultrasound-guided supraclavicular block using a curvilinear probe in 104 day-case hand surgery patients. Can J Anaesth 2009;56(1): 46–51.

[33] Liu SS, Zayas VM, Gordon MA, et al. A prospective, randomized, controlled trial comparing ultrasound versus nerve stimulator guidance for interscalene block for ambulatory shoulder surgery for postoperative neurological symptoms. Anesth Analg 2009;109(1):265–71.

[34] Liu SS, Gordon MA, Shaw PM, et al. A prospective clinical registry of ultrasound-guided regional anesthesia for ambulatory shoulder surgery. Anesth Analg 2010;111(3): 617–23.

[35] Kapral S, Greher M, Huber G, et al. Ultrasonographic guidance improves the success rate of interscalene brachial plexus blockade. Reg Anesth Pain Med 2008;33(3):253–8.

[36] Salinas FV, Neal JM. A tale of two needle passes. Reg Anesth Pain Med 2008;33(3): 195–8.

[37] Beach ML, Sites BD, Gallagher JD. Use of a nerve stimulator does not improve the efficacy of ultrasound-guided supraclavicular nerve blocks. J Clin Anesth 2006;18(8):580–4.

[38] Brull R, Lupu M, Perlas A, et al. Compared with dual nerve stimulation, ultrasound guidance shortens the time for infraclavicular block performance. Can J Anaesth 2009;56(11): 812–8.

[39] Taboada M, Rodriguez J, Amor M, et al. Is ultrasound guidance superior to conventional nerve stimulation for coracoid infraclavicular brachial plexus block? Reg Anesth Pain Med 2009;34(4):357–60.

[40] Sauter AR, Dodgson MS, Stubhaug A, et al. Electrical nerve stimulation or ultrasound guidance for lateral sagittal infraclavicular blocks: a randomized, controlled, observer-blinded, comparative study. Anesth Analg 2008;106(6):1910–5.

[41] Gurkan Y, Hosten T, Solak M, et al. Lateral sagittal infraclavicular block: clinical experience in 380 patients. Acta Anaesthesiol Scand 2008;52(2):262–6.

[42] Dingemans E, Williams SR, Arcand G, et al. Neurostimulation in ultrasound-guided infraclavicular block: a prospective randomized trial. Anesth Analg 2007;104(5):1275–80 [tables of contents].

[43] Koscielniak-Nielsen ZJ, Stens-Pedersen HL, Lippert FK. Readiness for surgery after axillary block: single or multiple injection techniques. Eur J Anaesthesiol 1997;14(2):164–71.

[44] Morros C, Perez-Cuenca MD, Sala-Blanch X, et al. [Contribution of ultrasound guidance to the performance of the axillary brachial plexus block with multiple nerve stimulation]. Rev Esp Anestesiol Reanim 2009;56(2):69–74 [in Spanish].

[45] Chan VW, Perlas A, McCartney CJ, et al. Ultrasound guidance improves success rate of axillary brachial plexus block. Can J Anaesth 2007;54(3):176–82.

[46] Casati A, Danelli G, Baciarello M, et al. A prospective, randomized comparison between ultrasound and nerve stimulation guidance for multiple injection axillary brachial plexus block. Anesthesiology 2007;106(5):992–6.

[47] Koscielniak-Nielsen ZJ, Rotboll-Nielsen P, Rassmussen H. Patients' experiences with multiple stimulation axillary block for fast-track ambulatory hand surgery. Acta Anaesthesiol Scand 2002;46(7):789–93.

[48] Frederiksen BS, Koscielniak-Nielsen ZJ, Jacobsen RB, et al. Procedural pain of an ultrasound-guided brachial plexus block: a comparison of axillary and infraclavicular approaches. Acta Anaesthesiol Scand 2010;54(4):408–13.

[49] Bloc S, Mercadal L, Garnier T, et al. Comfort of the patient during axillary blocks placement: a randomized comparison of the neurostimulation and the ultrasound guidance techniques. Eur J Anaesthesiol 2010;27(7):628–33.

[50] Salinas FV. Ultrasound and review of evidence for lower extremity peripheral nerve blocks. Reg Anesth Pain Med 2010;35(Suppl 2):S16–25.

[51] Gurnaney H, Kraemer F, Ganesh A. Ultrasound and nerve stimulation to identify an abnormal location of the femoral nerve. Reg Anesth Pain Med 2009;34(6):615.

[52] Sites BD, Beach ML, Chinn CD, et al. A comparison of sensory and motor loss after a femoral nerve block conducted with ultrasound versus ultrasound and nerve stimulation. Reg Anesth Pain Med 2009;34(5):508–13.

[53] Nader A, Malik K, Kendall MC, et al. Relationship between ultrasound imaging and eliciting motor response during femoral nerve stimulation. J Ultrasound Med 2009;28(3):345–50.

[54] Casati A, Baciarello M, Di Cianni S, et al. Effects of ultrasound guidance on the minimum effective anaesthetic volume required to block the femoral nerve. Br J Anaesth 2007;98(6):823–7.

[55] Mariano ER, Loland VJ, Sandhu NS, et al. Ultrasound guidance versus electrical stimulation for femoral perineural catheter insertion. J Ultrasound Med 2009;28(11):1453–60.

[56] Danelli G, Ghisi D, Fanelli A, et al. The effects of ultrasound guidance and neurostimulation on the minimum effective anesthetic volume of mepivacaine 1.5% required to block the sciatic nerve using the subgluteal approach. Anesth Analg 2009;109(5):1674–8.

[57] Bruhn J, Moayeri N, Groen GJ, et al. Soft tissue landmark for ultrasound identification of the sciatic nerve in the infragluteal region: the tendon of the long head of the biceps femoris muscle. Acta Anaesthesiol Scand 2009;53(7):921–5.

[58] Di Benedetto P, Casati A, Bertini L, et al. Posterior subgluteal approach to block the sciatic nerve: description of the technique and initial clinical experiences. Eur J Anaesthesiol 2002;19(9):682–6.

[59] Wadhwa A, Tlucek H, Sessler D. A simple approach to the sciatic nerve that does not require geometric calculations or multiple landmarks. Anesth Analg 2010;110(3):958–63.

[60] Abbas S, Brull R. Ultrasound-guided sciatic nerve block: description of a new approach at the subgluteal space. Br J Anaesth 2007;99(3):445–6 [author reply: 445–6].

[61] Danelli G, Fanelli A, Ghisi D, et al. Ultrasound vs nerve stimulation multiple injection technique for posterior popliteal sciatic nerve block. Anaesthesia 2009;64(6):638–42.

[62] Mariano ER, Cheng GS, Choy LP, et al. Electrical stimulation versus ultrasound guidance for popliteal-sciatic perineural catheter insertion: a randomized controlled trial. Reg Anesth Pain Med 2009;34(5):480–5.

[63] Perlas A, Brull R, Chan VW, et al. Ultrasound guidance improves the success of sciatic nerve block at the popliteal fossa. Reg Anesth Pain Med 2008;33(3):259–65.

[64] van Geffen GJ, van den Broek E, Braak GJ, et al. A prospective randomised controlled trial of ultrasound guided versus nerve stimulation guided distal sciatic nerve block at the popliteal fossa. Anaesth Intensive Care 2009;37(1):32–7.

[65] Vloka JD, Hadzic A, April E, et al. The division of the sciatic nerve in the popliteal fossa: anatomical implications for popliteal nerve blockade. Anesth Analg 2001;92(1):215–7.

[66] Schwemmer U, Markus CK, Greim CA, et al. Sonographic imaging of the sciatic nerve division in the popliteal fossa. Ultraschall Med 2005;26(6):496–500.

[67] Currie JM. Measurement of the depth to the extradural space using ultrasound. Br J Anaesth 1984;56(4):345–7.

[68] Wallace DH, Currie JM, Gilstrap LC, et al. Indirect sonographic guidance for epidural anesthesia in obese pregnant patients. Reg Anesth 1992;17(4):233–6.

[69] Bonazzi M, Bianchi De Grazia L, Di Gennaro S, et al. [Ultrasonography-guided identification of the lumbar epidural space]. Minerva Anestesiol 1995;61(5):201–5 [in Italian].

[70] Grau T, Leipold RW, Conradi R, et al. Efficacy of ultrasound imaging in obstetric epidural anesthesia. J Clin Anesth 2002;14(3):169–75.

[71] Grau T, Leipold RW, Conradi R, et al. Ultrasound imaging facilitates localization of the epidural space during combined spinal and epidural anesthesia. Reg Anesth Pain Med 2001;26(1):64–7.

[72] Grau T, Leipold RW, Conradi R, et al. Ultrasound control for presumed difficult epidural puncture. Acta Anaesthesiol Scand 2001;45(6):766–71.

[73] Grau T, Bartusseck E, Conradi R, et al. Ultrasound imaging improves learning curves in obstetric epidural anesthesia: a preliminary study. Can J Anaesth 2003;50(10):1047–50.

[74] Greher M, Scharbert G, Kamolz LP, et al. Ultrasound-guided lumbar facet nerve block: a sonoanatomic study of a new methodologic approach. Anesthesiology 2004;100(5):1242–8.

[75] Renes SH, Rettig HC, Gielen MJ, et al. Ultrasound-guided low-dose interscalene brachial plexus block reduces the incidence of hemidiaphragmatic paresis. Reg Anesth Pain Med 2009;34(5):498–502.

[76] Renes SH, Spoormans HH, Gielen MJ, et al. Hemidiaphragmatic paresis can be avoided in ultrasound-guided supraclavicular brachial plexus block. Reg Anesth Pain Med 2009;34(6):595–9.

[77] Jack NT, Renes SH, Bruhn J, et al. Phrenic nerve-sparing ultrasound-guided interscalene brachial plexus block in a patient with a contralateral pneumonectomy. Reg Anesth Pain Med 2009;34(6):618.

[78] Barrington MJ, Watts SA, Gledhill SR, et al. Preliminary results of the Australasian Regional Anaesthesia Collaboration: a prospective audit of more than 7000 peripheral nerve and plexus blocks for neurologic and other complications. Reg Anesth Pain Med 2009;34(6): 534–41.

[79] Gnaho A, Eyrieux S, Gentili M. Cardiac arrest during an ultrasound-guided sciatic nerve block combined with nerve stimulation. Reg Anesth Pain Med 2009;34(3):278.

[80] Loubert C, Williams SR, Helie F, et al. Complication during ultrasound-guided regional block: accidental intravascular injection of local anesthetic. Anesthesiology 2008;108(4):759–60.

[81] Auroy Y, Narchi P, Messiah A, et al. Serious complications related to regional anesthesia: results of a prospective survey in France. Anesthesiology 1997;87(3):479–86.

[82] Moayeri N, Bigeleisen PE, Groen GJ. Quantitative architecture of the brachial plexus and surrounding compartments, and their possible significance for plexus blocks. Anesthesiology 2008;108(2):299–304.

[83] Fredrickson MJ, Ball CM, Dalgleish AJ. A prospective randomized comparison of ultrasound guidance versus neurostimulation for interscalene catheter placement. Reg Anesth Pain Med 2009;34(6):590–4.

[84] Mariano ER, Loland VJ, Ilfeld BM. Interscalene perineural catheter placement using an ultrasound-guided posterior approach. Reg Anesth Pain Med 2009;34(1):60–3.

[85] Silvestri E, Martinoli C, Derchi LE, et al. Echotexture of peripheral nerves: correlation between US and histologic findings and criteria to differentiate tendons. Radiology 1995;197(1):291–6.

[86] Eichenberger U, Stockli S, Marhofer P, et al. Minimal local anesthetic volume for peripheral nerve block: a new ultrasound-guided, nerve dimension-based method. Reg Anesth Pain Med 2009;34(3):242–6.

[87] Marhofer P, Eichenberger U, Stockli S, et al. Ultrasonographic guided axillary plexus blocks with low volumes of local anaesthetics: a crossover volunteer study. Anaesthesia 2010;65(3):266–71.

[88] Sandhu NS, Bahniwal CS, Capan LM. Feasibility of an infraclavicular block with a reduced volume of lidocaine with sonographic guidance. J Ultrasound Med 2006;25(1):51–6.

[89] Sandhu NS, Maharlouei B, Patel B, et al. Simultaneous bilateral infraclavicular brachial plexus blocks with low-dose lidocaine using ultrasound guidance. Anesthesiology 2006;104(1):199–201.

[90] Soeding PE, Sha S, Royse CE, et al. A randomized trial of ultrasound-guided brachial plexus anaesthesia in upper limb surgery. Anaesth Intensive Care 2005;33(6):719–25.

[91] Dhir S, Ganapathy S. Use of ultrasound guidance and contrast enhancement: a study of continuous infraclavicular brachial plexus approach. Acta Anaesthesiol Scand 2008;52(3):338–42.

[92] De Tran QH, Bertini P, Zaouter C, et al. A prospective, randomized comparison between single- and double-injection ultrasound-guided infraclavicular brachial plexus block. Reg Anesth Pain Med 2010;35(1):16–21.

[93] Liu FC, Liou JT, Tsai YF, et al. Efficacy of ultrasound-guided axillary brachial plexus block: a comparative study with nerve stimulator-guided method. Chang Gung Med J 2005;28(6):396–402.

[94] Sites BD, Spence BC, Gallagher JD, et al. On the edge of the ultrasound screen: Regional anesthesiologists diagnosing nonneural pathology. Reg Anesth Pain Med 2006;31(6): 555–62.

[95] Yu WP, Xu XZ, Wu DZ, et al. [Efficacy of axillary approach brachial plexus blocking by ultrasound-guided four points via one-puncture technique]. Zhonghua Yi Xue Za Zhi 2007;87(11):740–5 [in Chinese].

[96] Domingo-Triado V, Selfa S, Martinez F, et al. Ultrasound guidance for lateral midfemoral sciatic nerve block: a prospective, comparative, randomized study. Anesth Analg 2007;104(5):1270–4.

[97] Orebaugh SL, Williams BA, Kentor ML. Ultrasound guidance with nerve stimulation reduces the time necessary for resident peripheral nerve blockade. Reg Anesth Pain Med 2007;32(5):448–54.

Advances in Anesthesia 28 (2010) 211–244

ADVANCES IN ANESTHESIA

SEVIER
MOSBY

The Anesthetic Management of Adult Patients with Organ Transplants Undergoing Nontransplant Surgery

Laura Hammel, MD[a],*, Joshua Sebranek, MD[b],
Zoltan Hevesi, MD[b]

[a]Department of Anesthesiology and Critical Care, University of Wisconsin Hospital and Clinics, 600 Highland Avenue, Madison, WI 53792, USA
[b]Department of Anesthesiology, University of Wisconsin Hospital and Clinics, 600 Highland Avenue, Madison, WI 53792, USA

T he United Network for Organ Sharing reports that in 2008 and 2009 there were more than 54,000 organs transplanted in the United States. Survival rates have continued to increase in the past several decades as surgical techniques, immunosuppressive therapy, and infection prophylaxis have improved. On October 31, 2009 there were nearly 280,000 surviving organ recipients who underwent transplantation between 1987 and 2009 (Table 1). Several organ types now have 1-year survival rates of 85% or greater, with some approaching 95%, and 3-year survival rates of 80% or better. Living donor kidney transplants, for example, have 1-year survival rates of 95% and 10-year survival rates greater than 75% [1]. As the number of people surviving organ transplant steadily increases, more of these patients are likely to present for nontransplant-related surgery, either elective or emergent, in centers that are not normally involved in transplant procedures. This population may be more likely to present for surgery than those without previous transplant for many reasons. Laparotomy for small bowel obstruction, hip arthroplasty given the increased risk of fracture and avascular necrosis as a result of chronic steroid use, lymph node excision and biopsy because of increased risk of lymphoproliferative disease, ureteral stent placement and removal and native nephrectomy in kidney transplant recipients, bronchoscopy in lung recipients, and biliary tract interventions in liver recipients are just a few of the increased surgical needs in this population. Incisional hernias rates are increased because of the effects of immunosuppressive drugs on wound healing and, abscess drainage because of increased risk of infection are additional problems requiring surgical intervention [2,3].

Many transplant recipients live relatively normal and productive lives, but often have limited physical reserves. A successful transplant abolishes the

*Corresponding author. E-mail address: Hammel@wisc.edu.

0737-6146/10/$ – see front matter
doi:10.1016/j.aan.2010.09.001

Table 1
United Network for Organ Sharing: patients transplanted in the United States,[a] 1 October 1987 to 31 October 2009 by organ received and most recent status[b]

Organ	Number of recipients (1 Oct 1987 to 31 Oct 2009)	Number of recipients reported with a failed graft but not reported dead[b]	Number of recipients reported dead[b]	Number of recipients not reported dead or with failed graft[b]
Kidney	261492	25135	80223	156134
Kidney-pancreas	16449	3186	4777	8486
Pancreas	5933	1195	1573	3165
Intestine	1694	8	767	919
Liver	90713	176	33164	57373
Heart	46214	34	22289	23891
Lung	18850	15	10735	8100
Heart-lung	1012	2	729	281
Total[c]	427689	29358	149368	248963

[a]The number of unique people who received each type of transplant between 1 October 1987 and 31 October 2009.
[b]The patient status is based on a combination of the most recent follow-up data received for each patient and any information found from the Social Security Death Master File (SSDMF). A patient is known to be dead when a death follow-up is received or a death is found in the SSDMF data. It is not known that all other patients are alive. This assumption could be false in cases where the patient is lost to follow-up, or the notification of death was not entered into the Organ Procurement and Transplantation Network data before January 1, 2010. Similarly, a graft is known to have failed when a graft loss follow-up is received. However, it is not known that all other grafts are currently functioning. For kidney and kidney-pancreas grafts, the availability of the US Center for Medicare & Medicaid Services medical evidence data was also examined to determine whether dialysis was performed after the date of the kidney transplant.
[c]The total does not equal the sum of all organs because some patients received more than 1 type of organ transplant during the time period.

symptoms and replaces function of the failed organ, but often there are persistent abnormalities from the underlying or preexisting illness that may have caused the organ failure or chronic physiologic abnormalities resulting from the organ failure itself [4]. Kidney recipients whose renal failure was caused by diabetic nephropathy and pancreas recipients still have persistent complications of diabetes such as gastropathy and neuropathy. Heart recipients whose heart failure resulted from ischemic cardiomyopathy often have extracardiac vascular disease. Cardiovascular disease is also frequently present in patients with chronic kidney disease and those with previous kidney transplant [5,6]. In addition, although immunosuppressive drug use is essential in this population to prevent allograft rejection and protect its function, these drugs have many adverse effects and can lead to renal dysfunction, bone marrow suppression, increased risk of infection, lymphoproliferative disorders, adrenal insufficiency, and pharmacologic interactions. Graft function can deteriorate with time because of chronic rejection and vasculopathy, but at any time graft function can be compromised or suboptimal as a result of acute rejection.

GENERAL CONSIDERATIONS FOR PREANESTHETIC EVALUATION

When a patient with a previous transplant presents for nontransplant surgery, a comprehensive evaluation and survey by the anesthesiologist should include the following key factors: evaluation of the graft function, health and function of other organ systems or the presence of concomitant diseases, presence of infection, and performance or functional status, during the preanesthetic evaluation. Adherence to the fundamental principles of preoperative evaluation along with a high level of vigilance is required [4,7,8]. Information and medical history should be gathered from the medical record, interview with the patient, next of kin or guardian. If medical information is unavailable locally, attempts should be made to contact the transplant center for pertinent history, especially with regard to previous anesthetics. Other useful information from the transplant center includes their most recent evaluations and recent data on graft function and general health of the patient. Close communication with the transplant team may be the single most important step in preparing the patient for surgery and developing a perioperative anesthetic plan [7].

A thorough review of systems along with a physical examination is essential in this population. Findings such as recent weight gain, edema, dyspnea, sweats, malaise, fever, rashes, abdominal pain, abnormal breath sounds on auscultation, and changes in stool or urine output are just some of the potential signs and symptoms of infection or rejection. It is crucial to remember that this population often does not exhibit typical signs and symptoms of infection and high index of suspicion and vigilance is required. Both infection and rejection are late causes of mortality in transplant patients and it is imperative to rule out these 2 processes before elective surgery.

Preoperative laboratory testing in this population should include evaluation of renal function with electrolytes and creatinine, as well as a complete blood count given the adverse effects immune-suppressant medications may have on these organ systems. Serum glucose should also be considered in those patients on corticosteroids or with diabetes mellitus. If neuraxial anesthesia is planned, consideration should be given to obtaining coagulation studies. Focused and functional testing of the transplanted organ is an important part of the preanesthetic evaluation to assess graft function and exclude active rejection. Table 2 suggests tests that may be required to optimize the safe delivery of anesthesia, although preoperative testing need not be limited to these guidelines. Each preoperative evaluation and testing should be considered individually based on the target organ system(s) to be evaluated, the patient's medical history, and the inherent risks of the upcoming surgical procedure.

Cardiovascular disease is a major cause of mortality and morbidity among organ transplant recipients, especially in those with chronic kidney disease or previous heart transplant, making the risk of a perioperative cardiovascular event a legitimate concern [6,7,9]. After kidney transplantation, a progressive increase in the incidence of ischemic cardiovascular, cerebrovascular, and peripheral vascular events has been documented in epidemiologic studies [5].

Table 2
Preoperative tests on transplant patients

Test target	Essential tests	Consider also
Blood	Total cell count	Hematocrit
	Hemoglobin	
Kidney	Creatinine	Urea
	Urine analysis	Creatinine clearance
Blood electrolytes	Na^+, K^+, Mg^{2+}, Ca^{2+}	
Liver	Prothrombin time	Full coagulation status
	Partial thromboplastin time	Ammonia
	Bilirubins	Albumin
	Aminotransferases	Prealbumin
	Alkaline phosphatase	Cholesterol
		Lactate dehydrogenase
		Galactose elimination capacity
Pancreas	Amylase	Lipase
Lung	Radiography	Spirometry
	Spirometry for lung and marrow	Sputum microbiology
	transplant patients	Blood gas analysis
Heart	Electrocardiography	Echocardiography
		Coronary angiography
Drugs	Cyclosporine or tacrolimus	
	concentration, if applicable	
Infections		C-reactive protein
		Targeted samples
Other	Blood glucose	
	Blood pressure	
	Pulse	
	Temperature	
	Respiratory rate	

Data from Toivonen HJ. Anaesthesia for patients with a transplanted organ. Acta Anaesthiol Scand 2000;44:819.

Many transplant recipients have undergone complete cardiac testing and in some cases, interventions, before their transplant surgery. Records of the testing and interventions can be easily obtained from the transplant center to be used for comparison and consideration before the upcoming surgery. The question that remains is how long a time period may be allowed to pass before additional cardiac testing should be performed before an upcoming elective surgery. There is, unfortunately, no clear or easy single answer or guideline. Each evaluation should proceed on an individual basis with thorough documentation of the patient's exercise capacity and functional status along with an electrocardiogram (ECG), taking into consideration any changes, as well as the inherent risk of the surgery itself and the patient's known cardiovascular history, keeping in mind that many of these patients may have asymptomatic coronary disease as a result of diabetes or the transplant itself. It may be prudent to discuss the upcoming surgery, need for testing, and perioperative optimization, such as initiation of beta-blocker therapy, with the patient's transplant team or cardiologist, especially if there is documented cardiovascular disease or previous cardiac intervention.

Posttransplantation diabetes mellitus (PTDM) is a common metabolic consequence of the agents of immunosuppressive therapy. PTDM is defined as sustained hyperglycemia that meets the diagnostic criteria of the American Diabetic Association (ADA) in any posttransplant patient who was not previously diabetic [10,11]. PTDM is generally assigned to the classification of type 2 diabetes because its pathophysiology is a combination of insulin resistance and insulin secretion defects. Risk factors for PTDM include age, nonwhite ethnicity, increased body mass index (BMI, calculated as weight in kilograms divided by the square of height in meters), chronic hepatitis C infection, pretransplant glucose intolerance, and use of glucocorticoids and calcineurin inhibitors. The incidence of PTDM is reported to be as high as 25% and possibly higher in patients with hepatitis C [4,11]. Unfortunately, PTDM has a negative effect on graft survival. Preexisting diabetes has implications for perioperative complications and morbidity, especially increased infection risk and poor wound healing. It is imperative to institute a plan of glycemic control before surgery with close attention to intraoperative and postoperative glucose management. Hyperglycemia suppresses various aspects of immune function, causes endothelial dysfunction and altered vascular reactivity, increases circulating inflammatory mediators, and is associated with a procoagulant state. If hyperglycemia is identified during the preoperative evaluation, the patient's primary care provider may be contacted to assist in the effort to achieve glycemic control before elective surgery. It is not within the scope of this document to debate the literature and the issues surrounding intensive glycemic control. Most of the information gathered is taken from studies of glycemic control in the intensive care unit and has been extrapolated to the perioperative period. The actual level of hyperglycemia that is predictive of adverse outcome is debated, but perioperative serum glucose levels greater than 200 mg/dL seem to be consistently associated with adverse outcomes including stroke, myocardial infarction, poor wound healing, infection, and death [12,13]. Maintaining perioperative glucose between 120 and 180 mg/dL is a conservative approach that might avoid the perils of intensive glucose control yet control hyperglycemia. If the patient has a serum glucose level of greater than 300 mg/dL documented on 2 or more consecutive checks, consideration should be given to postponing elective surgery until adequate glycemia is achieved.

If unexpected abnormal findings are identified on physical examination or laboratory testing, symptomatic changes outside the patient's baseline are documented, or suspicion for rejection or infection exists during the preanesthetic evaluation, consideration should be given to postponing any surgery that is nonurgent or elective. The patient should also be expeditiously referred back to the transplant center, cardiologist, or other consulting physician as indicated.

GENERAL CONSIDERATIONS OF ANESTHETIC MANAGEMENT

There is no ideal or generic anesthetic plan that can be used for all transplant recipients undergoing nontransplant surgery. There are no prospective studies comparing anesthesia techniques, but most anesthetics have been used with success including general (inhalational, balanced, and total intravenous), neuraxial, regional, and monitored anesthesia. A successful anesthetic plan requires a clear understanding of the medical and pharmacologic problems that accompany this population, the function and physiology of the allograft, functionality and general health of the patient, the underlying surgical condition, and proposed surgical procedure [4,14].

Monitoring

As a general rule, special equipment is not needed and anesthesia should be performed using standard American Society of Anesthesiology's monitoring guidelines. The decision to use invasive hemodynamic monitors, placement of central venous access, pulmonary artery catheters or other procedures such as transesophageal echocardiography should be made on a case by case basis. This decision should be guided by consideration of the patient's comorbidities, hemodynamic stability, the expertise of the anesthesiologist in placing the invasive device and interpreting the data, the inherent risk of the surgery, and the overall risk to benefit ratio of the proposed monitor [15]. It is important to consider that central venous access may be difficult as many of these patients have had long-standing illnesses with the need for central venous catheters for parenteral nutrition, hemodialysis, esophageal variceal hemorrhage, sepsis, and other clinical problems that required central venous access. These may have been complicated by thrombosis, stenosis, and infection making reaccessing these veins difficult or impossible [14]. Meticulous hygiene practice and aseptic technique are of utmost importance to minimize exposure to infectious organisms and bacteremia when attempting any invasive procedures in this population [4,8,16].

Airway Management

Airway management of transplant patients may pose a concern for several reasons. Many patients may have preexisting diabetes mellitus before transplant or acquire diabetes after transplant (PTDM). Diabetic patients can develop limitations in joint mobility caused by glycosylation of the connective tissue within their joints. Several retrospective and prospective evaluations performed at transplant institutions in patients with diabetes mellitus undergoing kidney and/or pancreas transplantation report increased rates of difficult laryngoscopy, including a retrospective analysis from our institution [17–19]. The airway management plan should be formulated after careful airway examination and review of previous anesthetic records. If recent records are not available locally, they may be obtained from the transplant center keeping in mind that if extended time has elapsed since the last anesthetic, the ongoing effects of diabetes on the mandibular and atlanto-occipital joints may result in a difficult intubation not previously reported. Graft-versus-host disease can also create limited joint mobility creating a similar scenario. This population is also at increased risk for lymphoproliferative disorders secondary to immune-suppressant drugs, and lymphoproliferative growth may compromise any part of the airway or mediastinum and cause life-threatening airway obstruction during sedation and anesthesia. Aspiration risk may be increased in transplanted patients as a result of delayed gastric emptying and gastropathy [4,8]. These potential problems should all be taken into consideration when constructing the anesthetic plan for airway management.

Oral endotracheal tubes are preferred over nasal tubes because of the increased potential for infection from the nasal route in this immune-compromised population. Early postoperative extubation is preferred if possible to prevent the development of nosocomial or ventilator-associated pneumonia.

Antibiotic Prophylaxis

Antibiotic prophylaxis has not been studied extensively in transplant recipients undergoing nontransplant surgery. Although transplant patients are considered at-risk hosts for infection because of their immune status, there is no evidence to suggest different bacteriology of surgical site infections than for the general population. However, the use of prophylaxis even for clean cases in this higher risk population is advocated and has some supporting evidence [20,21]. It is recommended that the guidelines for surgical antibiotic prophylaxis from the National Surgical Infection Project be followed and should be given before incision.(Table 3). Antimicrobial coverage need not be expanded to include atypical or opportunistic organisms as long as active infection with such an organism is not present or suspected [7,21,22].

General Anesthesia

All inhalational and intravenous anesthetics have been used with success in transplant recipients. The choice of anesthetics and adjunctive drugs should be determined by the type of surgery and condition of the patient. As a general guideline, if hepatic and renal functions are normal, all standard anesthetic medications and adjuncts may be used. Some special considerations for each type of organ transplant are discussed in the section on organ-specific considerations.

Intravenous Anesthetics

Premedication with benzodiazepines is acceptable, keeping in mind that most are metabolized by the liver and may have active metabolites that are cleared via the kidneys. Caution should be used in patients with hepatic or renal insufficiency as effects may be prolonged. Benzodiazepines should be avoided in patients who are somnolent or if there is a concern of respiratory depression or obstruction, as with any anesthetic that is performed. Some centers avoid them to facilitate extubation, but this is probably not justified in most surgeries. The intended effect of anxiolysis augments a smooth and more tolerated anesthetic.

Table 3
Antimicrobial prophylaxis for selected surgical procedures

Operation	Recommended antibiotic prophylaxis	Comments
Cardiothoracic surgery	Cefazolin, cefuroxime, or cefamandole. If patient has a β-lactam allergy: vancomycin or clindamycin	Most of the guidelines agree that prophylaxis for cardiac surgery should be administered for >24 h after surgery. The ASHP suggests continuation of prophylaxis for cardiothoracic surgery up to 72 h; however, its authors suggest that prophylaxis for <24 h may be appropriate. Cefamandole is not available in the United States
Vascular surgery	Cefazolin or cefuroxime. If patient has a β-lactam allergy: vancomycin with or without gentamycin, or clindamycin	Currently, none of the guidelines address antimicrobial prophylaxis for those patients with β-lactam allergy. Cefmetazole is not available in the United States. Although a recent study indicates that the combination of oral prophylaxis with parenteral antibiotics may result in lower wound infection rates, this is not specified in any of the published guidelines
Colon surgery	Oral: neomycin plus erythromycin base, or neomycin plus metronidazole. Parenteral: cefoxitin or cefotetan, or cefazolin plus metronidazole	
Hip or knee arthroplasty	Cefazolin or cefuroxime. If the patient has a β-lactam allergy: vancomycin or clindamycin	Although not addressed in any of the published guidelines, the workgroup recommends that prophylactic antimicrobial be completely infused before inflation of the tourniquet. Cefuroxime is recommended as a choice for patients undergoing total hip arthroplasty
Vaginal or abdominal hysterectomy	Cefazolin, cefotetan, cefoxitin, or cefuroxime	Metronidazole monotherapy is recommended in the ACOG Practice Bulletin as an alternative to cephalosporin prophylaxis for patients undergoing hysterectomy. Trovafloxin, although still available in the United States, is recommended only for serious infections

Abbreviations: ACOG, American College of Obstetricians and Gynecologists; ASHP, American Society of Health-System Pharmacists.
Data from Bratzler DW, Houck PM. Antimicrobial prophylaxis for surgery: an advisory statement from the National Surgical Infection Prevention Project. Clin Infect Dis 2004;38:1706–15.

The selection and administration of intravenous anesthetics should be guided by the patient's hemodynamic status, the drug's cardiovascular effects and pharmacokinetic properties, especially the biotransformation and elimination profiles of the drug. Drugs that undergo primarily hepatic metabolism, such as barbiturates, should be dose adjusted if administered to avoid prolonged effects in patients with hepatic insufficiency. Care should be taken when using barbiturates as cardiac output and mean arterial pressures can decrease precipitously as a result of venous pooling and loss of cardiac preload. Propofol is extensively metabolized by the liver to inactive glucuronic acid metabolites that are excreted by the kidneys. Despite the known mechanisms of biotransformation, there seems to be no need for dose adjustments in patients with hepatic or renal failure indicating an extrahepatic route of elimination as well [23]. Care should be used in patients with cardiovascular compromise as propofol can worsen cardiac contractility, compromise cardiac preload, cause bradycardia, and lower systemic vascular resistance culminating in diminished cardiac output and mean arterial pressure. Etomidate does not have the cardiac depressant effect of barbiturates and propofol. Etomidate is metabolized rapidly by hydrolysis within the liver and by plasma esterases, and also does not require dosage adjustment in renal or hepatic disease. One unique characteristic of etomidate is its ability to inhibit the 11-β-hydroxylase, an enzyme necessary for the synthesis of cortisol, for 5 to 8 hours after administration. The clinical significance in patients who already have adrenal suppression as a result of exogenous steroid use is unclear, but heightened attention should be paid to the need for perioperative stress-dose corticosteroids [23]. Ketamine is metabolized via the hepatic cytochrome P-450 system to norketamine, which has approximately one-third of the clinical activity of its parent and therefore the clinical effects of ketamine are prolonged in the presence of hepatic insufficiency. The metabolites of norketamine are excreted by the kidneys. The usual cardiac stimulating effects caused by central stimulation of the sympathetic system are not present in the denervated heart, but ketamine can still increase systemic vascular tone. Ketamine has neuroexcitatory effects and is known to cause myoclonic activity, although its ability to actually cause seizures is debated [23]. However, there are case reports of seizures after its administration in patients who have previously had liver transplant and in the presence of cyclosporine, an immunosuppressant drug with the potential for neurotoxicity [24]. Table 4 is an abbreviated list of drugs commonly used in the perioperative period that have active metabolites that require renal excretion and accumulate in patients with renal insufficiency.

Inhalational Anesthetics

All inhaled anesthetics have been used in transplanted patients with success. Among the inhaled anesthetics currently used, only halothane requires a truly cautionary note given its potential for hepatotoxicity and direct cardiac depressant effects. Of the most commonly used volatile anesthetics in the United States today, isoflurane, desflurane, and sevoflurane, there does not seem to

Table 4
Drugs with renally excreted active metabolites and their actions

Morphine	Morphine 6-glucuronide	Antianalgesic
	Morphine 3-glucuronide	Potent sedative-analgesic
	Normorphine	Neuroexcitatory and seizures
Meperidine	Normeperidine	Neuroexcitatory and seizures
Diazepam	Oxazepam	Sedative
Midazolam	1-Hydroxymidazolam	Sedative
Vecuronium	Desacetyl-vecuronium	Neuromuscular blockade
Ketamine	Norketamine	Neuroexcitatory and psychomimmetic actions

Data from Littlewood K. The immunocompromised adult and surgery. Best Pract Res Clin Anaesth 2008; 22(3):585–609.

be a significant clinical advantage or disadvantage of one over the others. The choice of inhaled anesthetic can be dictated by the anesthesiologist's preference, experiences, and comfort with the anesthetic [25]. The decision whether or not to use a volatile anesthetic need not be imposed by the presence of a transplanted organ, but should be guided by other patient factors, such as hemodynamic stability and history or risk of malignant hyperthermia. The theoretic risk of nephrotoxicity caused by the liberation of free fluoride and Compound A following sevoflurane metabolism does not seem to be a true clinical concern outside of laboratory animals [4,25]. The decision to use nitrous oxide (N_2O) as part of the anesthetic should be considered with caution. Whether or not to use N_2O as part of the anesthetic should be based on clinical findings of the patient and type of surgical procedure, such as the potential for postoperative nausea and for expanding air-filled cavities such as pneumothorax, intestinal obstruction, and tympanic membrane grafts. It is probably prudent to avoid prolonged use of N_2O because of the potential risk of bone marrow suppression and the potential for altered immunologic response (impaired chemotaxis and motility of polymorphonuclear leukocytes) [25]. Although these effects were seen in laboratory animals receiving N_2O for more than 24 hours, they may be potentiated in immune-compromised patients. N_2O can also worsen preexisting pulmonary hypertension, which may be present in patients who have undergone lung, heart, or liver transplant, by increasing pulmonary vascular resistance and potentiating hypoxemia. N_2O is best avoided in patients who have known or suspected pulmonary hypertension. Although there is little data on the use of N_2O in the transplanted population, the brief use of N_2O during induction or emergence is probably acceptable and without clinical consequence but may be best avoided if there are alternatives [25,26].

Neuromuscular Blockade

The decision to use neuromuscular blockade should be based on the type of surgery and actual need for muscle relaxation during the procedure or the need to optimize intubating conditions. The choice of specific neuromuscular blocking agent to be used should be dictated by length of surgery, underlying medical illnesses such as myasthenia or other neuromuscular disorders, history of malignant hyperthermia, and the functional state of the patient's kidney and liver. Of the nondepolarizing agents, the metabolism and clearance of mivacurium, a short-acting agent, and cisatracurium and atracurium, intermediate-acting agents, are independent of kidney and liver function (Table 5). In the presence of a normally functioning kidney or liver graft, other nondepolarizing agents, such as vecuronium, rocuronium, and pancuronium, exhibit normal clinical activity, but can have prolonged effects in the face of hepatic or renal insufficiency and require dose adjustments and close neuromuscular monitoring and evidence of full reversal before extubation [27]. Some immune-suppressant drugs can have effects on neuromuscular blockade. Azathioprine can increase the dose required to achieve and maintain muscle relaxation and cyclosporine can prolong the action of the neuromuscular blocking agents [28]. Succinylcholine, the only depolarizing agent available in the United States currently, is used frequently in this population given the need for rapid sequence intubation and rapid airway control. There are no contraindications in patients who have undergone organ transplant with the possible exception of previous cardiac transplant, in which its actions can be complex. Otherwise, succinylcholine should be avoided only if there are other clinical reasons, such as hyperkalemia, muscular dystrophy, or history of malignant hyperthermia [27,28].

Regional and Neuraxial Anesthesia

There are few contraindications to performing a regional or neuraxial anesthetic in previously transplanted patients. The consideration of spinal or epidural anesthesia is appropriate in this population as long as there is no increased risk for bleeding complications. There may be several advantages to choosing a neuraxial or regional technique in this population. Superior analgesia over systemic opioids, especially in patients who may have narcotics tolerance as a result of long-term opioid use, reduced pulmonary complications, decreased incidence of graft occlusion, and improved joint mobility are just a few of the benefits of regional and neuraxial anesthesia [29]. Clinically relevant doses of bupivicaine and ropiviciane, which are commonly used local anesthetics for neuraxial anesthesia, do not seem to result in toxic levels or

Table 5	
Drugs not solely dependent on renal and/or hepatic elimination	
Drug	Metabolism
Succinylcholine	Pseudocholinesterase
Propofol	Extrahepatic and hepatic metabolism
Esmolol	Red cell esterase
Remifentanil	Nonspecific esterases
Cisatracurium	Hofmann elimination
Mivacurium	Pseudocholinesterase
Atracurium	Non specific plasma esterase
Etomidate	Plasma esterases and hepatic metabolism

increased risk of toxic effects in renal and liver transplant recipients [8,14]. However, it is important to be prepared for the risk of hypotension because of preexisting autonomic neuropathy and cardiac denervation in this population when performing a neuraxial anesthetic [9,29]. Concurrent hemodynamic monitoring is imperative during the procedure. Direct and indirect-acting adrenergic agonists should be readily available along with emergency airway supplies. Cautious correction of hypovolemia before epidural or spinal anesthesia may help to attenuate the hypotension.

Although the risk of epidural abscess complicating epidural anesthesia is low (about 1 in 2000 or less), there seems to be a very slight increase of the incidence in immunocompromised patients in many epidemiologic series. *Staphylococcus aureus* is isolated in approximately two-thirds of the epidural abscesses indicating infection from normal skin flora. Meningitis after spinal anesthesia seemingly does not have a greater disposition for immunocompromised hosts compared with healthy patients. When meningitis occurs after spinal anesthesia, the organism cultured is usually an oropharyngeal bacteria implying iatrogenic infection from the proceduralist [29,30]. Therefore, if a neuraxial block is included in the anesthetic plan, it is imperative that strict aseptic technique is practiced and a mask should be worn. Although the risk of infectious complications is very low, it is important to be highly vigilant when monitoring these patients after a neuraxial anesthetic as the attenuated inflammatory response may diminish the typical signs and symptoms of epidural abscess or meningitis [29].

There is limited information available on the incidence of infectious complications after peripheral nerve block procedures in immunocompromised patients, other than a few case reports and series. Overall, the incidence of infectious complications seems to be extremely low, even in immune-suppressed patients. When they do occur, the organisms cultured are similar to those found in infections after neuraxial anesthesia, *Staphylococcus aureus* and mouth organisms, indicating skin or mouth flora from the anesthesiologist or patient as the source [31]. Again, aseptic technique and a mask should be considered essential when performing these procedures.

There may be other, albeit less well understood benefits of using a neuraxial or regional anesthetic technique in this population. There is consistent evidence that surgical stress suppresses both cellular and humoral immune function for several days after surgery. This effect may be exaggerated or prolonged in patients with preexisting immune dysfunction. General anesthetics alone do not diminish the surgical stress response [20,29]. Neuraxial anesthesia and postoperative analgesia are associated with some preservation of cell-mediated immunity and attenuated inflammatory response. Local anesthetics themselves lessen the inflammatory response to stress and injury [20,32]. The risk to benefit ratio of neuraxial anesthesia or regional block may, therefore, be altered in previously transplanted patients. The decision to perform a regional or neuraxial anesthetic technique in a previously transplanted patient must be made on an individual basis. Anesthetic alternatives, the risks of the technique that may be increased, balanced with the potential for greater benefit should all be carefully considered when constructing the anesthetic plan in this population.

Postoperative Pain Management

In addition to the use of neuraxial anesthesia and peripheral nerve blocks, opiates are also reasonable options for intraoperative and postoperative analgesia, keeping in mind the patient's renal and hepatic function. Delayed clearance of opioids can result in prolonged sedation in patients with underlying hepatic or renal insufficiency. Several of the narcotics have active metabolites that are renally excreted and can accumulate, such as morphine 3-glucuronide, which is 40 times as potent as morphine, and morphine 6-glucuoronide. Normeperidine, a metabolite of meperidine, is neuroexcitatory and has the potential to cause seizures as a result of delayed clearance in patients with renal insufficiency [9,33]. Remifentanil, which is cleared by plasma ester hydrolysis, is not affected by hepatic or renal function and may be an acceptable choice of opioid in this population (see Table 5) [33]. In the presence of a normally functioning kidney or liver graft, these drugs are metabolized and eliminated in a normal fashion and in usual clinical doses there should be no prolonged effects. Nonsteroidal antiinflammatory drugs are best avoided or used cautiously in this population of patients given their potential for hepatotoxicity and nephrotoxicity [4,8].

PERIOPERATIVE MANAGEMENT OF IMMUNOSUPPRESSIVE REGIMEN

Almost all survivors of organ transplant are immunocompromised, whether by the antirejection drugs or underlying illness such as an autoimmune disease or diabetes mellitus that caused their organ failure or both. Their immune competence can be further altered by a period of acute illness, the stress of surgery, and disruption of their immunosuppressive regimen by inexperienced providers. This instability can readily result in acute rejection, acute infection, or both [16]. The first step in perioperative planning requires a call to the transplant center to discuss the perioperative management of the patient's immunesuppressant drug regimen. In all instances, a transplant coordinator or other member of the transplant team will assist in devising the perioperative management plan for the immune-suppressant regimen.

It is helpful to have a basic understanding of the drugs most commonly used and their side-effect profile and drug interactions. Standard maintenance immunosuppression regimens usually consist of a combination of 2 or 3 drugs from the following classes: corticosteroids, calcineurin inhibitors, antiproliferatives, and inhibitors of the protein kinase mTOR. The number of drugs used and variations of the regimen are based on the recipient's risk of rejection, immunogenicity of the allograft (liver being the least allogeneic), and adverse reactions or toxicities that develop while on the drugs [20,28]. Corticosteroids are a key component of most maintenance regimens and are associated with numerous well-known adverse effects including hypertension, central obesity, hyperlipidemia, diabetes mellitus, and osteoporosis. Adrenal suppression occurs as the result of chronic use of exogenous corticosteroids and can manifest as overt adrenal insufficiency during times of stress, illness, surgery, or abrupt withdrawal. The decision to give stress-dose steroid prophylaxis is controversial. Despite the lack of data, most investigators recommend a preoperative augmentation of corticosteroids and in transplant recipients, a postoperative increase in the corticosteroid dose, with a rapid return to baseline dose based on the extent or stress of the surgery, time to recovery, and ability to take oral medications. In the transplant recipient, the prevention of postoperative allograft rejection is just as crucial as prevention of intraoperative adrenal crisis [7,21,28]. At our institution, dexamethasone 10 mg intravenously (IV) or hydrocortisone 50 to 100 mg IV is given at the time of surgery, followed by dexamethasone 3 mg IV every 12 hours for 2 or 3 days, or until the patient can resume their normal oral immunosuppressive regimen.

Calcineurin inhibitors have been an integral part of antirejection treatment since the 1980s. Tacrolimus is available in oral and intravenous preparations. Tacrolimus has replaced the use of cyclosporine in many instances. If the prospective surgical patient's regimen includes tacrolimus and the recommendation from the transplant center includes a course of IV tacrolimus, it is wise to communicate with your local pharmacy to determine if this drug is readily available. Monitoring of serum levels of tacrolimus is also required because of the narrow therapeutic index. It is also suggested to determine the turnaround time for this information as this drug level may not be immediately available at your institution, which may also pose a challenge in the care of these patients. The most common adverse effect of calcineurin inhibitors is nephrotoxicity. Other adverse effects include neurotoxicity and diabetes mellitus [28].

Azathioprine was the first immunosuppressive agent to be used with clinical success and is an inhibitor of purine nucleotide synthesis or an antiproliferative. It has been widely replaced by mycophenylate mofetil (MMF). The major side effects of MMF are gastrointestinal upset, leukopenia, anemia, and increased incidence of invasive cytomegalovirus infections, especially the gastrointestinal tract. MMF does not require therapeutic drug monitoring [20,28].

Sirolimus was introduced in 2000 and complexes with the protein kinase mTOR causing an arrest in a certain phase of the cell cycle. Sirolimus is effective when used in combination with a calcineurin inhibitor or antiproliferative drug. When used in conjunction with a calcineurin inhibitor it allows lower doses of the calcineurin inhibitor to be used, decreasing the risk of nephrotoxicity. Its use is limited by the development of hepatic artery thrombosis immediately after liver transplant, and thrombotic microangiopathy when used with cyclosporine concomitantly in kidney and kidney-pancreas recipients. The most common side effects of sirolimus include thrombocytopenia, anemia, leukopenia, diarrhea, and mouth ulcers. It is also associated with wound complications. The most serious and potentially fatal complication is interstitial alveolar pneumonitis [20,28].

ORGAN-SPECIFIC CONSIDERATIONS FOR ANESTHETIC MANAGEMENT OF THE TRANSPLANTED PATIENT

Thoracic Organs: Heart and Lung

Anesthesia for patients after heart transplant

According to the International Society for Heart and Lung Transplantation (ISHLT), more than 80,000 heart transplants have been performed since the first in 1967. In the ISHLT's 25th Official Adult Heart Transplant Report, the total number of heart transplants performed annually is estimated at 5000 worldwide. This report highlights several interesting trends in heart transplantation. First, the primary indication for transplantation has shifted from a balance between both ischemic and nonischemic cardiomyopathy to most patients being transplanted for nonischemic cardiomyopathy (50%). Ischemic cardiomyopathy now accounts for only 34% of transplantations. Other indications include adult congenital heart disease (3%), retransplantation (2%), and valvular heart disease (2%). Second, the average age of transplant recipients is increasing. Currently, 25% of all heart transplant recipients are age 60 years or more. Third, survival of transplant recipients continues to improve. The projected half-life for the most recent cohort of recipients is approximately 11 years; recipients transplanted between 1982 and 1991 had a half-life of 8.8 years. Fourth, morbidity data show the incidence of hyperlipidemia, renal insufficiency, and diabetes in this patient population continues to increase. Fifth, mortality data highlight the difficulty in striking a balance between inadequate and excessive immunosuppression. Cardiac allograft vasculopathy (CAV), believed to be an immune-mediated process, and late graft failure accounted for 33% of deaths in patients surviving beyond 5 years. Malignancy (23%) and infection (11%), both unfortunate consequences of immunosuppression, continue to have a significant effect on morbidity in long-term survivors [34].

As the number of heart transplant recipients increases, so does their average age, average life expectancy, and number of significant comorbidities. Anesthesiologists can expect to see them with increasing frequency in the operating room. A single-center study from the University of Toronto followed 86 heart transplant patients for 4 years and found that 18 of them returned to the operating room for a total of 32 noncardiac operations requiring anesthesia. Surgical cases included 9 cataract surgeries; 3 pacemaker insertions and laparotomies; 2 central line insertions, dental extractions, cholecystectomies, and inguinal herniorrhaphies; and 1 scleral buckle, brain tumor biopsy, thrombectomy, osteotomy, ileostomy, bronchoscopy, lung resection, and transurethral resection of prostate [35].

No randomized, double-blinded, controlled trial has been performed to determine the most appropriate choice of anesthetic for noncardiac surgery after heart transplantation. There is, however, a growing body of anecdotal reports, case reports, review articles, retrospective studies, and small case series addressing this patient population. Cumulatively, these reports and investigations suggest that with thoughtful and thorough preoperative evaluation, intraoperative vigilance, and attention to the special needs of these patients postoperatively; sedation, regional blocks, neuraxial blocks, and general anesthetics can be safely administered to the cardiac transplant patient for nontransplant surgery.

Surgical technique. The classic technique of heart transplantation continues to be used in modern-day operations. A median sternotomy is followed by exposure of the native heart and cannulation of the great vessels. Bicaval cannulation and institution of cardiopulmonary bypass (CPB) allows for removal of the native heart. A cuff of native, posterior right atrial tissue, surrounding both the inferior vena cava (IVC) and superior vena cava (SVC) ostia, along with a portion of the intraatrial septum and a cuff of posterior left atrial tissue, surrounding the ostia of the 4 pulmonary veins, is saved. The donor heart is inserted and an anastomosis is made between the donor left atrial free wall and the native left atrial tissue (containing the pulmonary vein ostia), continuing with an anastomosis to the intraatrial septum, and finally anastomosing the recipient's native right atrial tissue (containing the SVC and IVC ostia) to the donor right atrium. This is followed by both aortic and pulmonary artery anastomoses.

This technique is associated with significant morphologic changes of the right atrium and subsequent changes in tricuspid annular morphology. This results in significant tricuspid regurgitation (TR) in a high percentage of posttransplant patients. Unfortunately, tricuspid regurgitation is associated with decreased long-term survival in this patient population. As a result, several modifications to the classic technique have been proposed including the addition of a tricuspid annular ring or replacement of the tricuspid valve at the time of surgery. More recently, interest has shifted to a technique requiring bicaval anastomoses rather than the anastomosis of a right atrial cuff to the donor heart. Investigations of this technique show a significant decrease in the incidence of TR (31% vs 70%), no stenosis at the level of the venous anastomoses, and fewer atrial arrhythmias (15% vs 55%). This does not lead to significant increase in CPB time or donor organ ischemic time [36].

Immunosuppression. The ISHLT's 25th Official Adult Heart Transplant Report follows trends in posttransplant immunosuppression. These patients receive a course of induction immunosuppression followed by a separate regimen of maintenance immunosuppression. Maintenance therapy typically involves 2 immunosuppressive drugs with or without the addition of a corticosteroid (prednisone). The ISHLT reports there is no standardized regimen for immunosuppressive therapy for patients after heart transplantation. The most commonly used therapy is the combination of tacrolimus and mycophenolate mofetil (MMF) with or without corticosteroids (46%); 30% of patients were on the combination of cyclosporine and MMF with or without corticosteroids. Other common immunosuppressive drugs used in maintenance therapy include rapamycin and azathioprine [34].

Each immunosuppressive drug is associated with its own specific side effects. Anesthesia providers must be aware of these side effects. There are a few relevant interactions between immunosuppressive drugs and anesthetic drugs.

Corticosteroids are renowned for their side-effect profile. Of particular importance for the anesthesia provider is their propensity to cause adrenal suppression, hypokalemia, hypocalcemia, and hyperglycemia. Corticosteroids can also contribute to fluid retention, poor wound healing, obesity, osteoporosis, and steroid myopathy.

Cyclosporine is a highly nephrotoxic drug. It can also cause hypertension, hepatotoxicity, tremors, and seizures. The gingival hyperplasia and gastric atony, as well as the hyperkalemia and hypomagnesemia caused by cyclosporine can have obvious anesthetic implications. Cyclosporine has been reported to dramatically increase the duration of action of vecuronium and pancuronium [8]. It is available as an intravenous drug for patients unable to take the parenteral form. Cyclosporine blood levels should be closely monitored in the perioperative period.

Azathioprine's most significant side effects are myelosuppression and hepatotoxicity. Laboratory investigations suggest a slight antagonistic effect with nondepolarizing neuromuscular blockers, but this has been deemed clinically insignificant [37]. Tacrolimus is both nephrotoxic and neurotoxic. It has also been shown to cause hypertension, hyperlipidemia and hyperglycemia. MMF causes leukopenia and a variety of gastrointestinal symptoms. Rapamycin is known to cause myelosuppression and hyperlipidemia.

Posttransplant physiology. There are several, notable physiologic differences between a native heart and a transplanted heart. The most remarkable difference, and arguably that with the most anesthetic implications, is denervation. Efferent denervation ablates the resting parasympathetic tone responsible for maintaining baseline heart rate. Because of this, transplanted patients generally have an increased baseline heart rate of 90 to 100 beats per minute [38]. The loss of direct sympathetic innervation means that the cardiac response to physiologic stressors (exercise, hypovolemia, vasodilatation, pain, light anesthesia) is mediated by circulating catecholamines and, as a result, tends to occur much less quickly. Predominantly parasympathetic responses (visceral traction, abdominal insufflation, oculocardiac reflex, vasovagal bradycardia, hypertension-induced bradycardia, cardiac response to carotid massage, Valsalva maneuvers) are absent. Denervation also has pharmacologic ramifications. The denervated heart no longer responds normally to indirect-acting medications (medications that mediate effects via the autonomic nervous system). Administration of drugs such as neostigmine, physostigmine, pyridostigmine, edrophonium, glycopyrrolate, atropine, digoxin, and nifedipine no longer produce their anticipated heart rate effects. Indirect-acting drugs such as ephedrine have a decreased effect. Direct-acting drugs such as glucagon, norepinephrine, epinephrine, isoproterenol, dopamine, and beta-blockers are effective choices for managing hemodynamics in these patients. Reflex responses such as the bradycardia expected after administration of phenylephrine may not be present. Also, there is no evidence for alpha and beta receptor upregulation or denervation hypersensitivity after heart transplant [35]. There are several case reports suggesting reinnervation months to years after heart transplantation [39]. One dramatic report describes asystole after administration of neostigmine [40]. It is recommended that a muscarinic antagonist be administered in conjunction with an anticholinesterase in all heart transplant patients. Hemodynamically significant bradycardia will still respond to isoproterenol and transcutaneous pacing.

Afferent denervation in heart transplant patients is most notable for eliminating anginal symptoms. These high-risk patients will not reliably experience or report anginal symptoms with ischemia; complicating preoperative evaluation and decision making. As previously mentioned, there is evidence of reinnervation in patients months to years after transplant. There are several case reports of transplanted patients suffering anginal symptoms years after surgery [39]. Afferent denervation has also been shown to blunt renin-angiotensin-aldosterone regulation and vascular responses to changes in filling pressures.

Other physiologic changes in the transplanted heart include a mild decrease in ventricular function (by 3 months most recipients have returned to New York Heart Association (NYHA) class I functional capacity [35]), mild to moderate diastolic dysfunction, a dependence on preload for maintenance of cardiac output, and an increase in resting coronary blood flow as a result of loss of adrenergic tone. Surprisingly, several physiologic factors remain intact or unchanged; myocardial metabolism is normal, contractile reserve is normal, autoregulation of coronary blood flow remains intact, and the Frank-Starling mechanism is normal [37].

Early posttransplant patients can have significant ECG abnormalities. If a portion of the patient's native right atrium was retained during surgery, the ECG may demonstrate 2 P waves: 1 from the native atria (not conducted beyond the suture line) and another from the donor SA node (conducted normally via the AV node) [38]. Ventricular ectopy is common in the first several weeks after transplant, but usually diminishes. Supraventricular dysrhythmias (atrial premature beats, atrial fibrillation, and atrial flutter) are common after transplantation, but are also associated with episodes of acute rejection. New-onset supraventricular dysrhythmias, therefore, should heighten suspicion for rejection. First-degree atrioventricular block is common, as is either incomplete or complete right bundle branch block. Several studies quote a significant incidence of bradyarrythmias requiring pacemaker insertion (3.5%–20%) [41]. Antiarrythmic drugs such as verapamil, procainamide, and quinidine are useful for the treatment of supraventricular tachyarrythmias from atrial flutter and atrial fibrillation. Because of its negative inotropic effects, lidocaine should be used with caution in these patients.

Posttransplant morbidities. Heart transplant patients suffer significant posttransplant morbidities. The most ominous of these morbidities is rejection. There are 3 types of cardiac allograft rejection: hyperacute, acute vascular, and acute cellular rejection [37]. Most rejection episodes occur within the first 6 months after transplant. Most commonly, the severity of rejection episodes decreases with time. There are no specific clinical signs or symptoms associated with acute rejection, however, suspicion is increased with any of the following: fatigue, lethargy, nausea, fever, anorexia, hypotension, peripheral edema, dyspnea, S3 gallop, increased jugular venous pressure, decreased systolic function, worsening diastolic dysfunction, pericardial effusion, and new-onset ventricular or supraventricular dysrhythmias. There is evidence to show that acute allograft rejection significantly increases intraoperative morbidity [35]. All transplant recipients are rigorously screened for evidence of rejection. Endomyocardial biopsies, the gold standard for evaluating rejection, are performed weekly for the first 4 weeks after transplant, every other week for the second month after transplant, monthly from 2 to 6 months postoperatively, and then every 3 months through the first postoperative year. Screening is continued at least annually from then on.

CAV is the major manifestation of chronic rejection in heart transplant patients and is one of the leading late causes of death after heart transplant. The diffuse, concentric intimal thickening of the coronary arteries in CAV is believed to be caused by a combination of both immune-mediated and nonimmunologic risk factors [42]. At 1 year after transplant, angiographically significant coronary disease is present in 10% to 20% of patients, and at 5 years more than 50% of patients have angiographically significant disease [34]. The lack of afferent innervation can eliminate anginal symptoms causing silent ischemia in these patients.

Infection, another significant posttransplant morbidity, is a constant threat to heart transplant patients on immunosuppressive therapy. The highest incidence of infection occurs in the first several months postoperatively. This coincides with aggressive induction immunosuppression. Within the first year after transplant, non-CMV infection accounted for 33% of deaths in heart transplant recipients. After 5 years, infection accounted for 11% of deaths [34]. Infection can be difficult to diagnose in this population. Immunosuppressive therapy can mask the normal signs and symptoms (leukocytosis, fever, peritonitis) so one must have a high index of suspicion.

Malignancy is another unfortunate consequence of immunosuppression. It accounts for 23% of deaths in heart transplant patients at 5 years. At 10 years after transplant, 33% of patients had some form of malignancy, mostly skin cancers [34].

The ISHLT has reported that the incidence of renal insufficiency, hyperlipidemia, and diabetes has been increasing in this patient population. By 10 years after transplantation, 99% of recipients have hypertension, 14% have severe renal insufficiency (creatinine >2.5 in 8%, chronic dialysis in 5%, and renal transplant in 1%), 93% have hyperlipidemia, and 37% have diabetes. In their report, the ISHLT caution that because their analysis focused only on surviving recipients, the incidence of these morbidities is likely underestimated [34].

Preoperative evaluation. The preoperative evaluation of heart transplant recipients should start with a general history and physical examination. It is important to understand the indication for heart transplantation as some disease processes may have extracardiac implications. Knowing how far the patient is from surgery helps in determining which morbidities are most likely. Recently transplanted patients are at greater risk for arrhythmia, infection, ventricular dysfunction, and acute rejection. Patients further removed from surgery have a higher risk of CAV, malignancy, diabetes, and renal insufficiency. Knowing the date of a patient's most recent posttransplant evaluation and the results of any studies performed (endomyocardial biopsies, coronary angiography, ECG) is important. The patient's primary cardiologist, transplant surgeon, and even transplant anesthesiologist can be useful references for any questions regarding the patient's history.

Understanding the patient's functional status is the most important part of the preoperative evaluation. Exercise tolerance and functional status are excellent preoperative screening tools. By 3 months postoperatively, most recipients have returned to NYHA Class I. Any recent decrease in exercise tolerance or any current functional status greater than NYHA Class I should raise suspicion. A recent transthoracic or transesophageal echocardiogram helps to evaluate left ventricular function and is mandatory if there is any recent change in the patient's functional status. Echocardiography should also be considered if the patient describes any signs or symptoms suspicious for rejection, as acute episodes of rejection can significantly decrease ventricular function and can cause significant worsening of diastolic dysfunction.

CAV can cause significant ischemia without angina. The anesthesiologist caring for a heart transplant recipient should have a high index of suspicion for ischemia. An ECG can help to rule out acute ischemia and is useful in looking for evidence of old infarcts (Q waves). These patients are routinely screened for CAV. The transplant cardiologist should have copies of the most recent coronary angiogram. If there is any question about the progression of CAV, stress testing or coronary angiography should be performed if time allows.

Dysrhythmias are common in this patient population. A preoperative ECG is necessary. Ventricular dysrhythmias are prevalent in the early postoperative period and decrease with time. Supraventricular dysrhythmias are also common postoperatively. The new onset of any dysrhythmia, especially supraventricular in origin should raise suspicion for an episode of acute rejection. Right bundle branch blocks are common and are of no real significance [41]. Several patients require pacemaker placement for bradyarrhythmias after transplant. The presence of a pacemaker warrants its interrogation, an understanding of its current settings, and possible adjustment of those settings for surgery. Biphasic or 2 separate P waves are a common finding on ECG and are of no anesthetic significance.

The preoperative evaluation should also include a chest radiograph to look for pneumonia or other signs of cardiopulmonary disease. Laboratory evaluation should include a complete blood count to rule out anemia, myelosuppression, leukocytosis, and thrombocytopenia. Blood urea nitrogen and creatinine can help to evaluate renal function in the presence of probable hypertension and potentially renal-toxic immunosuppressive therapy. Electrolytes and glucose should also be evaluated in light of possible renal dysfunction and/or diabetes mellitus.

The preoperative physical examination should focus on the patient's airway, heart, and lungs. Evidence of volume overload suggesting ventricular failure (increased jugular venous pressure, S3 gallop, peripheral edema, hepatomegaly) should also be looked for.

Particular attention should be paid to nonspecific or constitutional findings (fever, sweating, rigors, and cachexia) that may suggest infection, acute, or chronic rejection.

Intraoperative care. No single anesthetic technique has been proven to be superior in caring for heart transplant patients having nontransplant surgery [43]. Spinal anesthesia, epidural anesthesia, regional anesthesia, general anesthesia, and sedation have all been safely performed in these patients. Because of their strict dependence on preload for cardiac output, the literature suggests that general anesthesia is preferred over neuraxial techniques. When a neuraxial technique is used, epidural anesthesia is preferred over spinal anesthesia. Anesthesiologists should consider careful preoperative volume loading when planning a neuraxial technique.

Another goal in caring for these patients is to minimize invasive techniques that increase the risk for infection. Oral intubation is preferred over nasal intubation. One should carefully consider the need for invasive monitoring (arterial lines, central lines). If needed, these lines should be placed with strict adherence to aseptic technique and should be removed as soon as possible. Groin sites should be avoided whenever possible because of the high risk of infection. Preoperative antibiotics should be given as per guidelines and before invasive line placement if possible. If large fluid shifts are expected, consider the use of a pulmonary artery catheter and/or transesophageal echocardiography. All other standard monitors are indicated. Intraoperative ECG is especially helpful for detecting ischemic events and dysrhythmias [44].

Immunosuppression should be continued with minimal interruption throughout the perioperative period. Consultation with pharmacy professionals can help with conversions from oral to intravenous medications. Transplant center physicians are also available to help with perioperative immunosuppression questions should they arise. This becomes especially important in patients expected to be intubated or sedated for significant amounts of time; also in patients expected to have a prolonged postoperative ileus. Stress-dose steroids should be considered in patients receiving corticosteroids as part of their immunosuppressive regimen.

Intraoperative drug administration should take into consideration the physiology of the transplanted heart. As mentioned previously, drugs that exert their cardiac effects via the autonomic nervous system do not have an effect on transplanted hearts. However, there are several reports of reinnervation in patients months to years after transplantation. Direct-acting agents (alpha and beta agonists and antagonists) are still effective. Consider having syringes of dilute epinephrine and isoproterenol immediately available.

Vagally mediated reflexes are absent (Valsalva, oculocardiac, carotid massage). The stress response is blunted (dependent on circulating catecholamines rather than direct innervation), so the tachycardic response to pain, light anesthesia, hypercarbia, hypoxia, and other stressors is slowed and blunted. Because of their effect on preload, potent vasodilators such as nifedipine, nitroglycerine, and nitroprusside may cause an exaggerated decrease in blood pressure because of the lack of baroreceptor-mediated reflex tachycardia.

Immunosuppressive therapy can be associated with significant morbidities that require intraoperative attention. Diabetes mellitus requires careful attention to blood glucose levels, the possibility of a difficult airway, and microcirculatory issues. Chronic steroid use may lead to osteoporosis and adrenal insufficiency requiring attention to patient positioning and stress-dose steroids, respectively. Renal insufficiency caused by some of the agents can prolong the effects of morphine (reducing the excretion of pharmacologically active metabolites). The use of nonsteroidal antiinflammatory drugs is relatively contraindicated in patients with renal insufficiency. Immunosuppressive drugs can alter the action of anesthetic drugs. Cyclosporine can enhance the effects of pentobarbital and fentanyl as well as prolong the action of vecuronium and pancuronium. Azathioprine can antagonize the effects of nondepolarizing muscle relaxants, although this may not be of clinical significance. Several drugs given during anesthesia can also have significant effects on plasma drug levels of immunosuppressants (particularly cyclosporine and tacrolimus). Plasma levels of these drugs should be followed closely in the perioperative period.

Postoperative care. Postoperative care in heart transplant patients requires continued vigilance. Careful attention should be paid to volume status, monitoring for signs of infection, monitoring for ischemia, and a quick return to the patient's normal immunosuppression regimen. Postoperative discharge criteria remain the same as for any other patient.

Anesthesia for patients after lung transplant
According to the ISHLT, nearly 26,000 lung transplants have been performed since the first in 1983. In the ISHLT's 25th Official Adult Lung and Heart/Lung Transplant Report, the total number of lung transplants performed annually is estimated at nearly 2200 worldwide. This report highlights several interesting trends in lung transplantation. First, chronic obstructive pulmonary disease (COPD) continues to be the primary indication for single lung transplantation (SLT) (50%). Other indications for SLT include idiopathic pulmonary fibrosis (IPF) (28%) and alpha-1 antitrypsin disease (A1AT) (7.1%). The primary indication for double lung transplantation (DLT) is cystic fibrosis (CF) (28%). Other indications for DLT include COPD (24%) and IPF (14%). Second, the average age of the lung transplant recipient is increasing. Currently, 24.1% of lung transplant recipients are aged 60 years or older and 3.7% are age 65 years or older. Third, survival

of transplant recipients continues to improve. The half-life of an SLT recipient is now 4.5 years and the conditional half-life (half-life of those recipients alive 1 year after transplant) is 6.4 years. The half-life of a DLT recipient is 6.2 years and the conditional half-life of a DLT recipient is 8.8 years. Fourth, 5-year morbidity analysis shows continued prevalence of hypertension (85.3%), hyperlipidemia (53%), renal dysfunction (37%), diabetes (35%), and bronchiolitis obliterans (BO) (33.7%). Malignancy is another common morbidity among transplant recipients. At 5 years after transplant, 17% of recipients reported a malignancy and at 10 years after transplant 34% of recipients had reported a malignancy. Fifth, mortality analysis continues to show that BO, believed to be a manifestation of acute and chronic rejection, accounts for 28.5% of deaths in patients surviving 3 to 5 years. Other causes of death include noncytomegalovirus infection (19.2%), graft failure (19%), and nonlymphoma malignancy (7.9%) [45].

As the number of SLT and DLT recipients continues to increase and their posttransplant outcomes continue to improve, we can expect to see them with increasing frequency in the operating room. An understanding of the physiology of the transplanted lung, the implications of immunosuppression, and the comorbidities that frequently affect this population is necessary to appropriately manage these patients.

Surgical technique. Because of its association with significant postoperative morbidity, the classic en bloc technique of DLT is no longer performed. This technique involved an en bloc resection of the donor's lungs, main-stem bronchi, carina, and distal trachea. It not only required a tracheal anastomosis, which was prone to dehiscence and stenosis but also extensive paratracheal dissection in the recipient, which occasionally led to denervation of the recipient's heart. Today both SLTs and DLTs are performed with main-stem bronchial anastomoses. The dated technique of creating an omental wrap around the bronchial anastomosis, to protect the suture line and aid in healing, is no longer performed.

Immunosuppression. Most lung transplant recipients receive a course of induction (high-dose) immunosuppression followed by a maintenance phase of lower-dose therapy. The ISHLT reports that maintenance therapy for most recipients consists of a 3-drug regimen. A corticosteroid (prednisone) is usually combined with either tacrolimus or cyclosporine and either MMF or azathioprine. The most common 3-drug combination for maintenance is prednisone, tacrolimus, and MMF [45]. All these drugs and their anesthetic implications are discussed in the section on anesthesia for noncardiac surgery after heart transplantation.

Posttransplant physiology. At the time of transplantation, the donor lung is denervated. This denervation is arguably the most significant physiologic difference between a transplanted and a native lung. It results in the loss of the cough reflex distal to the site of the bronchial anastomosis. This, of course, places the recipient at risk for both aspiration and infection. In the normal lung, autonomic innervation is responsible for regulating airway tone, however, there seems to be no clinically significant change in bronchomotor tone after transplantation nor is there an increase in the incidence of airway hyperreactivity [46]. Bronchodilators continue to be effective although some investigations suggest their effect is slightly decreased. Studies have also shown that denervation has little, if any, effect on respiratory rate or tidal volume. Evidence suggests that hypoxic pulmonary vaso-constriction (HPV) is unaffected by denervation [47].

In DLT recipients, pulmonary blood flow is normal. In SLT recipients, the transplanted lung receives 60% to 70% of pulmonary perfusion. In patients transplanted for primary pulmonary hypertension (PPH) blood flow to the transplanted lung can increase to as much as 99% of cardiac output [48].

In DLT patients, pulmonary function tests (PFTs), arterial blood gases (ABGs) and alveolar-arterial oxygen gradient return to normal within 9 months of transplant. Only a slight decrease in carbon dioxide diffusing capacity (DL$_{CO_2}$) remains. In SLT patients, PFTs continuously improve in the first 9 months after transplant. SLT recipients are generally left with a slight restrictive defect and a mildly decreased DL$_{CO_2}$ [48].

Mucociliary clearance is significantly decreased in lung transplant recipients. This has been shown in both short-term and long-term survivors. Together with the loss of the cough reflex, this places the lung transplant recipient at high risk for both mucus plugging and infection [49].

Lymphatic drainage is interrupted at the time of transplant, increasing the risk of interstitial edema, infiltrates on chest radiograph, and pneumonia. Bronchial circulation is also interrupted at the time of transplant. This can have a dramatic effect on anastomotic healing.

Posttransplant morbidities. Episodes of acute rejection are common among lung transplant recipients. During the first few months after transplant, most patients experience at least 1 episode of acute rejection. Nearly 60% of all rejection episodes occur within the first 3 months after transplant. Rejection is often hard to distinguish from infection. It often presents with cough, fever, malaise, dyspnea, hypoxia, wheezing, worsening PFTs, and infiltrates on chest radiograph. The clinical criteria for diagnosing rejection include increase in temperature 0.5°C above baseline, Pao$_2$ decrease of greater than 10 mmHg below baseline, new or changing infiltrates on chest radiograph, and a decrease in FEV1 (forced expiratory volume in the first second of expiration) of more than 10% below stable baseline [48]. Infection has to be excluded as a cause. Differentiating between rejection and infection is usually quite difficult and often only possible with bronchoscopy, bronchial-alveolar lavage, and cultures. Occasionally lung biopsy is required to make a definitive diagnosis. Treatment involves a prolonged burst of high-dose corticosteroids.

Infection is a significant cause of both morbidity and mortality in lung transplant recipients. It is the leading cause of death in the first year after transplant (39.5%) [45]. The high rate of infection in this period coincides with the administration of aggressive induction chemotherapy. In the 3- to 5-year posttransplant group, infection accounted for 19.5% of deaths [45]. As previously mentioned, it can be difficult to differentiate infection from rejection. In addition, immunosuppression often masks the clinical hallmarks of infection including fever and leukocytosis. Physicians caring for these patients must have a high index of suspicion for infection.

BO is a syndrome characterized by immune injury to the transplanted lung resulting in the obstruction of small airways with fibrous scar tissue. Patients with BO typically present with progressive cough, evidence of obstruction on PFTs, and interstitial infiltrates on chest radiograph [50]. Although exceedingly rare in the first year, BO is one of the leading causes of death in transplant recipients surviving beyond 1 year (21.5% of deaths in those surviving 1–3 years after transplant). At 5 years after transplant, 33.7% of recipients have a diagnosis of BO [45]. First-line treatment is generally corticosteroid therapy, but the only definitive treatment is retransplantation [51].

As with any group of immunosuppressed patients, malignancy rates in lung transplant recipients increase as duration of therapy increases. 3.6% of 1-year survivors have at least 1 form of malignancy. In those who survive 5 years, the incidence increases to 12.3%. In early survivors, lymphoma accounts for the greatest number of malignancies, whereas skin cancer leads in those surviving 5 years or more [45].

Other significant comorbidities reported by the ISHLT in 5-year survivors include hypertension (85.3%), hyperlipidemia (53.6%), renal dysfunction (37%), and diabetes (35.5%). The ISHLT's report looks only at survivors, and therefore may significantly underestimate the prevalence of these comorbidities [45].

Preoperative evaluation. A thorough history and physical examination is the cornerstone of the preoperative evaluation in these patients. It is important to understand the original indication for transplantation. In SLT recipients, 1 native, diseased lung is still present. This can present difficulties intraoperatively. Emphysematous lungs can be prone to bleb rupture and tension pneumothoraces. High airway pressures and differences in compliance may require lung isolation techniques in certain circumstances. The difference in compliance may also cause a biphasic end-title CO_2 tracing on capnography. Many of the indications for lung transplantation (A1AT, CF, sarcoidosis) have extrapulmonary effects that must be considered when caring for these patients.

Understanding the patient's posttransplant course is also helpful: prolonged postoperative intubation should increase suspicion for vocal cord dysfunction or airway narrowing, episodes of acute rejection suggest an increased exposure to corticosteroids, and progressively worsening PFTs may herald the onset of BO. Recently transplanted patients are at greater risk for episodes of rejection, infection, and interstitial edema, whereas patients further removed from surgery have a higher risk of BO, malignancy, diabetes, and renal insufficiency. Knowing the dates of a patient's most recent posttransplant evaluation and the results of any studies performed (PFTs, bronchoscopy, bronchioalveolar lavage, laboratory evaluation) is important. The patient's primary pulmonologist, transplant surgeon, and even transplant anesthesiologist can be useful references for questions regarding the patient's history, medication regimen, or plans for future care.

It is important to understand the indication for the present surgery. Surgical procedures, intraoperative positioning, the need for 1 lung ventilation, and the risk of septicemia all have implications in these patients. Postoperative pain and splinting can have deleterious effects as can iatrogenic diaphragmatic paralysis (brachial plexus blocks) and accessory muscle weakness (high spinal or high epidural).

As with any patient, understanding preoperative exercise tolerance and functional capacity is paramount. A recent decline in either should increase suspicion for rejection, infection, or BO. The presence of constitutional symptoms (fever, anorexia, malaise) increases concern. Any of these findings should prompt a more thorough investigation and consultation with the patient's transplant pulmonologist if time allows. One should also take time to understand the patient's immunosuppression medications and plan how to proceed with minimal interruption in the regimen. Several circumstances (bowel surgery, postoperative intubation) could require prolonged administration of intravenous, rather than oral, immunosuppressants. In these situations, a pharmacist and the patient's primary transplant team should be consulted.

In patients with a stable preoperative course, ordering up-to-date, baseline PFTs, ABG, ECG, and chest radiographs should be considered. Preoperative laboratory evaluation is warranted. A complete blood count including hemoglobin, white blood cells, and platelets can help rule out myelosuppression, anemia, thrombocytopenia, and leukocytosis. Renal function should be assessed with evaluation of blood urea nitrogen and creatinine. One should also evaluate electrolytes and glucose in light of possible renal dysfunction and possible diabetes mellitus.

Intraoperative care. No single anesthetic technique has been shown to be superior in lung transplant recipients. However, many investigators suggest the use of regional techniques whenever possible. Advantages of regional techniques in lung transplant recipients include a decreased requirement for systemic narcotic administration (and subsequent postoperative respiratory depression), improved postoperative analgesia (with less splinting and hypoventilation), and no need for airway manipulation, neuromuscular blockade, or positive-pressure ventilation. However, one must be careful to avoid iatrogenic diaphragmatic paralysis or accessory muscle weakness, which can accompany regional or neuraxial techniques. Regional techniques that place the patient at risk for a pneumothorax are not advised. Volume loading before the administration of a neuraxial block should be done cautiously as these patients are at risk for and extremely sensitive to pulmonary edema. Strict adherence to sterile technique is required, especially if long-term catheters are being placed.

Any sedation should be carefully titrated to avoid significant hypoventilation. Preoperative antibiotics should be administered as indicated. One should also consider the administration of stress-dose steroids in patients receiving corticosteroids as part of their immunosuppression. Standard American Society of Anesthesiology monitors should be used in all patients and careful consideration should be given to the placement of any invasive monitor. If an invasive monitor is planned, the use of sterile technique is paramount. Attempts should be made to avoid placement of any femoral lines given the high risk of infection. Internal jugular and subclavian lines should be placed cautiously to avoid a pneumothorax. Many investigators suggest placing these lines on the side of the patient's native diseased lung in SLT recipients. Pulmonary artery catheters (PAC) are not contraindicated in lung transplant recipients, however, fresh pulmonary artery suture lines are vulnerable to disruption with PAC insertion. Transesophageal echocardiography should be considered to aid in monitoring volume status and cardiac output.

General anesthesia can be safely performed in both SLT and DLT recipients. Airway manipulation is complicated by the possible presence of areas of stenosis and the risk of disruption of anastomoses. The use of a laryngeal mask airway can avoid these problems and should be considered in appropriate situations. If endotracheal intubation is planned, fiberoptic bronchoscopy can be used to visualize the anastomosis and ensure that the endotracheal tube is appropriately positioned. Larger endotracheal tubes allow for easier suctioning, either with a suction catheter or a bronchoscope. A larger tube also allows for the placement of an endobronchial blocker should lung isolation become necessary. Nasotracheal intubation should be avoided because of the risk of infection.

Positive-pressure ventilation can cause disruption of anastomotic suture lines, emphysematous bleb rupture or hyperinflation of the native, diseased lung. Increasing ventilatory pressures, therefore, raise concern for pneumothorax or hyperinflation of the native lung with subsequent compression of the transplanted lung and even cardiac compression resulting in hypotension [52]. An effort should be made to keep peak inspiratory pressures low. Because of differences in compliance between the native and transplanted lung, it is not unusual to see a biphasic capnography tracing in SLT recipients. The administration of humidified gases may help decrease mucus plugging in the perioperative period. Frequent, careful endotracheal tube suctioning and bronchodilator administration is also recommended.

NO_2, although not contraindicated, should be used with caution, especially in patients at risk for pneumothorax or emphysematous bleb rupture. Sevoflurane, because of its bronchodilatory properties, is an obvious choice for inhalational anesthetic. Other intraoperative anesthetics should be chosen with the goal of early emergence and minimal postoperative sedation. Propofol is potentially superior to thiopental as an induction agent, especially for short cases. One should also consider short-acting narcotics rather than hydromorphone. Intravenous and oral nonsteroidal antiinflammatory medications are also helpful in minimizing exposure to narcotics, but should be used with caution in patients with renal insufficiency. As previously mentioned, practitioners should be careful to avoid excess fluid administration as pulmonary edema is poorly tolerated in these patients.

Extubation criteria are no different for lung transplant recipients. As with any other patient, ensure complete reversal of neuromuscular blockade before extubation. Some suggest extubating SLT recipients with their diseased lung in the dependent position, as this may help to avoid aspiration pneumonia in the transplanted lung.

Postoperative care. Postoperative care in lung transplant recipients focuses on minimizing the risk of infection and encouraging an early return to the patient's baseline ventilatory status. Adequate pain control with careful attention to ventilatory depression along with bronchodilator therapy, incentive spirometry, and even physiotherapy can be helpful in this population. Minimizing any interruption in immunosuppression should be another primary goal.

Postoperative discharge criteria remain the same as for any other patient.

Abdominal Organs: Kidney, Liver, Pancreas, and Intestine
Kidney

As kidney transplant is the most commonly performed organ transplant, it is feasible that the nontransplant anesthesiologist will be required to perform an anesthetic on one of these patients. Many have preexisting multisystem diseases that persist after transplant. Diabetes mellitus, hypertension, hyperlipidemia, and cardiovascular disease are extremely common comorbidities in this patient subset [3,16].

When planning an anesthetic for this population, it is essential to assess kidney function preoperatively. After kidney transplant many patients experience a 20% reduction in the function of the transplanted organ as a result of chronic rejection, the toxic effects of immunosuppressive drugs, or both [3]. Although serum creatinine level is generally normal or near normal in an adequately functioning renal allograft, glomerular filtration rate may be diminished and drugs that require renal excretion, especially drugs with active metabolites, should be used judiciously with avoidance of repeated doses [3,9]. Table 4 is a list of potential perioperative medications with active metabolites that are cleared via the kidneys.

Renal allograft function is at risk from potentially nephrotoxic drugs, such as nonsteroidal antiinflammatory drugs and intravenous contrast agents. These medications are best avoided or used with extreme caution. A recent exposure to intravenous contrast should prompt a reevaluation of kidney function before proceeding to elective surgery [3,4,8]. The transplanted kidney is also vulnerable to other insults, such as ischemia, so it is important to maintain normovolemia and avoid intraoperative hypotension. Diuretics should not be given without careful consideration of the patient's intravascular volume status [3,9].

Pancreas

Pancreas transplantation has evolved slowly in the past 45 years to treat type 1 diabetes mellitus. In general, pancreas transplant takes place in 1 of 3 scenarios: simultaneous kidney transplantation (SPK), pancreas transplant in a patient who has previously received a kidney allograft or pancreas transplantation alone in a patient with preserved renal function. Emergence of superior surgical techniques and immune suppression in pancreas transplantation has improved outcomes since the first dismal attempts. Pancreatic graft survival rates at 5 years are best in the SPK group at about 69% [1]. Pancreas transplantation also continues to have the highest complication rates of solid organ transplants other than intestinal transplant [16].

Patients who have undergone pancreas transplant are often those with the most severe diabetic complications, which persist despite transplant and may negatively affect anesthetic management. The anesthetic plan should reflect that diabetic stiff joint syndrome, gastropathy and gastroparesis, and autonomic neuropathy persist after transplant [16,18]. Pancreas recipients are at high risk for coronary artery disease, which is frequently silent or asymptomatic. The results of previous cardiac testing and interventions, as well as a thorough evaluation of the patient's current ECG and functional status are imperative. Preoperative assessment should also include evaluation of metabolic status, serum glucose, renal function, including electrolytes and acid-base status, and volume status. Individuals with a functioning pancreatic graft should have effective glucose metabolism and intraoperative supplementation is likely not required [7,16]. In patients with failed or poorly functioning grafts, a plan for perioperative glucose control should be established. Intraoperative monitoring of glucose to detect hyperglycemia and hypoglycemia and treatment with insulin to avoid diabetic ketoacidosis is essential in patients with failed grafts. Previous abdominal surgery in this population increases the risk of intraoperative bleeding and adequate intravenous access, and up-to-date typing and screening should be considered an important part of the anesthetic management plan. One caveat of special concern in patients with bladder drainage of the exocrine pancreas is the potential for severe metabolic acidosis caused by bicarbonate losses. These patients may require intraoperative monitoring of acid-base status and possible bicarbonate replacement.

Liver

The first successful human liver transplantation was performed in 1967 [1]. In 2008 and 2009 there were nearly 13,000 liver transplants performed in more than 140 institutions in the United States with almost 57,500 recipients surviving at October 31, 2009 (see Table 1). After transplantation, tests of synthetic liver function and aminotransferases should normalize. The bilirubin level generally normalizes within 3 months and transaminases in 2 weeks after transplant if the allograft is functioning normally. Drug metabolism returns to normal soon after reperfusion of the allograft. Synthesis and clearance of coagulation factors, such as factors I, II, V, VII, VIII, IX, X, XI, XII, and XIII, and regulatory proteins, such as antithrombin III, protein C, protein S, and plasminogen, also return to normal soon after transplantation in a well-functioning allograft [53]. Platelet function normalizes after transplant, but platelet count may be persistently less than normal after transplant. However, the absolute platelet count is typically adequate for normal hemostasis. Some patients may undergo splenectomy after liver transplantation if severe thrombocytopenia and splenomegaly persist. Preoperative testing in this patient population should include evaluation of aspartate aminotransferase, alanine aminotransferase, γ-glutamyl transferase, internationalized normalized ratio, bilirubin, alkaline phosphatase, albumin, and platelet count. Evidence of abnormalities or inadequate hepatic function seen on basic testing may be indicators of rejection, infection, or biliary stasis, and communication with the transplant center is important along with postponement of elective surgery [4,16].

Intravenous anesthetics and other drugs that are hepatically metabolized or cleared can be safely administered as long as all evidence points to a well-functioning allograft without biliary stasis [3,54]. Both general and regional anesthesia techniques may be used with success and without deterioration in allograft function as long as there are no contraindications to the technique chosen and adequate hepatic perfusion is maintained throughout the procedure [54,55].

Abdominal operations in liver transplant recipients have the potential for major bleeding so it is important to have prepared adequately with at least large bore intravenous catheters and possibly central venous access, and an up-to-date type and cross. It is important to maintain adequate systemic blood pressure and volume as hypoperfusion and ischemic insult are poorly tolerated by the liver allograft because the normal physiologic mechanisms that maintain and control blood flow in the liver are blunted [16]. It may be necessary to communicate with the institutional blood bank to determine the availability of blood products before surgery. Many facilities may have limited available resources. Platelets are often not stored on site and must be transported from a regional center when needed. If intraoperative bleeding is considered a viable risk, then it is prudent to ensure availability of blood products before the day of surgery. Some transplanted patients may have had multiple transfusions previously and are at risk for acquiring antibodies that may further delay the ability to obtain blood products in an emergency. Therefore, adequate preparation should be given to the potential need for transfusion and blood products before the patient presents to the operating suite.

Liver recipients with pretransplant hepatopulmonary syndrome and portopulmonary hypertension usually have resolution of hypoxemia and pulmonary hypertension some time after transplant. However, some may have residual hypoxemia or persistent pulmonary hypertension. If a patient is on a long-term pulmonary vasodilator, such as sildenafil or epoprostenol, it should be continued in the perioperative period. Despite continuing the medications, pulmonary hypertension can be worsened perioperatively by hypoxemia, hypercapnia, or acidosis, and additional measures such as nitric oxide should be available to treat pulmonary hypertension. It may be prudent to contact the transplant center or the patient's pulmonologist for assistance in constructing a perioperative plan for management of the patient's pulmonary hypertension and to discuss possible supplemental measures during the operative procedure [16]. Intensive care admission following the surgical procedure should be strongly considered in this population for close respiratory and hemodynamic monitoring.

Intestinal

Since 1987 there have been approximately 1700 intestinal transplants with slightly more than 900 reported surviving with a functional graft (see Table 1). More than half of these are children. The transplanted bowel elicits a significant alloimmune response and rejection is an all too common problem with this type of transplant. There is also a significant incidence of graft-versus-host disease in this population [12,16]. This subset of transplanted patients requires a high level of multidisciplinary support. Other than absolute emergent situations, it is unlikely that these patients will present for surgery outside of a transplant center. Should an anesthesiologist be confronted with this particular transplanted patient, there are several important factors to consider when constructing the anesthetic plan. Gastric and intestinal motility are often significantly delayed, and this should be reflected in the plan for airway management [16]. Chronic liver dysfunction is a common finding. Chronic renal dysfunction is also frequently present as a result of multiple insults of hypovolemia, sepsis, need for immunosuppressants, and frequent therapy with antibiotics [12,16]. If abdominal surgery is necessary, the anesthesiologist should be prepared for a difficult surgical dissection and the potential for hemorrhagic complications. These patients have invariably been subjected to multiple central venous catheters for chronic parenteral nutrition and administration of medication. Recurrent episodes of infection and venous thromboses cause venous damage and the reality of difficult venous access should be anticipated [16]. Denervation and impaired lymphatic drainage of the transplanted intestine affect intestinal permeability and absorption [8]. These patients frequently have derangements in their acid-base status and electrolytes and suffer malnutrition. Hypoproteinemia is common and is associated with pleural effusions, ascites, and edema. Infection and sepsis are an unfortunate but common morbidity in this population because of bacteremia from bowel translocation, and the need for vasopressor support should also be anticipated [12,16].

Preoperative testing should include evaluation of electrolytes, acid-base status, glucose, liver and kidney function, complete blood count, and coagulation studies. As these patients are often weak and debilitated at baseline, postoperative mechanical ventilatory support may be necessary. Many of these patients required tracheostomy during the peritransplant period because of the need for prolonged mechanical ventilation, which may effect airway management. Although early extubation is desirable, extubation should not be attempted unless electrolyte, fluid, and acid-base status are optimal, oxygenation is adequate, there is hemodynamic stability, and pain management is optimal [12,16]. Communication with the intensive care staff before surgery to alert them to the possibility of admission to the unit will likely facilitate the patient's care. Open lines of communication with the transplant center during all phases of care should be established.

SUMMARY

Organ transplantation is the definitive therapy for end-stage organ failure and disease in many circumstances. As donor pools are expanded, surgical techniques improve, and immunosuppressive drugs become more sophisticated, the yearly numbers of organ transplants will likely continue to increase and survival rates will improve. There is increasing likelihood that the general anesthesiologist will care for these patients outside of transplant centers. Patients who have received organ allografts have traded an acute or chronic illness for other chronic conditions and will often present for other surgical interventions. The anesthesiologist must have the necessary skills and knowledge to adequately care for this often medically complex patient population.

References

[1] Bloom R, Goldberg L, Wang A, et al. An overview of solid organ transplantation. Clin Chest Med 2005;26:529–43.

[2] Leapman S, Vidne B, Butt K, et al. Elective and emergency surgery in renal transplant patients. Ann Surg 1976;183(3):266–70.

[3] Tran S. Anesthetic considerations for patients post-organ transplantation. Semin Anesth Periop Med Pain 2003;22(2):119–24.

[4] Toivonen H. Anaesthesia for patients with a transplanted organ. Acta Anaesthesiol Scand 2000;44:812–33.

[5] Kasiske B. Epidemiology of cardiovascular disease after renal transplantation. Transplantation 2001;72(suppl 6):5–8.

[6] Sarnak M, Levey A, Schoolworth A, et al. Kidney disease as a risk factor for development of cardiovascular disease. A statement from the American Heart Association Councils on Kidney in Cardiovascular Disease, High Blood Pressure Research, Clinical Cardiology, and Epidemiology and Prevention. Circulation 2003;108:2154–69.

[7] Gohh R, Warren G. The preoperative evaluation of the transplanted patient for non-transplant surgery. Surg Clin North Am 2006;86:1147–66.

[8] Kostopanagiotu G, Smyrniotis V, Arkadopoulos N, et al. Anesthetic and perioperative management of adult transplant recipients in nontransplant surgery. Anesth Analg 1999;89:613–22.

[9] Sladen R. Anesthetic considerations for the patient with renal failure. Anesthesiol Clin North America 2000;18(4):791–807.

[10] American Diabetes Association. Standards of medical care for patients with diabetes mellitus. Diabetes Care 2003;26(suppl):33–50.

[11] Mora P. Post-transplantation diabetes mellitus. Am J Med Sci 2005;329(2):86–94.

[12] Akhtar S, Barash P, Inzucchi S. Scientific principles and clinical implications of perioperative glucose regulation and control. Anesth Analg 2010;110(2):478–97.

[13] The NICE-SUGAR Study Investigators. Intensive versus conventional glucose control in critically Ill patients. N Engl J Med 2009;360(13):1283–97.

[14] Kostopanagiotu G, Sidiropoulou T, Pyrsopoulos N, et al. Anesthetic and perioperative management of intestinal and multi-visceral allograft recipient in nontransplant surgery. Transpl Int 2008;21:415–27.

[15] Sandham J, Hall R, Brant R, et al. A randomized, controlled trial of the use of pulmonary artery catheters in high-risk surgical patients. N Engl J Med 2003;348(1):5–14.

[16] Keegan M, Plevak D. The transplant recipient for nontransplant surgery. Anesthesiol Clin North America 2004;22:827–61.

[17] Warner M, Contreras M, Warner MA, et al. Diabetes mellitus and difficult laryngoscopy in renal and pancreatic transplant patients. Anesth Analg 1998;86:516–9.

[18] Hogan K, Rusy D, Springman S. Difficult laryngoscopy and diabetes mellitus. Anesth Analg 1988;67:1152–5.

[19] Reissal E, Orko R, Maunuksela L, et al. Predictability of difficult laryngoscopy in patients with long term diabetes mellitus. Anaesthesia 1990;45:1024–7.

[20] Littlewood K. The immunocompromised adult and surgery. Best Pract Res Clin Anaesthesiol 2008;22(3):585–609.

[21] Whiting J. Perioperative concerns for transplant recipients undergoing nontransplant surgery. Surg Clin North Am 2006;86(5):1185–94, vi–vii.

[22] Bratzler HP. Antimicrobial prophylaxis for surgery: an advisory statement from the National Surgical Infection Prevention Project. Am J Surg 2005;189:395–404.

[23] White P, Romero G. Nonopioid intravenous anesthesia. In: Barash PG, Cullen BF, Stoelting RK, editors. Clinical anesthesiology. 5th edition. Philadelphia: Lippincott Williams & Wilkins; 2006. p. 334–52.

[24] Agarwal A, Raza M, Dhiraaj S, et al. Is ketamine a safe anesthetic for percutaneous liver biopsy in a liver transplant recipient immunosuppressed with cyclosporine? Anesth Analg 2005;100:85–6.

[25] Ebert T. Inhalational anesthesia. In: Barash PG, Cullen BF, Stoelting RK, editors. Clinical anesthesiology. 5th edition. Philadelphia: Lippincott Williams & Wilkins; 2006. p. 384–420.

[26] Morgan G Jr, Mikhail M, Murray M. Inhalational anesthetics. In: Barash PG, Cullen BF, Stoelting RK, editors. Clinical anesthesiology. 4th edition. New York: Lange Medical Books/McGraw-Hill; 2006. p. 155–78.

[27] Donati F, Bevan D. Neuromuscular blocking agents. In: Barash PG, Cullen BF, Stoelting RK, editors. Clinical anesthesiology. 5th edition. Philadelphia: Lippincott Williams & Wilkins; 2006. p. 421–52.

[28] Lin S, Cosgrove C. Perioperative management of immunosuppression. Surg Clin North Am 2006;86:1167–83.

[29] Horlocker T, Wedel D. Regional anesthesia in the immunocompromised patient. Reg Anesth Pain Med 2006;31(4):334–45.

[30] Moen V, Dahlgren N, Irestedt L. Severe neurological complications after central neuraxial blockades in Sweden, 1990–1999. Anesthesiology 2004;101:950–9.

[31] Cuvillon P, Ripart J, Lalourcey L, et al. The continuous femoral nerve block catheter for postoperative analgesia: bacterial colonization infection rate and adverse effects. Anesth Analg 2001;93:1045–9.

[32] Liu S, Carpenter R, Neal J. Epidural anesthesia and analgesia. Their role in postoperative outcome. Anesthesiology 1995;82:1474–506.

[33] Coda B. Opioids. In: Barash PG, Cullen BF, Stoelting RK, editors. Clinical anesthesiology. 5th edition. Philadelphia: Lippincott Williams & Wilkins; 2006. p. 353–83.

[34] Taylor D, Edwards L, Aurora P, et al. Registry of the International Society for Heart and Lung Transplantation: twenty-fifth official adult heart transplant report – 2008. J Heart Lung Transplant 2008;27:943–56.

[35] Cheng D, Ong D. Anaesthesia for non-cardiac surgery in heart-transplanted patients. Can J Anaesth 1993;40:981–6.

[36] Lakse A, Carrel T, Niederhäuser U, et al. Modified operation technique for orthotopic heart transplantation. Eur J Cardiothorac Surg 1995;9(3):120–6.

[37] Ashary N, Kaye A, Hegazi A, et al. Anesthetic considerations in the patient with a heart transplant. Heart Dis 2002;4:191–8.

[38] Blasco L, Parameshwar J, Vuylsteke A. Anaesthesia for noncardiac surgery in the heart transplant recipient. Curr Opin Anaesthesiol 2009;22:109–13.

[39] Csete M, Glas K. Anesthesia for organ transplantation. In: Barash P, Cullen B, Stoelting R, editors. Clinical anesthesia. Philadelphia: Lippincott Williams & Wilkins; 2006. p. 1358–76.

[40] Bjerke RJ, Mangione MP. Asystole after intravenous neostigmine in a heart transplant recipient. Can J Anaesth 2001;48(3):305–7.

[41] Ng V, Cassorla L. Cardiac transplant recipient undergoing noncardiac surgery. In: Bready L, Dillman D, Parameshwar J, editors. Decision making in anesthesiology: an algorithmic approach. Philadelphia: Mosby Elsevier; 2007. p. 468–71.

[42] Dong C, Redenbach D, Wood S, et al. The pathogenesis of cardiac allograft vasculopathy. Curr Opin Cardiol 1996;11:183–90.

[43] Baker J, Yost C, Niemann C. Organ transplantation. In: Miller R, editor. Anesthesia. Philadelphia: Elsevier Churchill Livingstone; 2005. p. 2263–73.

[44] Fontes M, Rosenbaum S. Noncardiac surgery after heart transplantation. Anesthesiol Clin North Am 1997;15:207–20.

[45] Christie J, Edwards L, Aurora P, et al. Registry of the International Society for Heart and Lung Transplantation: twenty-fifth official adult lung and heart/lung transplantation report – 2008. J Heart Lung Transplant 2008;27:957–69.

[46] Haddow GR, Brock-Utne JG. A non-thoracic operation for a patient with single lung transplantation. Acta Anaesthesiol Scand 1999;43:960–3.

[47] Robin E, Theodore J, Burke C, et al. Hypoxic pulmonary vasoconstriction persists in the human transplanted lung. Clin Sci (Lond) 1987;72:283–7.

[48] Haddow G. Anaesthesia for patients after lung transplantation. Can J Anaesth 1997;44:182–97.

[49] Herve P, Silbert D, Cerrina J, et al. Impairment of bronchial mucociliary clearance in long-term survivors of heart/lung and double lung transplantation. The Paris-Sud Lung Transplant Group. Chest 1993;103:59–63.

[50] Quinlan J, Murray A, Cerrina J. Anesthesia for heart, lung, and heart-lung transplantation. In: Kaplan J, editor. Kaplan's cardiac anesthesia. Philadelphia: Saunders Elsevier; 2006. p. 845–65.

[51] Stoelting R, Dierdorf S. Acute respiratory failure. In: Stoelting R, Dierdorf S, editors. Anesthesia and co-existing disease. Philadelphia: Churchill Livingstone; 2002. p. 217–32.

[52] Myles P. Pulmonary transplantation. In: Kaplan J, Slinger P, editors. Thoracic anesthesia. Philadelphia: Churchill Livingstone; 2003. p. 295–314.

[53] Kang Y, Audu P. Coagulation and liver transplantation. Int Anesthesiol Clin 2006;44(4):17–36.

[54] Feng Z-Y, Zhang J, Zhu SM, et al. Is there any difference in anesthetic management of different post-OLT stage patients undergoing nontransplant organ surgery? Hepatobiliary Pancreat Dis Int 2006;5(3):368–73.

[55] Zeyneloglu P, Pirat A, Sulemanji D, et al. Perioperative anesthetic management for recipients of orthotopic liver transplant undergoing nontransplant surgery. Exp Clin Transplant 2007;5:1–3.

Advances in Anesthesia 28 (2010) 245–267

ADVANCES IN ANESTHESIA

Perioperative Implications of Obstructive Sleep Apnea

Karen J. Roetman, MD*, Christopher Bernards, MD

Department of Anesthesiology, B2-AN 1100 9th Avenue, Virginia Mason Medical Center, Seattle, WA, USA

O bstructive sleep apnea (OSA) was first described by novelist Charles Dickens in *The Posthumous Papers of the Pickwick Club*, published in 1937. The character Joe was an obese boy who was constantly hungry, red in the face, and always falling asleep in the middle of his duties. Dickens [1] writes:

> The object that presented itself to the eyes of the astonished clerk was a boy—a wonderfully fat boy—habited as a serving lad, standing upright on the mat, with his eyes closed as if in sleep. 'Sleep!' said the old gentleman, 'he's always asleep. Goes on errands fast asleep, and snores as he waits at tables.' 'How very odd!' said Mr Pickwick. 'Ah! Odd indeed,' returned the old gentleman; 'I'm proud of that boy—wouldn't part with him on any account—he's a natural curiosity!'.

OSA is a common cause of daytime sleepiness for millions of Americans. It is estimated that in adults between the ages of 30 and 60 years, 9% of women and 24% of men have OSA, whereas 2% of women and 4% of men have OSA with daytime sleepiness [2]. The prevalence of OSA increases with age [3]. OSA is associated with an increased incidence of hypertension [4], coronary artery disease [5,6], cardiovascular morbidity and mortality [7], cor pulmonale [8], stroke [9,10], neurocognitive dysfunction [11], motor vehicle accidents [12], and a decreased quality of life [13].

DEFINITION OF OSA

OSA is clinically characterized by recurrent episodes of upper-airway obstruction that result in cessation (apnea) or reduction (hypopnea) in airflow during sleep, often accompanied by hypoxia and/or hypercarbia. The diagnosis of OSA is based on the apnea-hypopnea index (AHI), which is a count of the number of apneas and hypopneas per hour of sleep. Apnea is defined as the cessation of airflow for at least 10 seconds in the presence of thoracoabdominal ventilatory efforts and hypopnea as a 50% or more reduction in breathing

*Corresponding author. E-mail address: anekjr@vmmc.org.

0737-6146/10/$ – see front matter
doi:10.1016/j.aan.2010.09.002

amplitude. The occurrence of more or less frequent oxygen desaturations or electroencephalography (EEG) arousals is taken as an additional diagnostic tool to identify these conditions [14]. Obstruction is often inferred from thoracoabdominal paradox, the shape of the airflow signal, or when snoring intensity increases during the event [15].

Determinants of Upper-airway Patency

The upper airway begins at the nose and lips and ends at the larynx. The pharyngeal airway includes collapsible soft tissue such as the tongue and soft palate enclosed by bony structures such as the mandible and cervical vertebrae. The patency of this collapsible segment is likely dictated by the interaction between anatomic characteristics, effects of lung volume, and neural regulation of pharyngeal dilator muscles. Together, these mechanisms determine airway caliber.

Anatomic Factors

Numerous studies have shown that patients with OSA have structurally narrower and more collapsible airways than patients who do not have OSA who are matched in age and body mass index (BMI, calculated as weight in kilograms divided by the square of height in meters) [16,17]. Craniofacial and upper-airway abnormalities have been shown to predispose patients with OSA to upper-airway obstruction [18]. Micrognathia with an inferior-located hyoid bone has been shown to be a major risk factor for OSA in Japanese patients. This risk factor was most significant in obese patients with large tongues [19]. An anatomic imbalance between upper-airway soft-tissue volume and bony enclosure size may result in pharyngeal airway obstruction during sleep and general anesthesia. Tsuiki and colleagues [20] measured tongue cross-sectional area and craniofacial dimensions through lateral cephalograms in 50 adult male patients with OSA and 55 adult male individuals who did not have OSA and found that when maxillomandibular dimensions were matched, patients with OSA had a significantly larger tongue for a given maxillomandibular size compared with individuals who did not have OSA. Schwab and colleagues [21] used volumetric analysis techniques with magnetic resonance imaging to study the upper-airway soft-tissue structures in sleep apnea and control individuals with a variety of ethnic backgrounds. These investigators showed that the volume of soft-tissue structure surrounding the upper airway is enlarged in patients with OSA. They also showed a greater risk for sleep apnea the larger the volume of the tongue, lateral pharyngeal walls, and soft tissue.

Effect of Lung Volumes on Pharyngeal Patency

Lung volume normally decreases during sleep [22]. Obesity is associated with further reductions in lung volumes caused by increased elastic resistance and decreased compliance of the chest wall, resulting in reduced total respiratory compliance. Decreased pulmonary compliance leads to decreased expiratory reserve volume, functional residual capacity (FRC), vital capacity, and total lung capacity [23]. Whereas the decrease in FRC is responsible for the development of severe hypoxemia during obstructive episodes in obese patients with OSA, the decrease in lung volumes has been shown to contribute to pharyngeal airway obstruction. Van de Graaff [24] studied the effect of thoracic traction on upper-airway resistance during breathing. In anesthetized dogs with denervated upper airways, thoracic traction generated during inspiration reduced upper-airway resistance significantly. These findings indicate that tonic and phasic forces generated by the thorax can improve upper-airway patency. The increased patency during inspiration cannot be attributed solely to activity of upper-airway muscles. Likewise in humans, Heinzer [25] reported a significant decrease in respiratory events during non-rapid eye movement (REM) sleep in patients with OSA when lung volume was increased by negative extrathoracic pressure during sleep. Small changes in lung volume during sleep in patients with OSA have been shown to cause large changes in the continuous positive airway pressure (CPAP) required to prevent flow limitation in the upper airway [26]. Therefore, lung volume has an important effect on the upper airway in patients with OSA and is one factor that increases the risk of OSA in obese patients. Tagaito and colleagues [27] examined the structural interaction between a passive pharyngeal airway and lung volume before and during lung inflation in 8 anesthetized and paralyzed patients with sleep-disordered breathing. Increasing lung volume by applying negative extrathoracic pressure (thereby leaving the transpharyngeal pressure unchanged) improved pharyngeal collapsibility, especially in obese patients. Increased lung volume during inspiration is believed to provide caudal tracheal traction that increases the longitudinal tension on the upper airway independent of upper-airway muscle activity, causing unfolding of the pharyngeal mucosa and stiffening the airway. Traction on the trachea could be explained as a sum of mediastinal traction and the force generated by changes in intrathoracic pressure [28].

Neuromuscular Control

Neuromuscular control of the upper airway plays an important role in OSA pathogenesis. Because upper-airway dilator muscles are important in maintaining pharyngeal patency, reductions in activity of these muscles may be important in mediating REM-related obstructive apnea. Sauerland and Mitchell [29] showed that the electromyographic activity of the largest upper-airway dilator muscle, the genioglossus (GG), was increased during inspiration and markedly reduced during expiration. Mezzanotte and colleagues [30] reported that patients with OSA have significantly greater basal genioglossal activity during wakefulness compared with age and BMI-matched patients who do not have OSA. However, this augmented activity was significantly reduced during sleep. This finding suggests that the neuromuscular compensation present during wakefulness that is necessary to keep the anatomically compromised airway of patients with sleep apnea open is lost during sleep, leading to airway collapse. These investigators further showed that sleep onset is associated with significantly larger decrements in GG and tensor palatine muscle activity in patients with OSA compared with controls [31]. More recently Eckert and colleagues [32] studied the mechanisms of worsening OSA during REM sleep. When airway resistance and blood gas disturbances were minimized by CPAP, genioglossal activity was reduced during REM sleep to a similar extent in OSA and healthy individuals. This finding suggests a generalized reduction in genioglossal activity during REM, which likely renders individuals who are highly reliant on upper-airway dilator muscles vulnerable to pharyngeal collapse during REM sleep.

Ventilatory Control

Multiple feedback loops exist to control and stabilize breathing by adjusting arterial blood gas tensions [33]. Ventilation is constantly monitored and adjusted to maintain appropriate arterial pH and P_{CO_2}. That sleep can affect control of these feedback loops was first reported more than 50 years ago by Bulow [34], who observed that decreases in carbon dioxide sensitivity at sleep onset led to episodes of hypopnea or apnea with breathing instability. Sullivan [35] subsequently reported that suppression of respiratory stimuli (wakefulness, vagal, peripheral, and central chemoreceptors) results in near cessation of ventilation, suggesting that decreased metabolic control during sleep may explain the irregular breathing pattern characteristic of the sleep state. Several recent studies using a loop-gain model to measure respiratory system stability suggest that patients with OSA have less ventilatory stability. Loop gain is an engineering term that describes the stability of a system controlled by negative feedback loops. In the case of respiration, loop gain represents the sensitivity of the negative feedback loop that controls ventilation [36]. Younes and colleagues [37] reported that the chemical control system is more unstable in patients with severe OSA than in patients with milder OSA. In a follow-up study the same investigators confirmed chemical instability in patients with OSA and suggested that the mechanisms responsible for the instability may vary considerably among patients [38]. Wellman and colleagues [36] studied ventilatory instability in the context of airway collapsibility in patients with OSA and found a high correlation between loop gain in patients with pharyngeal closing pressure near atmospheric pressure, suggesting that this group may be highly susceptible to changes in ventilatory stability. However, whether loop gain is a cause or consequence of OSA has not been established. It is likely that a combination of upper-airway anatomic, neuromuscular, and ventilatory control mechanisms accounts for the pathogenesis of OSA.

MORBIDITY AND OSA

OSA is recognized as a contributor to the pathogenesis of multiple organ system diseases that may be as important as airway obstruction itself as a cause of perioperative morbidity and mortality.

OSA and Cardiovascular Diseases

The pathophysiology of OSA and cardiovascular disease is complex and multifactorial, involving mechanical, hemodynamic, inflammatory, autonomic, and neural stresses. The association between OSA and hypertension, coronary artery disease, and heart failure offers opportunity to improve cardiac outcomes by treating OSA.

Systemic Hypertension

Approximately 50% of patients with OSA are hypertensive and 30% of hypertensive patients have OSA [39]. The most convincing evidence to support OSA as a cause in the development of hypertension comes from epidemiologic data from the Wisconsin Sleep Cohort Study. This study evaluating the association between sleep-disordered breathing and hypertension showed a 3-fold increased risk of developing new-onset hypertension in patients with an AHI of 15 or more. This association was independent of age, gender, BMI, and antihypertensive medications [40]. The Sleep Heart Health Study also showed that sleep-disordered breathing is associated with systemic hypertension in middle-aged adults and older individuals even after controlling for demographics and anthropometric variables (BMI, neck circumference, waist/hip ratio, smoking, and alcohol intake) [4]. Subsequent analysis of the Sleep Heart Health data showed that there is a stronger association between sleep-disordered breathing and hypertension for those aged less than 60 years but no association was found for those more than 60 years of age [41]. In addition to human data, 2 animal models support a causal link between sleep-disordered breathing and increased arterial blood pressure. Fletcher and colleagues [42] showed that rats exposed to intermittent hypocapnic hypoxia for 8 hours each day showed significant increases in blood pressure compared with controls. Brooks and colleagues induced OSA in dogs by intermittent airway occlusion during nocturnal sleep. In this model OSA resulted in acute transient increases in nighttime blood pressure and eventually produced sustained daytime hypertension.

Although the physiologic studies provide strong evidence to support a causal relationship between OSA and hypertension, the mechanism by which OSA causes hypertension is less well established. A likely mechanism of increased arterial pressure is through sustained sympathetic nervous system excitation and vascular remodeling. Hypoxia and hypercapnia secondary to partial or complete closure of the upper airway during sleep result in oxygen desaturation and increased sympathetic nervous system activity in patients with OSA [43,44]. The primary role of the sympathetic nervous system is maintenance and regulation of blood pressure. The baroreceptors respond to stretching of the vessel wall (increased blood pressure) by decreasing sympathetic neural outflow, resulting in vasodilation and decreased blood pressure. Recent studies suggest that in addition to short-term regulation of blood pressure, the sympathetic neural system plays an important role in long-term regulation of blood pressure [45–47].

In addition to activation of the sympathetic nervous system, the repetitive hypoxemia-normoxia cycle results in activation of inflammatory pathways, which may be important in the molecular pathogenesis of cardiovascular disease [48] independent of increased sympathetic activity [49]. Hypoxia is a major stimulus of vascular endothelial growth factor, which is a potent angiogenic cytokine. Vascular endothelial growth factors are especially increased in patients with severe OSA [50,51]. Bokinsky and colleagues [51] showed that patients with OSA also have increased spontaneous platelet aggregation and activation, which may increase the risk of mural thrombus formation.

CPAP has been shown to attenuate the sympathetic response to obstructive respiratory events and to lower nocturnal blood pressure in patients with OSA [52,53], reduce platelet aggregation [51], and reduce vascular endothelial growth factor in patients with nocturnal hypoxia [54]. However, the effect of CPAP on daytime blood pressure is not so well established. Peppard and colleagues [40] found a small but significant reduction in systolic and diastolic blood pressure with therapeutic CPAP. Although these studies suffer from small sample size, with most patients normotensive at baseline, they do support considering OSA when evaluating all hypertensive patients.

Sleep Apnea and Heart Failure

Observational data support the association between OSA and heart failure [55–57]. Sustained respiratory effort against an occluded airway leads to negative intrathoracic pressure as low as -80 cm water. This negative intrathoracic pressure increases cardiac afterload by increasing the left ventricular transmural pressure, resulting in increased left ventricular wall stress/tension and impaired relaxation, causing decreased stroke volume and cardiac output [58,59]. Otto [60] compared cardiac structural and functional changes in obese adults with and without OSA and found that patients with OSA tended toward abnormal right ventricular filling and diastolic dysfunction suggesting that OSA, independent of obesity, may induce cardiac changes that predispose to atrial fibrillation and heart failure. This observation is important because OSA in patients with heart failure is associated with an increased risk of death independent of confounding factors [61]. Treatment of OSA with CPAP has been shown to improve left ventricular function in patients with congestive heart failure [62,63]. This evidence supports the use of CPAP in the perioperative period for patients with heart failure.

Cardiac Arrhythmias

Several studies show an association between OSA and nocturnal arrhythmias. Arrhythmias observed during sleep include atrial fibrillation, bradycardia, non-sustained ventricular tachycardia, sinus arrest, second-degree atrioventricular conduction block, and frequent premature ventricular contractions [64–67]. The recurrent apneic and hypopneic episodes resulting in arterial desaturation, hypercapnia, and increased sympathetic tone may acutely trigger nocturnal dysrhythmias, or chronically affect the electrical conduction system [66,68]. The Sleep Heart Health Study showed that patients with severe OSA (AHI>30 events/h) have a 4-fold increase in prevalence of atrial fibrillation [69]. Kanagala and colleagues [70] showed that treatment with appropriate levels of CPAP lowers the incidence of recurrent atrial fibrillation in patients with OSA following cardioversion. The bradycardic response to obstructive apnea is probably related to intrathoracic pressure swings, parasympathetic activity, hypoxia, and sleep phase. Changes in heart rate depend on a balance of sympathetic and parasympathetic tone. The stimulation of upper-airway receptors may increase parasympathetic activity, causing a decrease in heart rate [68,71]. In a study of nonsurgical patients with OSA, Becker and colleagues [72] found a 7.5% incidence of clinically significant (second- and third-degree atrioventricular block and sinus arrest of greater than 2 seconds' duration) heart block. The incidence of pathologically significant rhythm disturbances such as supraventricular tachycardia and ventricular arrhythmias is less clear. In addition, some studies found no causal relation between OSA and arrhythmias [73].

OSA and Coronary Artery Disease

Several studies have found a positive association between OSA and ischemic heart disease. Peker and colleagues [5] showed that middle-aged patients with OSA followed for 7 years showed an almost 5-fold increase in risk of developing coronary heart disease independent of age, sex, hypertension, diabetes, and current smoking. In patients without clinical coronary artery disease, the presence and severity of OSA has been shown to be independently associated with the presence and extent of coronary artery calcification [74]. Cardiac sudden death is increased during sleeping hours in patients with OSA and the degree of nocturnal hypoxemia is related to the risk of sudden cardiac death [75]. Kuniyoshi and colleagues [76] found that the diurnal variation in the onset of myocardial infarction (MI) in patients with OSA was strikingly different from the diurnal variation in patients without OSA. Patients with nocturnal onset of MI between 12 midnight and 6 AM had a high likelihood of having OSA. These findings suggest that OSA may be a trigger for MI.

Thus, OSA may increase cardiovascular risk by several different mechanisms. Repetitive hypoxemia and hypercapnia causing sympathetic activation, vascular endothelial dysfunction, increased oxidative stress, inflammation, increased platelet aggregation, and metabolic dysregulation are all implicated in the pathophysiology of cardiovascular disease associated with OSA [77].

OSA and Stroke

OSA is both a possible risk factor and a consequence of stroke [78,79]. Habitual snoring alone has been shown to increase the risk of cerebrovascular disease [80–82]. The Wisconsin Sleep Cohort Study reported that moderate OSA (defined as AHI>20) was associated with a 3-fold increment in the risk of developing a stroke [83]. Studies looking at patients following stroke report a 44% to 72% incidence of OSA (defined as AHI>10) [84,85]. Proposed mechanisms for the increased risk of OSA following stroke include hypertension, reduction in cerebral blood flow, altered cerebral blood flow, altered cerebral blood flow autoregulation, impaired endothelial function, accelerated atherogenesis, thrombosis, and paradoxic embolism [86].

CLINICAL PRESENTATION

Boxes 1 and 2 list physical characteristics and signs and symptoms frequently associated with OSA.

Box 1: Physical characteristics associated with OSA

Obesity

Large neck circumference

Craniofacial abnormalities

Anatomic nasal obstruction

Obesity and Neck Circumference

OSA is strongly correlated with obesity. A study of patients presenting for bariatric surgery reported a 71% to 77% prevalence of OSA in patients with a BMI of 35 to 59.9 kg/m^2 and 90% prevalence with BMI 60 kg/m^2 or greater [87]. Increases in weight have been shown to increase the prevalence of OSA, which is an independent risk factor for developing obesity. Young and colleagues [2] found that the prevalence of OSA increased 4-fold with each increase in the standard deviation of the BMI. In addition, an increase in weight has been shown to worsen OSA. An 11-year longitudinal study of 690 Wisconsin residents measuring the association between weight change and AHI showed that a 10% weight gain predicted an approximate 32% increase in the AHI and a 6-fold increase in the risk for developing moderate to severe OSA. A 10% weight loss predicted a 26% decrease in the AHI [88].

Several studies have reported that neck circumference is a better predictor of obstructive apnea than BMI [89–92]. Horner and colleagues [93] showed that more adipose tissue is present in those areas surrounding the collapsible segment of the pharynx in patients with OSA, compared with equally obese control subjects without OSA. Shelton and colleagues [94] performed magnetic resonance imaging and polysomnography on patients with and without OSA. They reported that all patients had a collection of adipose tissue adjacent to the pharynx, the volume of which correlated with the severity of OSA. Weight loss resulted in fewer apneas and hypopneas and a marked decrease in the

Box 2: Signs and symptoms of OSA with daytime sleepiness

Fatigue

Cognitive difficulties

Nocturnal awakenings

Nocturnal choking/gagging

Insomnia

Snoring

Observed apnea

Sexual dysfunction

pharyngeal adipose tissue volume, suggesting that the volume of pharyngeal adipose tissue is causally related to OSA. Similarly, Mortimer [95] studied fat distribution in obese and nonobese patients with OSA and found that both groups have excess fat deposition, especially anterolateral to the upper airway, when compared with weight-matched controls.

Recent data suggest that intraabdominal body fat distribution may be even more significant than fat accumulation in the pharyngeal region as a predictor of OSA. Shafer [96] reported that regional body fat distribution predicts the presence and severity of OSA, but fat accumulation in the neck and parapharyngeal region are of minor importance. Martinez-Rivera and colleagues [97] showed that truncal obesity was significantly better than BMI at predicting OSA. Vgontzas and colleagues [98] showed that sleep-disordered breathing correlated with the amount of visceral fat, but not BMI, total fat, or subcutaneous fat. Deegan and McNicholas [99] suggested a gender difference in the effect of fat distribution. After controlling for BMI and age, waist circumference correlated more closely with AHI than neck circumference among men, whereas the opposite was true for women.

Leptin, a hormone that is made in adipose tissue, is involved in controlling body weight, energy expenditure, and body fat distribution [98]. Serum leptin is increased in obese people and patients with OSA, suggesting the potential of leptin resistance in the development of obesity [96]. Chin [100] showed that CPAP reduced visceral fat accumulation and decreased serum leptin levels. Evidence showing a correlation between leptin levels and hypoxemia and arterial carbon dioxide levels suggests that further research is needed in this area [87,101,102].

Snoring

Snoring occurs in up to 30% to 50% of adults more than 50 years old, and subjective sleepiness occurs in more than 30% of adults [15,103,104]. Although snoring and daytime hypersomnolence are common in patients with sleep-disordered breathing, not all patients with these symptoms have the disorder. Deegan and McNicholas [99] evaluated with full polysomnography 250 consecutive patients referred to a sleep laboratory because of suspicion of sleep-disordered breathing and found that although snoring was strongly associated with the presence of OSA, it had a positive predictive value of only 63% and a negative predictive value of 56%.

Screening for OSA

It is estimated that 80% of men and 93% of women with moderate to severe sleep apnea are undiagnosed [105]. Thus, identifying patients with OSA before surgery and anesthesia cannot rely on history alone. Prospectively identifying patients with OSA may be important because of data suggesting that they are at greater risk of perioperative morbidity [106]. For example, Gupta and colleagues [107] published a retrospective chart review in which they documented that patients with OSA were more likely to require unplanned admission to the intensive care unit (ICU) after joint replacement surgery than were patients without OSA. However, an important limitation of this study is that there was no reliable indication that it was the patients' OSA (not other associated disease) that was responsible for the higher incidence of unplanned ICU admission. Blake and colleagues [108] showed that patients with OSA had more respiratory obstructive events per hour and more oxygen desaturation than controls without OSA during a 12-hour period on the first postoperative night. Liao and colleagues [109] published a retrospective review of postoperative complications in patients with OSA. Their data showed that patients with OSA had a higher incidence of postoperative complications compared with controls (39% vs 18%) primarily related to oxygen desaturation. The American Society of Anesthesiologists (ASA) guidelines for perioperative management of patients with OSA recommend that anesthesiologists should work to identify patients and consider obtaining sleep studies on patients at risk for OSA. However, the screening tool devised by the ASA task force has not been validated. Polysomnography remains the gold standard for the diagnosis of OSA. However, there are numerous barriers to obtaining sleep studies on patients before surgery. These studies are expensive and time-consuming and patients are often reluctant to comply with recommended testing. For example, Fidan and colleagues [110] screened 433 patients and recommended sleep studies for 41 of the patients based on symptoms. Only 18 of the patients agreed to undergo polysomnography.

Subjective clinical evaluation is probably the most common tool used to screen patients for OSA. However, this method of screening has serious limitations. Viner and colleagues [111] found that in patients with a high predicted probability of sleep apnea, subjective impression alone correctly identified only 52% of patients with sleep apnea and had a specificity of 70%. However, in patients with a low predicted probability of sleep apnea, the use of clinical data is sufficiently sensitive to permit about a 30% reduction in the number of unnecessary sleep studies. Hoffstein and Szalai [112] found that subjective impression of the examining clinician provided a sensitivity of 60% and a specificity of 63%. Clinical impression alone is not sufficient to reliably identify patients with or without sleep apnea.

Numerous screening tools have been developed to identify patients at risk for OSA. However, there is no consensus as to the best screening test.

The Berlin Questionnaire consists of 3 categories related to the risk of having sleep apnea. Patients can be classified into high risk or low risk based on their responses to individual questions about smoking, weight, snoring, observed apnea, and daytime hypersomnolence. This questionnaire has been validated in the primary care population with a sensitivity and specificity of 0.89 and 0.71 [113].

The STOP Questionnaire developed by Chung and colleagues condenses the Berlin Questionnaire into a 4-question OSA screening tool for surgical patients. The STOP questions include:

1. S: Do you snore loudly, loud enough to be heard through a closed door?
2. T: Do you feel tired or fatigued during the daytime almost every day?

3. O: Has anyone observed that you stop breathing during sleep?
4. P: Do you have a history of high blood pressure with or without treatment?

The sensitivity of the STOP questionnaire with an AHI greater than 5, greater than 15, and greater than 30 as cutoffs was 65.6%, 74.3%, and 79.5%. Specificity for this tool was 60%, 53%, and 48%, respectively. When BMI, age, neck circumference, and gender were incorporated, the sensitivities were increased to 83.6%, 92.9%, and 100% with specificity of 56.4%, 43%, and 37% [114].

More recently Ramachandran and colleagues [115] developed the Perioperative Sleep Apnea Prediction (P-SAP) score for the diagnosis of OSA, which incorporates airway screening tools normally used during a preoperative anesthetic assessment. The investigators identified independent clinical predictors of OSA including age greater than 43 years, male gender, obesity, snoring, diabetes type 2, hypertension, thick neck, Mallampati class 3 or 4, and reduced thyromental distance. A P-SAP score of 2 or greater resulted in high sensitivity (93%) at the expense of specificity (32%), whereas a P-SAP score of 6 or greater resulted in low sensitivity (23%) with high specificity (91%).

Thus far, none of the current screening tools offers both a high sensitivity (low false-negative rate) and high specificity (low false-positive rate). In addition, the current screening tools focus on the ability of screening tests to accurately identify patients with OSA but not the risk for adverse postoperative outcome.

OSA IN THE PERIOPERATIVE PERIOD

As noted earlier, OSA is associated with multiple chronic diseases, including cardiovascular disease, cerebrovascular disease, and morbid obesity, any one of which may increase perioperative risks. Consequently, one of the difficulties in interpreting studies that show an association between OSA and perioperative morbidity/mortality is distinguishing those caused by the underlying chronic morbidity (eg, coronary artery disease) from those related to acute OSA exacerbation. One might reasonably question whether this distinction makes any difference. We argue that it does to the extent that monitoring and prevention of morbidity secondary to exacerbation of OSA-induced cardiovascular disease (eg, postoperative electrocardiogram telemetry, perioperative β-blockers) is different from what is required to prevent acute morbidity/mortality from exacerbation of airway obstruction (eg, continuous oximetry, supplemental O_2). In this section we discuss only the issue of perioperative exacerbation of airway obstruction.

OSA is a disease in which the normal decrease in airway muscle tone associated with sleep causes airway obstruction, which in turn causes hypoxic and hypercarbic episodes that are terminated by arousal, restoration of awake levels of airway muscle tone, and subsequent hyperventilation to reestablish normoxia and normocarbia until the next obstructive episode. Thus, it is reasonable to be concerned that anything that either decreases the ability to arouse in response to obstruction or that impairs the response to hypercarbia or hypoxia may put patients at increased risk of morbidity or mortality.

The issue of whether patients suffer morbidity or mortality from acute episodes of airway obstruction is important because if they do not then our concerns that we may acutely worsen the risk of obstruction are misplaced. However, the available evidence suggests that this risk is all too real. For example, Gami and colleagues [75] examined death certificates for 112 persons who were diagnosed with OSA at the Mayo Clinic and who died suddenly from cardiac causes. They compared these patients with individuals in the general population who also died a sudden cardiac death. They found that in the general population the timing of sudden cardiac death peaked between 6 AM and noon and was lowest during the hours of sleep, from midnight to 6 AM. In contrast, the patients with diagnosed OSA were most likely to die during the hours of sleep (midnight to 6 AM). In addition, the risk of dying between midnight and 6 AM was directly correlated with OSA severity. This finding is not proof that OSA episodes can precipitate sudden cardiac death, but it is strong suggestive evidence.

Consistent with this study, Hanly and colleagues [116] reported that the occurrence of ST-segment depression during sleep in patients with OSA without a history of coronary artery disease was positively correlated with OSA severity, arousal index (number of arousals per hour), and time spent with O_2 saturation less than 90%. Again, this study is not proof, but it is suggestive evidence that anything that acutely increases OSA severity, arousals, and/or desaturations may put patients at risk of morbid cardiac events. Our study of opioid effects in patients with OSA showed that opioid administration increased arousals, increased the amount of time spent with O_2 saturations less than 90%, and increased OSA severity as measured by the AHI [117]. We found that opioids increase all of the risk factors that Hanley and colleagues found were associated with ST-segment depression in patients with OSA.

Although these findings provide only indirect evidence that OSA can acutely cause morbidity/mortality, there is one clear example of death caused by OSA. Specifically, Pearce and Saunders [118] published a case report in which a patient suffered cardiorespiratory arrest during a sleep study. The investigators attributed the arrest to the fact that the patient did not arouse sufficiently to reestablish a patent airway during an obstructive episode. (NB At the institution where this occurred, polysomnography was not monitored, ie, nobody was watching the woman who died. That is not the case at many institutions where sleep studies are continuously supervised and monitored by registered polysomnographic technologists.) The patient could not be resuscitated and postmortem examination revealed no clear cause of death. The coroner attributed death to OSA and entered this on the death certificate.

Thus, we are probably being appropriately cautious in assuming that anything we do in the perioperative period that increases the severity of OSA symptoms may increase the risk of acute morbidity and mortality. We might increase OSA severity by decreasing airway muscle tone, decreasing the ability to arouse from sleep during obstruction, or by decreasing the ability to respond to hypoxia/hypercarbia following arousal.

Preoperative Period

Risks to patients with OSA in the preoperative period largely involve preoperative sedation. The risks associated with sedation in turn are presumably related to the drug class(es) used (eg, opioids, benzodiazepines), drug dose(s), monitoring provided, and use of supplemental oxygen. As in much of this medical area, the available data are limited.

Berry and colleagues [119] used a blinded observer study design to examine the dose-dependent effects of a targeted propofol infusion on the frequency of airway obstruction in a group of patients with suspected sleep-disordered breathing and a group of control subjects. They found that all patients suspected of having sleep-disordered breathing experienced partial or complete obstruction at one or more propofol concentrations and that the frequency of obstruction was dose-related. In contrast, none of the control group experienced airway obstruction. The goal of these investigators' study was to determine whether propofol sedation could be used as a provocative test for sleep apnea so they did not examine whether propofol sedation impaired arousal mechanisms in response to obstruction. However, because propofol can prevent arousal in response to surgery it is clear that there are propofol doses at which patients do not arouse and clear their obstructed airway. What that dose may be is unknown.

The effect of sedative doses of benzodiazepines on airway patency has also been investigated. Drummond [120] examined the effect of midazolam on airway patency and airway muscle tone in nonobese individuals of unknown OSA status. Midazolam was titrated to produce light sedation but with the retained ability to respond to a loud voice (median dose 5 mg). Tongue muscle tone decreased to 42% of baseline as measured by electromyography, and 10 of 12 patients developed airway obstruction. Drummond observed that muscle tone increased to 69% of baseline during obstruction but this increased muscle tone was insufficient to alleviate obstruction in any patient.

Although by no means exhaustive, the available data suggest that sedative-hypnotic drugs commonly used for preoperative or procedural sedation increase the risk of airway obstruction in all patients and this risk is greater in patients with OSA.

Opioids are another class of drugs commonly used for sedation. They carry the double risk of both generalized depression of the central nervous system and a potent depression of respiratory drive. Bernards and colleagues [117] examined the effect of remifentanil on sleep and respiration in patients with moderate OSA (AHI = 15–30) in a double-blind, randomized, single-dose, polysomnography study. These investigators found that in this group of patients receiving this remifentanil dose (0.075 µg/kg/h) remifentanil decreased the number of obstructive apneas, and did not impair arousal in response to obstruction. Arousals were increased. However, oxygen saturation was decreased on average and the number of events in which saturation decreased to less than 90% was markedly increased. The decrease in obstructive episodes was attributed to the near complete abolition of REM sleep, which is a previously described effect of opioids on human sleep pattern [121–123]. Decreased oxygen saturation was attributed not to a worsening of OSA but to opioid-mediated hypoventilation.

The investigators also observed that a subset of patients with OSA developed a marked incidence of central sleep apnea in response to remifentanil infusion (from an average of 0.4/h to 17/h). The investigators were unable to identify the cause or clinical significance of this opioid-emergent central sleep apnea pattern.

Thus, this study suggests that acute administration of modest opioid doses does not pose a markedly greater risk to patients with moderate OSA than to those without. However, one cannot draw conclusions about patients with more severe OSA or larger opioid doses. There are opioid doses that can be fatal in any patient, and patients with more severe OSA may behave differently. Thus, although this study suggests that a wholesale admonition against opioid administration to patients with OSA is unwarranted it does not represent a free pass to unfettered opioid use. Caution is advised.

There are no data examining the combination of opioids and sedative-hypnotics, a common sedative regimen. Thus, one should be particularly cautious when combining both drug classes. The suggestion regarding caution raises the obvious question of what constitutes appropriate caution. We argue that these patients should not be left unattended or unmonitored following sedation and that monitoring should include continuous pulse oximetry. These patients should probably receive supplemental oxygen while sedated, and equipment and expertise for emergency airway management should be immediately at hand.

OSA represents a difficult challenge for the clinician caring for these patients in the perioperative period because there are virtually no data from which we can define appropriate clinical practices. For example, in 2003 the Clinical Practice Review Committee of the American Academy of Sleep Medicine (AASM) addressed the question of how best to ameliorate the risks of OSA in the perioperative period and concluded, "Scientific literature regarding the perioperative risk and best management techniques for obstructive sleep apnea patients is scanty and of limited quality. There is insufficient information to develop AASM standards of practice recommendation" [124]. Several years later (2006) the ASA Task Force on Perioperative Management of Patients with Obstructive Sleep Apnea addressed the same issue and essentially agreed with the AASM in concluding that there was insufficient scientific information to provide evidence-based recommendations for the care of patients with OSA [125]. The absence of data did not prevent the ASA from promulgating numerous recommendations, some of which are unhelpful and possibly dangerous (see later discussion).

This point is not to suggest that there is no reason to be concerned about the perioperative risks to patients with OSA. There are valid theoretic reasons to believe that these patients may be at greater risk of ventilatory complications in the perioperative period than they are at baseline. What follows is a review of some of those risks and potential methods to reduce them.

Intraoperative Management

There is no evidence to support a choice of one anesthetic technique or anesthetic drug over another. However, given the concern for residual sedation (see later discussion) it seems prudent to choose techniques and/or drugs that minimize this issue. Thus, a spinal or epidural anesthetic may offer advantages over a general anesthetic but not if it is administered with a long-acting sedative regimen.

Airway management

Airway management is a paramount concern in the anesthetic management of all surgical patients. Because OSA is a disease of airway patency, it is reasonable to be concerned that these patients pose a greater risk of difficult airway management than do patients without OSA. However, given that a large proportion of patients with OSA are obese it is difficult to separate difficulties resulting from obesity from those resulting from OSA. A recent study by Neligen and colleagues [126] was able to distinguish OSA versus obesity-related reasons for difficult endotracheal intubation. In a group of 180 consecutive morbidly obese patients (BMI average 49.4 kg/m²) these investigators found a difficult laryngoscopy rate of 8.3% (Cormack and Lehane grade 3 or 4 view) and a difficult intubation rate of 3.3 % (3 or more intubation attempts). However, there was no correlation between the diagnosis or severity of OSA and difficulty with laryngoscopy or intubation. The only correlate with difficult laryngoscopy was neck circumference, but neck circumference did not correlate with difficult intubation. Only male gender and Mallampati score of 3 or 4 predicted difficult intubation. Thus, in this study of morbidly obese patients positioned on a ramp for intubation, OSA was not a predictor of difficult laryngoscopy or intubation.

Chung and colleagues [127] and Hiremath and colleagues [128] took a slightly different approach to addressing the issue of OSA and airway management. These investigators referred patients who were difficult to intubate for polysomnography to determine whether they had OSA. Both of these studies suffer from an unavoidable selection bias because not all patients who were difficult to intubate agreed to undergo polysomnography. However, of those who did agree to undergo polysomnography, both studies found that a significant percentage of patients who were difficult to intubate also had OSA (Chung and colleagues = 66%; Hiremath and colleagues = 28%). In both of these studies the average BMI (30 and 32 kg/m²) was in the obese range, thus it is not possible to determine whether intubation difficulties were related to obesity or OSA.

The currently available data suggest that patients with OSA may be at greater risk of difficult intubation but whether this results from obesity or OSA is unclear. However, it seems prudent to consider that airway difficulties may be more likely in patients with OSA and to plan accordingly. Thus, it seems reasonable to pay strict attention to head positioning (Isono and colleagues [129] have shown that the sniffing position is optimal for a patent airway in patients with OSA) and immediate availability of ancillary airway devices (eg, nasal and pharyngeal airways, laryngeal mask airway, fiberoptic bronchoscope).

Many of these patients are obese and the associated decrease in FRC means that they tolerate episodes of inadequate ventilation poorly. This situation makes adequate preoxygenation and denitrogenation even more important than in nonobese patients.

Intraoperative management

There are currently no appropriately controlled, randomized, prospective studies examining the most appropriate anesthetic technique for patients with OSA. As a general rule it may be reasonable to choose drugs and techniques that minimize the risk of residual sedation or respiratory depression in the postoperative period.

Postoperative Care

Arguably, the primary concern regarding the perioperative care of patients with OSA is how best to care for them out of the operating room when a clinician experienced in airway management and ventilatory support is no longer continuously present. Likewise, the recovery room is not a grave concern because intensive monitoring and care from nurses trained in patient evaluation and airway support are routine. The real question is how best to care for these patients when they leave the recovery room and how to judge when they are ready to leave the recovery room and go to a less monitored setting like the hospital ward or home.

The practice guidelines promulgated by the ASA task force on the care of patients with OSA addressed this issue. The guidelines state, "These patients should not be discharged from the recovery room to an unmonitored setting until they are no longer at risk for postoperative respiratory depression." Given the chronic nature of their disease one is left to wonder whether patients with OSA are ever "no longer at risk of respiratory depression", postoperative or otherwise. The ASA practice guidelines go on to define criteria by which risk of postoperative respiratory depression can be assessed: "Adequacy of post-operative respiratory function may be documented by observing patients in an unstimulated environment, *preferably while they seem to be asleep*, to establish that they are able to maintain their baseline oxygen saturation while breathing room air." In evaluating this recommendation it is worth keeping in mind that these patients suffer from OSA not "preferably while they seem to be asleep" apnea. OSA is a state-dependent disease that is manifest only during sleep. Therefore, it is not reasonable to assume one can make any judgments about ventilatory adequacy in the absence of documented sleep, which is why the electroencephalography is recorded during polysomnographic diagnosis of OSA. In addition, observing a period of adequate ventilation and assuming, based on that observation, that the patient is no longer at risk is like assuming that a single normal blood sugar reading documents that a diabetic is no longer at risk of diabetic ketoacidosis. In addition, adequate ventilation at discharge from the recovery room tells one nothing about what happens when the patient begins self-administering opioids to treat postoperative pain. In addition, although the work by Bernards and colleagues [117] suggests that moderate opioid doses do not pose unique risks to patients with moderate OSA their study was performed during a single night in which remifentanil markedly suppressed REM sleep. Because many patients' OSA is worse during REM sleep, REM suppression may increase their risk on following nights. Specifically, REM suppression is generally followed by REM rebound over subsequent nights [130–132]. The confluence of REM rebound, sleep deprivation, and ongoing opioid use may represent an important risk that does not occur until several days after patients leave the recovery room.

The medical literature is insufficient to guide our postoperative care of these patients. Although the ASA guidelines are well intentioned they are not a substitute for relevant data. Some readers may think that in the absence of data, following the ASA guidelines is potentially helpful and certainly not harmful. Perhaps a historical observation will dissuade readers of this notion. In the 1950s the American Academy of Pediatricians recommended that infants be put to sleep in the prone position to prevent aspiration and occipital flattening, among other perceived risks. However, we now recognize that prone positioning is a major contributor to sudden infant death syndrome and contributed to the death of tens of thousands of infants and the horrible suffering of their families. Thus, the best approach to the perioperative care of patients with OSA is not the ASA practice guideline but an informed and observant physician evaluating an individual patient and their individual circumstances.

References

[1] Dickens C, Seymour R, Browne HK. The posthumous papers of the Pickwick Club. London: Chapman and Hall; 1837.

[2] Young T, Palta M, Dempsey J, et al. The occurrence of sleep-disordered breathing among middle-aged adults. N Engl J Med 1993;328(17):1230–5.

[3] Duran J, Esnaola S, Rubio R, et al. Obstructive sleep apnea-hypopnea and related clinical features in a population-based sample of subjects aged 30 to 70 yr. Am J Respir Crit Care Med 2001;163(3 Pt 1):685–9.

[4] Nieto FJ, Young TB, Lind BK, et al. Association of sleep-disordered breathing, sleep apnea, and hypertension in a large community-based study. Sleep Heart Health Study. JAMA 2000;283(14):1829–36.

[5] Peker Y, Carlson J, Hedner J. Increased incidence of coronary artery disease in sleep apnoea: a long-term follow-up. Eur Respir J 2006;28(3):596–602.

[6] Shahar E, Whitney CW, Redline S, et al. Sleep-disordered breathing and cardiovascular disease: cross-sectional results of the Sleep Heart Health Study. Am J Respir Crit Care Med 2001;163(1):19–25.

[7] Marin JM, Carrizo SJ, Vicente E, et al. Long-term cardiovascular outcomes in men with obstructive sleep apnoea-hypopnoea with or without treatment with continuous positive airway pressure: an observational study. Lancet 2005;365(9464):1046–53.

[8] Alchanatis M, Tourkohoriti G, Kosmas EN, et al. Evidence for left ventricular dysfunction in patients with obstructive sleep apnoea syndrome. Eur Respir J 2002;20(5):1239–45.

[9] Yaggi HK, Concato J, Kernan WN, et al. Obstructive sleep apnea as a risk factor for stroke and death. N Engl J Med 2005;353(19):2034–41.

[10] Munoz R, Duran-Cantolla J, Martinez-Vila E, et al. Severe sleep apnea and risk of ischemic stroke in the elderly. Stroke 2006;37(9):2317–21.

[11] Alchanatis M, Zias N, Deligiorgis N, et al. Comparison of cognitive performance among different age groups in patients with obstructive sleep apnea. Sleep Breath 2008;12(1):17–24.

[12] Yee B, Campbell A, Beasley R, et al. Sleep disorders: a potential role in New Zealand motor vehicle accidents. Intern Med J 2002;32(7):297–304.

[13] Lacasse Y, Godbout C, Series F. Health-related quality of life in obstructive sleep apnoea. Eur Respir J 2002;19(3):499–503.

[14] Sleep-related breathing disorders in adults: recommendations for syndrome definition and measurement techniques in clinical research. The Report of an American Academy of Sleep Medicine Task Force. Sleep 1999;22(5):667–89.

[15] Kushida CA, Littner MR, Morgenthaler T, et al. Practice parameters for the indications for polysomnography and related procedures: an update for 2005. Sleep 2005;28(4):499–521.

[16] Isono S, Remmers JE, Tanaka A, et al. Anatomy of pharynx in patients with obstructive sleep apnea and in normal subjects. J Appl Physiol 1997;82(4):1319–26.

[17] Haponik EF, Smith PL, Bohlman ME, et al. Computerized tomography in obstructive sleep apnea. Correlation of airway size with physiology during sleep and wakefulness. Am Rev Respir Dis 1983;127(2):221–6.

[18] Lowe AA, Ono T, Ferguson KA, et al. Cephalometric comparisons of craniofacial and upper airway structure by skeletal subtype and gender in patients with obstructive sleep apnea. Am J Orthod Dentofacial Orthop 1996;110(6):653–64.

[19] Endo S, Mataki S, Kurosaki N. Cephalometric evaluation of craniofacial and upper airway structures in Japanese patients with obstructive sleep apnea. J Med Dent Sci 2003;50(1):109–20.

[20] Tsuiki S, Isono S, Ishikawa T, et al. Anatomical balance of the upper airway and obstructive sleep apnea. Anesthesiology 2008;108(6):1009–15.

[21] Schwab RJ, Pasirstein M, Pierson R, et al. Identification of upper airway anatomic risk factors for obstructive sleep apnea with volumetric magnetic resonance imaging. Am J Respir Crit Care Med 2003;168(5):522–30.

[22] Hudgel DW, Devadatta P. Decrease in functional residual capacity during sleep in normal humans. J Appl Physiol 1984;57(5):1319–22.

[23] Jubber AS. Respiratory complications of obesity. Int J Clin Pract 2004;58(6):573–80.

[24] Van de Graaff WB. Thoracic influence on upper airway patency. J Appl Physiol 1988;65(5):2124–31.

[25] Heinzer RC, Stanchina ML, Malhotra A, et al. Effect of increased lung volume on sleep disordered breathing in patients with sleep apnoea. Thorax 2006;61(5):435–9.

[26] Heinzer RC, Stanchina ML, Malhotra A, et al. Lung volume and continuous positive airway pressure requirements in obstructive sleep apnea. Am J Respir Crit Care Med 2005;172(1):114–7.

[27] Tagaito Y, Isono S, Remmers JE, et al. Lung volume and collapsibility of the passive pharynx in patients with sleep-disordered breathing. J Appl Physiol 2007;103(4):1379–85.

[28] Van de Graaff WB. Thoracic traction on the trachea: mechanisms and magnitude. J Appl Physiol 1991;70(3):1328–36.

[29] Sauerland EK, Mitchell SP. Electromyographic activity of intrinsic and extrinsic muscles of the human tongue. Tex Rep Biol Med 1975;33(3):444–55.

[30] Mezzanotte WS, Tangel DJ, White DP. Waking genioglossal electromyogram in sleep apnea patients versus normal controls (a neuromuscular compensatory mechanism). J Clin Invest 1992;89(5):1571–9.

[31] Mezzanotte WS, Tangel DJ, White DP. Influence of sleep onset on upper-airway muscle activity in apnea patients versus normal controls. Am J Respir Crit Care Med 1996;153(6 Pt 1):1880–7.

[32] Eckert DJ, Malhotra A, Lo YL, et al. The influence of obstructive sleep apnea and gender on genioglossus activity during rapid eye movement sleep. Chest 2009;135(4):957–64.

[33] Isono S. Obstructive sleep apnea of obese adults: pathophysiology and perioperative airway management. Anesthesiology 2009;110(4):908–21.

[34] Bulow K. Respiration and wakefulness in man. Acta Physiol Scand Suppl 1963;209: 1–110.

[35] Sullivan CE, Kozar LF, Murphy E, et al. Primary role of respiratory afferents in sustaining breathing rhythm. J Appl Physiol 1978;45(1):11–7.

[36] Wellman A, Jordan AS, Malhotra A, et al. Ventilatory control and airway anatomy in obstructive sleep apnea. Am J Respir Crit Care Med 2004;170(11):1225–32.

[37] Younes M, Ostrowski M, Thompson W, et al. Chemical control stability in patients with obstructive sleep apnea. Am J Respir Crit Care Med 2001;163(5):1181–90.

[38] Younes M, Ostrowski M, Atkar R, et al. Mechanisms of breathing instability in patients with obstructive sleep apnea. J Appl Physiol 2007;103(6):1929–41.

[39] Fletcher EC, DeBehnke RD, Lovoi MS, et al. Undiagnosed sleep apnea in patients with essential hypertension. Ann Intern Med 1985;103(2):190–5.

[40] Peppard PE, Young T, Palta M, et al. Prospective study of the association between sleep-disordered breathing and hypertension. N Engl J Med 2000;342(19):1378–84.

[41] Haas DC, Foster GL, Nieto FJ, et al. Age-dependent associations between sleep-disordered breathing and hypertension: importance of discriminating between systolic/diastolic hypertension and isolated systolic hypertension in the Sleep Heart Health Study. Circulation 2005;111(5):614–21.

[42] Fletcher EC, Lesske J, Qian W, et al. Repetitive, episodic hypoxia causes diurnal elevation of blood pressure in rats. Hypertension 1992;19(6 Pt 1):555–61.

[43] Carlson JT, Hedner J, Elam M, et al. Augmented resting sympathetic activity in awake patients with obstructive sleep apnea. Chest 1993;103(6):1763–8.

[44] Waradekar NV, Sinoway LI, Zwillich CW, et al. Influence of treatment on muscle sympathetic nerve activity in sleep apnea. Am J Respir Crit Care Med 1996;153(4 Pt 1):1333–8.

[45] Joyner MJ, Charkoudian N, Wallin BG. A sympathetic view of the sympathetic nervous system and human blood pressure regulation. Exp Physiol 2008;93(6): 715–24.

[46] Osborn JW. Hypothesis: set-points and long-term control of arterial pressure. A theoretical argument for a long-term arterial pressure control system in the brain rather than the kidney. Clin Exp Pharmacol Physiol 2005;32(5–6):384–93.

[47] Fink GD. Arthur C. Corcoran Memorial Lecture. Sympathetic activity, vascular capacitance, and long-term regulation of arterial pressure. Hypertension 2009;53(2): 307–12.

[48] Ryan S, Taylor CT, McNicholas WT. Selective activation of inflammatory pathways by intermittent hypoxia in obstructive sleep apnea syndrome. Circulation 2005;112(17): 2660–7.

[49] Vongpatanasin W, Thomas GD, Schwartz R, et al. C-reactive protein causes downregulation of vascular angiotensin subtype 2 receptors and systolic hypertension in mice. Circulation 2007;115(8):1020–8.

[50] Imagawa S, Yamaguchi Y, Higuchi M, et al. Levels of vascular endothelial growth factor are elevated in patients with obstructive sleep apnea–hypopnea syndrome. Blood 2001;98(4):1255–7.

[51] Bokinsky G, Miller M, Ault K, et al. Spontaneous platelet activation and aggregation during obstructive sleep apnea and its response to therapy with nasal continuous positive airway pressure. A preliminary investigation. Chest 1995;108(3):625–30.

[52] Somers VK, Dyken ME, Clary MP, et al. Sympathetic neural mechanisms in obstructive sleep apnea. J Clin Invest 1995;96(4):1897–904.

[53] Ali NJ, Davies RJ, Fleetham JA, et al. The acute effects of continuous positive airway pressure and oxygen administration on blood pressure during obstructive sleep apnea. Chest 1992;101(6):1526–32.

[54] Lavie L, Kraiczi H, Hefetz A, et al. Plasma vascular endothelial growth factor in sleep apnea syndrome: effects of nasal continuous positive air pressure treatment. Am J Respir Crit Care Med 2002;165(12):1624–8.

[55] Usui K, Parker JD, Newton GE, et al. Left ventricular structural adaptations to obstructive sleep apnea in dilated cardiomyopathy. Am J Respir Crit Care Med 2006;173(10):1170–5.

[56] Sin DD, Fitzgerald F, Parker JD, et al. Risk factors for central and obstructive sleep apnea in 450 men and women with congestive heart failure. Am J Respir Crit Care Med 1999;160(4):1101–6.

[57] Laaban JP, Pascal-Sebaoun S, Bloch E, et al. Left ventricular systolic dysfunction in patients with obstructive sleep apnea syndrome. Chest 2002;122(4):1133–8.

[58] Shiomi T, Guilleminault C, Stoohs R, et al. Leftward shift of the interventricular septum and pulsus paradoxus in obstructive sleep apnea syndrome. Chest 1991;100(4):894–902.

[59] Hall MJ, Ando S, Floras JS, et al. Magnitude and time course of hemodynamic responses to Mueller maneuvers in patients with congestive heart failure. J Appl Physiol 1998;85(4):1476–84.

[60] Otto ME, Belohlavek M, Romero-Corral A, et al. Comparison of cardiac structural and functional changes in obese otherwise healthy adults with versus without obstructive sleep apnea. Am J Cardiol 2007;99(9):1298–302.

[61] Wang H, Parker JD, Newton GE, et al. Influence of obstructive sleep apnea on mortality in patients with heart failure. J Am Coll Cardiol 2007;49(15):1625–31.

[62] Kaneko Y, Floras JS, Usui K, et al. Cardiovascular effects of continuous positive airway pressure in patients with heart failure and obstructive sleep apnea. N Engl J Med 2003;348(13):1233–41.

[63] Mansfield DR, Gollogly NC, Kaye DM, et al. Controlled trial of continuous positive airway pressure in obstructive sleep apnea and heart failure. Am J Respir Crit Care Med 2004;169(3):361–6.

[64] Hoffstein V, Mateika S. Cardiac arrhythmias, snoring, and sleep apnea. Chest 1994;106(2):466–71.

[65] Guilleminault C, Connolly SJ, Winkle RA. Cardiac arrhythmia and conduction disturbances during sleep in 400 patients with sleep apnea syndrome. Am J Cardiol 1983;52(5):490–4.

[66] Gami AS, Somers VK. Implications of obstructive sleep apnea for atrial fibrillation and sudden cardiac death. J Cardiovasc Electrophysiol 2008;19(9):997–1003.

[67] Mehra R, Benjamin EJ, Shahar E, et al. Association of nocturnal arrhythmias with sleep-disordered breathing: the Sleep Heart Health Study. Am J Respir Crit Care Med 2006;173(8):910–6.

[68] Madden BP, Shenoy V, Dalrymple-Hay M, et al. Absence of bradycardic response to apnea and hypoxia in heart transplant recipients with obstructive sleep apnea. J Heart Lung Transplant 1997;16(4):394–7.

[69] Baldwin CM, Griffith KA, Nieto FJ, et al. The association of sleep-disordered breathing and sleep symptoms with quality of life in the Sleep Heart Health Study. Sleep 2001;24(1):96–105.

[70] Kanagala R, Murali NS, Friedman PA, et al. Obstructive sleep apnea and the recurrence of atrial fibrillation. Circulation 2003;107(20):2589–94.

[71] Bonsignore MR, Marrone O, Insalaco G, et al. The cardiovascular effects of obstructive sleep apnoeas: analysis of pathogenic mechanisms. Eur Respir J 1994;7(4):786–805.

[72] Becker HF, Koehler U, Stammnitz A, et al. Heart block in patients with sleep apnoea. Thorax 1998;53(Suppl 3):S29–32.

[73] Flemons WW, Remmers JE, Gillis AM. Sleep apnea and cardiac arrhythmias. Is there a relationship? Am Rev Respir Dis 1993;148(3):618–21.

[74] Sorajja D, Gami AS, Somers VK, et al. Independent association between obstructive sleep apnea and subclinical coronary artery disease. Chest 2008;133(4):927–33.

[75] Gami AS, Howard DE, Olson EJ, et al. Day-night pattern of sudden death in obstructive sleep apnea. N Engl J Med 2005;352(12):1206–14.

[76] Kuniyoshi FH, Garcia-Touchard A, Gami AS, et al. Day-night variation of acute myocardial infarction in obstructive sleep apnea. J Am Coll Cardiol 2008;52(5): 343–6.

[77] Shamsuzzaman AS, Gersh BJ, Somers VK. Obstructive sleep apnea: implications for cardiac and vascular disease. JAMA 2003;290(14):1906–14.

[78] Mohsenin V. Sleep-related breathing disorders and risk of stroke. Stroke 2001;32(6): 1271–8.

[79] Dyken ME, Im KB. Obstructive sleep apnea and stroke. Chest 2009;136(6):1668–77.

[80] Palomaki H, Partinen M, Erkinjuntti T, et al. Snoring, sleep apnea syndrome, and stroke. Neurology 1992;42(7 Suppl 6):75–81 [discussion: 82].

[81] Partinen M. Ischaemic stroke, snoring and obstructive sleep apnoea. J Sleep Res 1995;4(S1):156–9.

[82] Neau JP, Meurice JC, Paquereau J, et al. Habitual snoring as a risk factor for brain infarction. Acta Neurol Scand 1995;92(1):63–8.

[83] Arzt M, Young T, Finn L, et al. Association of sleep-disordered breathing and the occurrence of stroke. Am J Respir Crit Care Med 2005;172(11):1447–51.

[84] Parra O, Arboix A, Bechich S, et al. Time course of sleep-related breathing disorders in first-ever stroke or transient ischemic attack. Am J Respir Crit Care Med 2000;161(2 Pt 1): 375–80.

[85] Bassetti CL, Milanova M, Gugger M. Sleep-disordered breathing and acute ischemic stroke: diagnosis, risk factors, treatment, evolution, and long-term clinical outcome. Stroke 2006;37(4):967–72.

[86] Yaggi H, Mohsenin V. Sleep-disordered breathing and stroke. Clin Chest Med 2003;24(2):223–37.

[87] Lopez PP, Stefan B, Schulman CI, et al. Prevalence of sleep apnea in morbidly obese patients who presented for weight loss surgery evaluation: more evidence for routine screening for obstructive sleep apnea before weight loss surgery. Am Surg 2008;74(9): 834–8.

[88] Peppard PE, Young T, Palta M, et al. Longitudinal study of moderate weight change and sleep-disordered breathing. JAMA 2000;284(23):3015–21.

[89] Davies RJ, Ali NJ, Stradling JR. Neck circumference and other clinical features in the diagnosis of the obstructive sleep apnoea syndrome. Thorax 1992;47(2):101–5.

[90] Katz I, Stradling J, Slutsky AS, et al. Do patients with obstructive sleep apnea have thick necks? Am Rev Respir Dis 1990;141(5 Pt 1):1228–31.

[91] Hoffstein V, Mateika S. Differences in abdominal and neck circumferences in patients with and without obstructive sleep apnea. Eur Respir J 1992;5(4):377–81.

[92] Davies RJ, Stradling JR. The relationship between neck circumference, radiographic pharyngeal anatomy, and the obstructive sleep apnoea syndrome. Eur Respir J 1990;3(5):509–14.

[93] Horner RL, Mohiaddin RH, Lowell DG, et al. Sites and sizes of fat deposits around the pharynx in obese patients with obstructive sleep apnoea and weight matched controls. Eur Respir J 1989;2(7):613–22.

[94] Shelton KE, Woodson H, Gay S, et al. Pharyngeal fat in obstructive sleep apnea. Am Rev Respir Dis 1993;148(2):462–6.

[95] Mortimore IL, Marshall I, Wraith PK, et al. Neck and total body fat deposition in nonobese and obese patients with sleep apnea compared with that in control subjects. Am J Respir Crit Care Med 1998;157(1):280–3.

[96] Schafer H, Pauleit D, Sudhop T, et al. Body fat distribution, serum leptin, and cardiovascular risk factors in men with obstructive sleep apnea. Chest 2002;122(3):829–39.

[97] Martinez-Rivera C, Abad J, Fiz JA, et al. Usefulness of truncal obesity indices as predictive factors for obstructive sleep apnea syndrome. Obesity (Silver Spring) 2008;16(1):113–8.

[98] Vgontzas AN, Papanicolaou DA, Bixler EO, et al. Sleep apnea and daytime sleepiness and fatigue: relation to visceral obesity, insulin resistance, and hypercytokinemia. J Clin Endocrinol Metab 2000;85(3):1151–8.

[99] Deegan PC, McNicholas WT. Predictive value of clinical features for the obstructive sleep apnoea syndrome. Eur Respir J 1996;9(1):117–24.

[100] Chin K, Shimizu K, Nakamura T, et al. Changes in intra-abdominal visceral fat and serum leptin levels in patients with obstructive sleep apnea syndrome following nasal continuous positive airway pressure therapy. Circulation 1999;100(7):706–12.

[101] Tatsumi K, Kasahara Y, Kurosu K, et al. Sleep oxygen desaturation and circulating leptin in obstructive sleep apnea-hypopnea syndrome. Chest 2005;127(3):716–21.

[102] O'Donnell CP, Schaub CD, Haines AS, et al. Leptin prevents respiratory depression in obesity. Am J Respir Crit Care Med 1999;159(5 Pt 1):1477–84.

[103] Young T, Shahar E, Nieto FJ, et al. Predictors of sleep-disordered breathing in community-dwelling adults: the Sleep Heart Health Study. Arch Intern Med 2002;162(8):893–900.

[104] Netzer NC, Hoegel JJ, Loube D, et al. Prevalence of symptoms and risk of sleep apnea in primary care. Chest 2003;124(4):1406–14.

[105] Young T, Evans L, Finn L, et al. Estimation of the clinically diagnosed proportion of sleep apnea syndrome in middle-aged men and women. Sleep 1997;20(9):705–6.

[106] Benumof JL. Obstructive sleep apnea in the adult obese patient: implications for airway management. Anesthesiol Clin North America 2002;20(4):789–811.

[107] Gupta RM, Parvizi J, Hanssen AD, et al. Postoperative complications in patients with obstructive sleep apnea syndrome undergoing hip or knee replacement: a case-control study. Mayo Clin Proc 2001;76(9):897–905.

[108] Blake DW, Chia PH, Donnan G, et al. Preoperative assessment for obstructive sleep apnoea and the prediction of postoperative respiratory obstruction and hypoxaemia. Anaesth Intensive Care 2008;36(3):379–84.

[109] Liao P, Yegneswaran B, Vairavanathan S, et al. Postoperative complications in patients with obstructive sleep apnea: a retrospective matched cohort study. Can J Anaesth 2009;56(11):819–28.

[110] Fidan H, Fidan F, Unlu M, et al. Prevalence of sleep apnoea in patients undergoing operation. Sleep Breath 2006;10(3):161–5.

[111] Viner S, Szalai JP, Hoffstein V. Are history and physical examination a good screening test for sleep apnea? Ann Intern Med 1991;115(5):356–9.

[112] Hoffstein V, Szalai JP. Predictive value of clinical features in diagnosing obstructive sleep apnea. Sleep 1993;16(2):118–22.

[113] Netzer NC, Stoohs RA, Netzer CM, et al. Using the Berlin Questionnaire to identify patients at risk for the sleep apnea syndrome. Ann Intern Med 1999;131(7):485–91.

[114] Chung F, Yegneswaran B, Liao P, et al. STOP questionnaire: a tool to screen patients for obstructive sleep apnea. Anesthesiology 2008;108(5):812–21.

[115] Ramachandran SK, Kheterpal S, Consens F, et al. Derivation and validation of a simple perioperative sleep apnea prediction score. Anesth Analg 2010;110(4):1007–15.

[116] Hanly P, Sasson Z, Zuberi N, et al. ST-segment depression during sleep in obstructive sleep apnea. Am J Cardiol 1993;71(15):1341–5.

[117] Bernards CM, Knowlton SL, Schmidt DF, et al. Respiratory and sleep effects of remifentanil in volunteers with moderate obstructive sleep apnea. Anesthesiology 2009;110(1):41–9.

[118] Pearce S, Saunders P. Obstructive sleep apnoea can directly cause death. Thorax 2003;58(4):369.

[119] Berry S, Roblin G, Williams A, et al. Validity of sleep nasendoscopy in the investigation of sleep related breathing disorders. Laryngoscope 2005;115(3):538–40.

[120] Drummond GB. Comparison of sedation with midazolam and ketamine: effects on airway muscle activity. Br J Anaesth 1996;76(5):663–7.

[121] Cronin A, Keifer JC, Baghdoyan HA, et al. Opioid inhibition of rapid eye movement sleep by a specific mu receptor agonist. Br J Anaesth 1995;74(2):188–92.

[122] Farney RJ, Walker JM, Cloward TV, et al. Sleep-disordered breathing associated with long-term opioid therapy. Chest 2003;123(2):632–9.

[123] Shaw IR, Lavigne G, Mayer P, et al. Acute intravenous administration of morphine perturbs sleep architecture in healthy pain-free young adults: a preliminary study. Sleep 2005;28(6):677–82.

[124] Meoli AL, Rosen CL, Kristo D, et al. Upper airway management of the adult patient with obstructive sleep apnea in the perioperative period–avoiding complications. Sleep 2003;26(8):1060–5.

[125] Gross JB, Bachenberg KL, Benumof JL, et al. Practice guidelines for the perioperative management of patients with obstructive sleep apnea: a report by the American Society of Anesthesiologists Task Force on Perioperative Management of patients with obstructive sleep apnea. Anesthesiology 2006;104(5):1081–93 [quiz: 1117–1088].

[126] Neligan PJ, Porter S, Max B, et al. Obstructive sleep apnea is not a risk factor for difficult intubation in morbidly obese patients. Anesth Analg 2009;109(4):1182–6.

[127] Chung F, Yegneswaran B, Herrera F, et al. Patients with difficult intubation may need referral to sleep clinics. Anesth Analg 2008;107(3):915–20.

[128] Hiremath AS, Hillman DR, James AL, et al. Relationship between difficult tracheal intubation and obstructive sleep apnoea. Br J Anaesth 1998;80(5):606–11.

[129] Isono S, Tanaka A, Ishikawa T, et al. Sniffing position improves pharyngeal airway patency in anesthetized patients with obstructive sleep apnea. Anesthesiology 2005;103(3):489–94.

[130] Knill RL, Skinner MI, Novick T, et al. The night of intense REM sleep after anesthesia and surgery increases urinary catecholamines. Can J Anaesth 1990;37(4 Pt 2):S12.

[131] Knill RL, Moote CA, Skinner MI, et al. Anesthesia with abdominal surgery leads to intense REM sleep during the first postoperative week. Anesthesiology 1990;73(1):52–61.

[132] Endo T, Roth C, Landolt HP, et al. Selective REM sleep deprivation in humans: effects on sleep and sleep EEG. Am J Physiol 1998;274(4 Pt 2):R1186–94.

Advances in Anesthesia 28 (2010) 269–284

ADVANCES IN ANESTHESIA

EVIER
OSBY

An Update on Postoperative Cognitive Dysfunction

Tiffany L. Tsai, BA[a], Laura P. Sands, PhD[b],
Jacqueline M. Leung, MD, MPH[a],*

[a]Department of Anesthesia & Perioperative Care, Parnassus Avenue, University of California, San Francisco, CA 94143-0648, USA
[b]School of Nursing, Purdue University, North University Street, West Lafayette, IN 47907-2069, USA

P ostoperative cognitive dysfunction or decline (POCD) is increasingly recognized as a common phenomenon after major surgery [1–4]. Because older age is a strong preoperative risk factor of POCD [2,5], the incidence of POCD is expected to increase as the population of older surgical patients grows. Improving the measurement of POCD and identifying its etiology is clinically important, as recent studies have associated POCD with impairments in daily functioning [6], premature departure from the labor market [7], and dependency on government economic assistance after hospital discharge [7].

In this article, we review the definitions of POCD and discuss current methodological issues in this growing area of research. We also present relevant hypotheses on its pathophysiology and discuss the long-term significance of POCD.

Broadly speaking, POCD refers to problems in thinking and memory after surgery. POCD is not yet recognized in the International Classification of Diseases and is not listed as a diagnosis in the Diagnostic and Statistical Manual [8]. The term POCD is used mostly in literature to represent a decline in a variety of neuropsychological domains including memory, executive functioning, and speed of processing. POCD has been defined in a consensus statement as "a spectrum of postoperative central nervous system (CNS) dysfunction both acute and persistent ... including brain death, stroke, subtle neurologic signs and neuropsychological impairment [9]. "

POCD should be distinguished from delirium or dementia. Delirium describes an acute confusional state featuring disturbances in attention and decreased awareness of the environment [10,11]. Delirium symptoms fluctuate during the course of the day, and the patient often is disoriented. In addition, hallucinations and inappropriate communication or behavior may be observed

Supported in part by National Institutes of Health grant 1RO1AG031795-02.

*Corresponding author. E-mail address: leungj@anesthesia.ucsf.edu.

0737-6146/10/$ – see front matter
doi:10.1016/j.aan.2010.09.003

in the presence of delirium. In contrast, a typical patient with POCD is oriented but exhibits significant declines from his or her own baseline level of performance on one or more neuropsychological domains [12–15]. After surgery, changes in cognitive status may present in the form of a frank delirium or POCD, or both. POCD differs from dementia, which describes a chronic, often insidious, decline in cognitive function. Alzheimer's disease remains the most common form of dementia, but there is considerable overlap in neurodegenerative disease.

SELECTION OF NEUROCOGNITIVE TESTS TO MEASURE POCD

Most studies of POCD have focused on describing changes in brain functioning, and more specifically, have studied either performance-based or self-report perceptions of changes in memory, executive function, attention, learning, language, visual spatial skills, mathematics, motor function, and anxiety or depression [16]. The selection of neurocognitive tests to document these cognitive changes varies extensively between studies [16]. This variability in choice of tests may be because of the absence of a clear, theoretically derived, and empirically tested model that describes the causes and outcomes of cognitive changes associated with the surgical experience. Therefore, while a consensus-recommended battery of tests was established more than 10 years ago [9], it was not accompanied by this necessary model [17], nor did it have an explanation of how the tests within the battery met the consensus definition of POCD. Without the adoption of such a model, it is difficult to conclude whether tools intended to detect POCD are, in fact, assessing the presence of POCD.

Since the consensus guidelines were published in 1995, diagnostic criteria for POCD have been suggested. One stated criterion specified that there must be significant changes in neuropsychological tests involving several of the following domains: learning and memory, attention, executive functioning, and language [18]. Additional areas for assessment suggested by Deiner and Silverstein include declines in perception and abstract thinking [19]. Although these guidelines provide guidance for the selection of tools to assess for POCD, they were not accompanied with specific justification for the choice of cognitive domains that should be assessed when testing a patient for POCD [17].

Recent reviews of POCD after cardiac [16] and noncardiac [20] surgery reveal that the 2 most commonly assessed cognitive domains assessed were (1) learning and memory and (2) attention and concentration. Of the studies included in these reviews, 97% of studies including patients undergoing cardiac surgery included a memory and learning test and 70% of studies including patients undergoing noncardiac surgery included a memory and learning test. Similarly, 94% of studies including patients undergoing cardiac surgery included an attention and concentration test and 57% of studies including patients undergoing noncardiac surgery included an attention and concentration test. About one-third of studies included tests of verbal and language skills and tests of visual and spatial skills. Still fewer studies included tests of numerical reasoning (6% for both types of surgical subjects) or executive function (14% for cardiac surgery and 6% for noncardiac surgery subjects). Few studies reported the percentage of subjects who experienced significant decline in performance after surgery for each cognitive test. Consequently, it is difficult to determine whether patterns of deficits in specific domains emerge across studies. One review concluded that declines in memory and attention and psychomotor function were consistently found after coronary artery bypass graft (CABG), but cautioned that the domains of POCD detected are likely to be a function of the tests used to assess POCD [21]. Increased reporting of results for individual tests would help inform the development of a conceptual framework that explains which domains of cognitive functioning are expected to be affected by different surgical experiences.

Many studies have used composite measures of cognitive functioning to assess patients for the presence of POCD. Nearly a third of studies of POCD in patients undergoing noncardiac surgery incorporated composite measures of functioning in their protocol [20]. The most commonly used composite measure was the Mini Mental State Examination (MMSE); it was included in 21% of reviewed studies. An important debate is whether composite measures and composite scores should be used to detect POCD. Composite measures and composite scores do not differentiate which areas of neuropsychological functioning are affected by the surgical experience. Understanding the specific areas of neuropsychological functioning involved in POCD would not only advance conceptual models of POCD, but would also help in specifying which self-care activities are likely to be affected by POCD. In contrast, Rasmussen and colleagues [22] suggest that the use of composite tests or scores is not problematic because the purpose of the postoperative neuropsychological testing is to detect the presence of general, rather than specific, changes in cognitive functioning.

ADMINISTRATION OF NEUROPSYCHOLOGICAL TESTS

There are many procedural issues that should be considered when administering a neuropsychological protocol for the purpose of detecting POCD [22,23]. Those issues might be categorized into the following: test selection, test administration, and test scoring for the purpose of detection of POCD. Test selection should be guided by choosing tests that have validity for detecting change in functioning in those domains expected to be negatively affected by the surgical experience. In addition, there are several practical issues that should be considered when choosing tests for the assessment of POCD. For example, it is important to choose tests with difficulty levels that do not result in floor effects (many subjects scoring the lowest score possible) or ceiling effects (many subjects scoring the highest score possible) [23]. Tests that do not have floor or ceiling effects are likely to have greater sensitivity to detecting a change in functioning associated with surgery. Choosing tests with parallel versions reduces potential practice effects from remembering test stimuli from earlier administrations. This is particularly problematic for word-list learning tasks because some subjects are able to recall words from a prior administration of the task. The parallel versions should be administered in a different order between subjects (eg, ordered according to a Latin-square design) to avoid potential bias in estimates of change due to differential difficulty levels of different forms [24]. Tests should be validated for the language in which they will be administered. For example, the difficulty of word-list generation tasks that require the subject to list as many words as possible that begin with a specific letter varies depending on the letter specified [25]. Difficulty levels will vary across languages for the same letter.

Administration of tests used to detect POCD should be standardized across occasions and subjects. Consensus recommendations include that testing be conducted by "the same suitably qualified and trained individual and that the tests minimize subjectivity and be performed in a standardized manner" [9]. This recommendation is meant to reduce variance in subjects' tests scores that cannot be ascribed to the subjects' ability alone. Because preoperative performance may be negatively affected by surgery-associated anxiety [23], it has been suggested that the administration of mood and anxiety scales with the neuropsychological tests would allow for statistical adjustment of cognitive test scores by subjects' mood state [22].

Although a variety of scoring methods for the detection of POCD have been used across studies, investigators generally agree that scoring methods should consider (1) baseline performance, (2) practice effects, and (3) change on more than one neuropsychological test [9,17,23,26]. Baseline assessments allow determination of whether an actual change in cognitive functioning occurred subsequent to the surgical event. Nearly half of studies of POCD have been conducted in adults undergoing cardiac surgery, a population at risk for cognitive changes because of underlying heart or vessel disease [27]. Practice effects refer to improvement in performance because of familiarity with test procedures and can occur in patients with [28] and without existing cognitive impairment [29]. A common way of measuring practice effects is to measure the average improvement in performance for a group of matched controls. An important question is how well the matched controls truly match the surgical population to which they are compared. For example, studies that provide comparisons between subjects and controls reveal that controls differ from subjects, with fewer males [5,30], lower depression levels [5], lower rates of comorbidity [31], and lower attrition rates in the control group [30].

TIMING OF ASSESSMENT FOR POCD

Another methodology issue in the study of POCD is that no general consensus has been established thus far regarding the optimum timing of assessments after surgery. In previous studies, cognitive function was measured beginning 1 day to as long as 5 years after surgery. POCD can be broadly divided into acute, intermediate, and late or long-term changes based on information from previous studies. Specifically, acute POCD has been used to describe cognitive decline detected within 1 week after surgery, intermediate POCD for changes within 3 months, and long-term POCD for changes 1 to 2 years following surgery. However, the exact significance of detecting POCD at these various time points is unclear. The time interval at which a diagnosis of POCD holds the greatest clinical significance has not been determined, nor have any studies invalidated the importance of conducting assessments at a specific time point.

Early assessments of POCD likely capture a different phenomenon than what late assessments of POCD capture, and each are accompanied by a unique set of issues. Surgery-related factors may affect test performance in the immediate postoperative period, including acute pain [32–34], the use of drugs [24,35], nausea, limited mobility, and fatigue. Thus, it has been argued that patients should not be evaluated for POCD until at least 1 week postoperatively [9,14,36]. Recent evidence suggested this delay might be arbitrary, as negative outcomes are associated with POCD detected in the first week after surgery. In a 2008 study of patients undergoing noncardiac surgery, POCD detected at hospital discharge (mean duration of stay, <7 days) was associated with an increased risk of death within the first 3 months after surgery [5]. Restricting testing to only the later postoperative period is also problematic because many patients are already discharged within 1 week after surgery. In fact, recent data from the National Center for Health Statistics showed that the average lengths of stay for patients between the ages of 45 and 84 years are currently between 5.0 and 5.6 days [37]. It has been reported that the average length of stay of patients older than 50 years who underwent major noncardiac surgery with no postoperative complications was 4 days [38]. In our study, 88% of those identified with POCD were discharged within a week of surgery [34]. In addition, Rohan and colleagues [39] reported that 47% of patients undergoing minor noncardiac surgery were found to have POCD before discharge. These findings suggest that limiting screening for POCD to 7 days *after* surgery could result in missed recognition of POCD in many surgical patients. In-hospital patient education usually includes detailed instructions for wound care, administration of new medications, symptom monitoring, and details of needed restrictions in daily activities. If postsurgical patients are experiencing POCD at the time they are given self-care discharge instructions, their ability to understand and recall these instructions may be limited and may put them at risk for postsurgical complications.

The rate of patient attrition is noted to be lower in studies assessing for early rather than late POCD. Newman and colleagues [20] reported a 5.4% attrition rate for evaluations performed between 7 and 21 days after noncardiac surgery; 19% for evaluations between 22 days and 132 days; and 17% for evaluations beyond 6 months postoperatively. Patient attrition may be selective. In cohort studies, patients unavailable for follow-up were more likely to be older patients who had worse baseline cognitive performance [40] or were sicker [41]. If patients experiencing cognitive decline are more likely to decline assessment, this selective attrition will bias study results toward the null, obscuring the detection of cognitive changes postoperatively.

POCD assessments that occur in the immediate postoperative period are important for elucidating the relationship between POCD and delirium. Because POCD and delirium both feature deficits in attention, whether they are related events on a continuum or distinct conditions remains unclear. In a retrospective analysis of the International Study for Postoperative Cognitive Dysfunction (ISPOCD) research data, patients with postoperative delirium had a higher incidence of POCD 1 week postoperatively [40]. The ISPOCD study was not initially designed to measure postoperative delirium as a primary outcome, so validated measures of delirium were not incorporated into the study protocol. It is not clear whether detection of delirium via chart reviews and the Mini Mental State Examination (MMSE) performance has similar sensitivity and specificity for detecting delirium as that of commonly used measures such as the Confusion Assessment Methods (CAM) [11]. Although the ISPOCD results seem to suggest that postoperative delirium and POCD appear to be discrete events, other research provides support to the continuum hypothesis, specifically, that POCD is a subclinical from of delirium. For example, Monk and colleagues [5] found that patients who were delirious after major noncardiac surgery were also more likely to have POCD at hospital discharge. Furthermore, areas of cognitive functioning that show decline in patients with POCD such as attention are common with criteria for detecting delirium. In a study of older orthopedic patients, Lowery and colleagues [42] identified a group of patients with "subsyndrome delirium," defined as those not meeting the CAM criteria for delirium but showing a decline in global cognitive functioning as measured by the MMSE. These patients exhibited greater declines in performance on attention tasks than did nondelirious patients within the first week after surgery. Because most cases of delirium occur in the early postoperative period, an improved understanding of the relationship between POCD and delirium will be derived from additional studies that perform neurocognitive testing and delirium assessment simultaneously within the first several days after surgery.

PATHOPHYSIOLOGY OF POCD

The exact pathophysiology of POCD remains undefined. Previous studies of POCD have focused on investigating the risk factors associated with early POCD. Table 1 describes the variables that have been shown to be associated with early/intermediate POCD. In terms of patient-related baseline factors, or sometimes called predisposing factors, increasing age and lower levels of education have been identified as the main ones in the early study by the International Study on Postoperative Dysfunction (ISPOCD) [2]. In a subsequent study by Johnson and colleagues [3] that included only a subset of the population reported in the initial study, the avoidance of alcohol intake was determined to be a predisposing factor for POCD. A patient's preoperative cognitive status also has been shown to be associated with POCD [43].

Whether patients have a genetic predisposition for development of the POCD genotype is not well understood because findings from studies to

Table 1	
Patient-related risk factors for early/intermediate POCD	
Patient-related risk factors	Supporting evidence
Age	ISPOCD, Stockton, Ancelin, Monk [2,5,92,96]
Education	ISPOCD, Monk [2,5]
Burden of illness	Monk [5]
Preoperative depression	Leung (delirium only) [97]
Preoperative cognitive impairment	Johnson [3]
Preoperative habits and drug use	Monk [5]
Apolipoprotein E4	Heyer, Lelis, Leung, Tardiff [58–60,62]

Proposed patient-related risk factors of POCD and studies with supporting evidence.
Abbreviations: ISPOCD, International Study on Post-Operative Cognitive Dysfunction; POCD, postoperative cognitive dysfunction or decline.

date are conflicting. Genetic studies from population-based investigations [44,45] have demonstrated a relationship between certain genotypes and the risk of dementia and cognitive decline. Specifically, elevated risk of Alzheimer's disease has been demonstrated among individuals with the E4 allele of the apolipoprotein E (APOE) gene in many populations [46,47]. The E4 allele of APOE is associated with earlier onset of Alzheimer's disease [48]; however, the APOE4 genotype is neither necessary nor sufficient for the occurrence of Alzheimer's disease [48]. The APOE polymorphism also affects response to trauma, age-related cognitive decline, [49] and several other disorders [50–52]. APOE is a polymorphic protein associated with plasma lipoproteins. Three major isoforms can be recognized, designated as APOE2, APOE3, and APOE4, according to their relative position after isoelectric focusing [53]. APOE is unique among apolipoproteins in that it has a special relevance to nervous tissue [54]. APOE is involved in the mobilization and redistribution of cholesterol in repair, growth, and maintenance of myelin and neuronal membranes during development or after injury [55–57]. The 3 smaller studies that demonstrated an association between the APOE allele and cognitive decline were conducted in patients undergoing carotid endarterectomy and cardiac operations [58–60]. The largest study that failed to demonstrate an association between apolipoprotein E genotype and POCD measured at 1 week or 3 months after surgery was conducted in patients undergoing noncardiac surgery [61]. However, this study likely underestimated the incidence of POCD because the investigators considered any patients who were not "fit enough for testing" as not having POCD. Recently, McDonagh and colleagues [43] conducted a study in 394 older patients undergoing noncardiac surgery and similarly reported that apolipoprotein E4 was not associated with POCD measured at 6 weeks or at 1 year after surgery. Similarly, other biomarkers such as B-type natriuretic peptide, C-reactive protein, D-dimer, matrix mettaloproteinase-9, neuron-specific enolase, and S-100b also had no association with POCD measured at 6 weeks or at 1 year after surgery. The results on apolipoprotein E4 are in contrast to our work in 190 older patients undergoing noncardiac surgery, in which the presence of 1 copy of the E4 allele was associated with an increased risk of early postoperative delirium [62]. Even after adjusting for covariates, patients with 1 copy of the E4 allele were still more likely to have an increased risk of early postoperative delirium compared with those without the E4 allele. In contrast to the studies by Abildstrom and colleagues [61] and by McDonagh and colleagues [43], we measured delirium in the first few days after surgery, whereas the other investigators measured POCD at 6 weeks after surgery. One small study in critically ill patients corroborated our findings that apolipoprotein E4 was associated with a longer duration of delirium [63]. Methodological differences between delirium and cognitive assessments, difference in the timing of assessments, and potential differences in patient populations among different studies may result in differences in the findings. Nevertheless, the possible link between postoperative delirium and genetic predisposition is intriguing.

What is the possible mechanism between apolipoprotein and postoperative delirium? Previous studies suggest that the effects of APOE are mediated through alterations in lipid transport in regenerating neurons, proinflammatory cytokine release from activated microglia, amyloid precursor protein metabolism, increased blood brain carrier permeability, alterations in platelet function, and systemic inflammation [64–66]. One hypothesized mechanism is that APOE E4 allele diminishes the capacity for repair in cases of cerebral injury or capacity for homeostasis/maintenance. Whether this mechanism occurs to increase the likelihood of developing postoperative delirium remains to be proven.

In addition to predisposing risk factors, numerous potential precipitating risk factors for POCD have been investigated (Table 2). The early ISPOCD study reported that the duration of anesthesia, a second operation, postoperative infections, and pulmonary complications [2] increase the risk of POCD. In

Table 2
Precipitating factors for early/intermediate POCD

Precipitating factors	Supporting evidence	Refuting evidence
Second operation	ISPOCD [2]	Monk [5]
Postoperative infection	ISPOCD [2]	Monk [5]
Respiratory complications	ISPOCD [2]	Monk [5]
General anesthetic	?	ISPOCD, Williams-Russo [4,77]
Anesthetic type	?	Leung [98]
Anesthetic maintenance (hypotension)	?	Williams-Russo [1]
Pain management	Leung, Vaurio [99,100]	?

Proposed precipitating factors for early or intermediate POCD and studies with supporting or refuting evidence.

Abbreviations: ISPOCD, International Study on Post-Operative Cognitive Dysfunction; POCD, postoperative cognitive dysfunction or decline.

cardiac surgery, the use of cardiopulmonary bypass has been implicated as one of the precipitating factors [67,68]. During cardiopulmonary bypass, cannulation of the aortic root may result in cerebral microemboli, which could lead to POCD [69]. In addition, a profound systemic inflammatory response occurs with cardiopulmonary bypass, which may contribute to POCD [70]. However, despite the earlier reports that POCD is prevalent after cardiac surgery [67,68], studies in patients who underwent cardiac surgery without the use of cardiopulmonary bypass did not demonstrate a lower incidence of POCD, despite a smaller embolic load in the middle cerebral artery measured by Doppler in patients undergoing off-pump surgery [71,72]. Thus, it remains inconclusive how surgery type actually affects POCD. Similarly, whether the type of anesthesia affects POCD remains inconclusive. In experimental settings involving animals, general anesthetics produced neurotoxicity and subsequent cognitive impairment in young and aged animals, but whether these changes are reproducible in clinical studies has not been determined [73]. Most previous studies compared the cognitive outcomes between general versus regional anesthesia. Earlier studies suggested an association between general anesthesia and a higher incidence of cognitive dysfunction relative to epidural anesthesia [74,75]. However, recent studies concluded that there was no relationship between anesthetic techniques and the magnitude or pattern of postoperative cognitive dysfunction [1,2,4,76].

If anesthesia type did not seem to affect POCD, what about the conduct of anesthesia? The influence of intraoperative hypotension on POCD has also been evaluated. In a prospective, randomized study of older adults (age >50 years) undergoing total hip replacement, Williams-Russo and colleagues [77] demonstrated that patients who underwent epidural anesthesia and were rendered markedly hypotensive had a similar incidence of postoperative cognitive dysfunction as those who were maintained in the normotensive state. Taken together, to date, no single anesthetic type or technique has been identified to be superior in minimizing POCD for older surgical patients.

Given that the type of surgery and anesthetic type and management do not appear to influence rates of POCD, our group has focused on events in the postoperative period that may influence POCD, given that patients experience substantial pain postoperatively and are administered many medications with central nervous system effects. In 225 patients 65 years or older undergoing noncardiac surgery, we measured POCD in the first 2 postoperative days [34]. In patients without postoperative delirium, 13% of patients experienced POCD on day 1, 7% on day 2, and 15% had POCD on either day 1 or day 2 after the surgery. Multivariate regression analyses revealed that only postoperative analgesia was associated with the development of POCD. Compared with those receiving postoperative analgesia through a patient-controlled analgesia device that administered opioids intravenously, those who received postoperative analgesia orally were at significantly lower risk for the development of POCD. Our results demonstrate that older patients undergoing noncardiac surgery who are not delirious can experience significant declines in cognitive functioning postoperatively. Those at least risk of experiencing POCD were those who received postoperative analgesia orally. Opioid analgesics administered orally may result in a lower blood level of the drug because of first-pass effect when compared with intravenously administered narcotics, which may directly cross the blood brain barrier. Alternatively, the use of oral narcotics for postoperative analgesia may be a marker for a less painful state. However, this result remains significant even when adjusting for the level of pain.

In addition to studies targeting the identification of risk factors of POCD, recent investigations have focused on identifying the pathophysiology for POCD. Surgery can result in a complex systemic response, which includes neuroinflammation [78]. Systemic and neural inflammation, which occur as a result of surgery, may directly affect patient outcome. For example, blood loss and tissue injury in orthopedic procedures might affect the immune system to produce an inflammatory response [79]. Data from preclinical studies support the concept that inflammation is a possible pathogenic mechanism for POCD, and cytokines such as interluekin-1β have been implicated [80–82]; however, the clinical relevance of these experimental findings remains to be determined. Future studies using translational and multidisciplinary approaches are indicated to determine the role of inflammation as a possible causative factor in the pathophysiology of POCD.

Finally, cognitive reserve and a patient's propensity for developing adverse postoperative neurologic outcomes need to be considered when discussing the pathophysiology of POCD. A hypothetical construct coined "cognitive reserve" has been used to describe models of cognitive aging and situations where the brain sustains injury [83]. Surrogates of cognitive reserve have included education level, occupational attainment, and performance on tests of knowledge (such as vocabulary). Evidence that greater educational attainment is associated with a reduced relative risk of developing Alzheimer's disease has been demonstrated in many previous studies [84–86]. The association between lower occupational attainment and incident dementia has been found in a number of studies as well [87]. Although cognitive reserve is typically invoked as an important concept in dementia research, there is also evidence that cognitive reserve may play a protective role against POCD. As a result, future research targeting the role of cognitive reserve in POCD and postoperative delirium is an intriguing idea and should be pursued.

LONG-TERM SIGNIFICANCE OF POCD

The question of whether major surgery and anesthesia ultimately lead to long-term cognitive decline is controversial. In a population study, Dijkstra and colleagues [88] reported that the number of operations and the total duration of anesthesia were related to the number of subject health-related complaints but did not predict cognitive performance or memory complaints. Several other studies that included assessments more than 6 months after surgery similarly reported no decline in cognitive status from that measured before surgery [89–93]. However, 2 recent studies that included patients who had undergone noncardiac surgery reported that acute POCD was associated with increased mortality after surgery (for one study, at 1 year; and for the second study, at 3 months) [5,7]. Also, in cardiac surgical patients, Newman and colleagues [94] provided data showing that cognitive function at discharge was a significant predictor of long-term cognitive function. In contrast, a recent study by Avidan and colleagues [95] provides results to the contrary. In this study, the investigators enrolled participants from an Alzheimer's disease research center who had substantial pre-event data. The subjects were stratified into 3 groups based on whether they underwent surgery, were admitted to a hospital for a major illness not requiring surgery, or did not undergo surgery and had no major illness (control group). Subjects were assessed annually, and some were assessed for as many as 21 years. The battery of neuropsychological tests administered at each occasion was comprehensive of those domains of cognitive function known to be affected in the presence of drugs and other precipitating events. The sophisticated statistical methods used in this study allowed assessments of subjects' trajectory of cognitive performance before and after the event of interest. The study findings suggested that neither nondemented nor mildly demented individuals had accelerated long-term decline in cognitive function attributable to surgery or major illness compared with matched controls. Clearly, whether early POCD is related to accelerated long-term decline in cognitive function was not completely addressed by this study because cognitive assessments were not synchronized with hospitalization. Therefore, a definitive study to address the prognostic significance of cognitive dysfunction associated with surgery and/or hospitalization needs to include sufficient sample size and both short-term and long-term longitudinal assessments to more fully understand how major illness and surgery impacts quality of life and cognitive functioning, and to determine ultimately if there are reversible precipitating factors that are modifiable. Continuing research on POCD may also shed light about the pathophysiology of other neurodegenerative disease including Alzheimer's disease.

SUMMARY

Numerous studies over the past decade have reported an acute change in cognitive status in adult patients after major surgery. Most evidence suggests that these early cognitive changes are transitory and do not persist in the long term. However, the prognostic significance of POCD remains a hotly debated topic, especially in light of recent data showing that patients with early POCD were at higher risk of mortality after discharge.

Furthermore, whether patients with early POCD actually have preexisting mild cognitive impairment and experience a steeper downward cognitive trajectory independent of the effect of anesthesia and surgery is another question that warrants further investigation. We anticipate that future studies will elucidate better the pathophysiology of POCD through the use of large sample sizes and longitudinally collected patient data in both the early and late postoperative period. We also advocate for a theoretically derived and empirically tested model that describes the causes and outcomes of POCD. Such a model must be established to truly standardize the neurocognitive test battery and timing of administration in the study of POCD.

References

[1] Williams-Russo P, Sharrock N, Mattis S, et al. Cognitive effects after epidural vs general anesthesia in older adults. JAMA 1995;274:44–50.

[2] Moller J, Cluitmans P, Rasmussen L, et al. ISPOCD investigators: long-term postoperative cognitive dysfunction in the elderly: ISPOCD1 study. Lancet 1998;351:857–61.

[3] Johnson T, Monk T, Rasmussen LS, et al. Postoperative cognitive dysfunction in middle-aged patients. Anesthesiology 2002;96:1351–7.

[4] Rasmussen LS, Johnson T, Kuipers HM, et al. Does anaesthesia cause postoperative cognitive dysfunction? A randomised study of regional versus general anaesthesia in 438 elderly patients. Acta Anaesthesiol Scand 2003;47:260–6.

[5] Monk TG, Weldon BC, Garvan CW, et al. Predictors of cognitive dysfunction after major noncardiac surgery. Anesthesiology 2008;108:18–30.

[6] Phillips-Bute B, Mathew JP, Blumenthal JA, et al. Association of neurocognitive function and quality of life 1 year after coronary artery bypass graft (CABG) surgery. Psychosom Med 2006;68:369–75.

[7] Steinmetz J, Christensen KB, Lund T, et al. Long-term consequences of postoperative cognitive dysfunction. Anesthesiology 2009;110:548–55.

[8] American Psychiatric Association. American Psychiatric Association, Task Force on DSM-IV: diagnostic and statistical manual of mental disorders: DSM-IV-TR, 4th edition. Washington, DC, American Psychiatric Association, 2000.

[9] Murkin J, Newman S, Stump D, et al. Statement of consensus on assessment of neurobehavioral outcomes after cardiac surgery. Ann Thorac Surg 1995;59:1289–95.

[10] Lipowski Z. Delirium (acute confusional states). JAMA 1987;258:1789–92.

[11] Inouye S, vanDyck C, Alessi C, et al. Clarifying confusion: the confusion assessment method. Ann Intern Med 1990;113:941–8.

[12] Blumenthal J, Mahanna E, Madden D, et al. Methodological issues in the assessment of neuropsychologic function after cardiac surgery. Ann Thorac Surg 1995;59:1345–50.

[13] Makensen G, Gelb A. Postoperative cognitive deficits: more questions than answers. Eur J Anaesthesiol 2004;21:85–8.

[14] Hanning CD. Postoperative cognitive dysfunction. Br J Anaesth 2005;95:82–7.

[15] Wu C, Hsu W, Richman J, et al. Postoperative cognitive function as an outcome of regional anesthesia and analgesia. Reg Anesth Pain Med 2004;29:257–68.

[16] Rudolph J, Schreiber K, Culley D, et al. Measurement of post-operative cognitive dysfunction after cardiac surgery: a systematic review. Acta Anaesthesiol Scand 2010;54:663–77.

[17] Lewis M, Maruff P, Silbert B. Statistical and conceptual issues in defining post-operative cognitive dysfunction. Neurosci Biobehav Rev 2004;28:433–40.

[18] Bekker A, Weeks E. Cognitive function after anaesthesia in the elderly. Best Pract Res Clin Anaesthesiol 2003;17:259–73.

[19] Deiner S, Silverstein JH. Postoperative delirium and cognitive dysfunction. Br J Anaesth 2009;103(Suppl 1):i41–6.

[20] Newman S, Stygall J, Hirani S, et al. Postoperative cognitive dysfunction after noncardiac surgery. Anesthesiology 2007;106:572–90.

[21] Symes E, Maruff P, Ajani A, et al. Issues associated with the identification of cognitive change following coronary artery bypass grafting. Aust N Z J Psychiatry 2000;34:770–84.

[22] Rasmussen L, Larsen K, Houx P, et al. The assessment of postoperative cognitive function. Acta Anaesthesiol Scand 2001;45:275–89.

[23] Funder K, Steinmetz J, Rasmussen L. Methodological issues of postoperative cognitive dysfunction research. Semin Cardiothorac Vasc Anesth 2010;14:119–22.

[24] Sands L, Katz I, Doyle S. Detecting subclinical change in cognitive functioning in older adults. Part I: Explication of the method. Am J Geriatr Psychiatry 1993;1:1–13.

[25] Borkowski J, Benton A, Spreen O. Word fluency and brain damage. Neuropsychologia 1967;5:135–40.

[26] Sauer AM, Kalkman C, van Dijk D. Postoperative cognitive decline. J Anesth 2009;23:256–9.

[27] Rafnsson SB, Deary IJ, Smith FB, et al. Cardiovascular diseases and decline in cognitive function in an elderly community population: the Edinburgh Artery Study. Psychosom Med 2007;69:425–34.

[28] Sands LP, Phinney A, Katz IR. Monitoring Alzheimer's patients for acute changes in cognitive functioning. Am J Geriatr Psychiatry 2000;8:47–56.

[29] Sands L, Katz I, Doyle S. Detecting subclinical change in cognitive functioning in older adults: part 2 initial validation of the method. Am J Geriatr Psychiatry 1993;1:275–87.

[30] Keizer AM, Hijman R, Kalkman CJ, et al. The incidence of cognitive decline after (not) undergoing coronary artery bypass grafting: the impact of a controlled definition. Acta Anaesthesiol Scand 2005;49:1232–5.

[31] Silbert BS, Maruff P, Evered LA, et al. Detection of cognitive decline after coronary surgery: a comparison of computerized and conventional tests. Br J Anaesth 2004;92:814–20.

[32] Duggleby W, Lander J. Cognitive status and postoperative pain: older adults. J Pain Symptom Manage 1994;9:19–27.

[33] Heyer E, Sharma R, Winfree C, et al. Severe pain confounds neuropsychological test performance. J Clin Exp Neuropsychol 2000;22:633–9.

[34] Wang Y, Sands L, Vaurio L, et al. The effects of postoperative pain and its management on postoperative cognitive dysfunction. Am J Geriatr Psychiatry 2007;15:50–9.

[35] Ersek M, Cherrier MM, Overman SS, et al. The cognitive effects of opioids. Pain Manag Nurs 2004;5:75–93.

[36] Rasmussen L, Stygall J, Newman SP. Cognitive dysfunction and other long-term complications of surgery and anesthesia. In: Miller RD, editor. Miller's anesthesia. 7th edition. Philadelphia: Churchill Livingstone/Elsevier; 2009. p. 2v, xxii, 3084, I–89.

[37] National Center for Health Statistics (U.S.). Health, United States, 2009: With Special Feature on Medical Technology. Hyattsville (MD): Department of Health and Human Services, Centers for Disease Control and Prevention, National Center for Health Statistics; 2010.

[38] Fleischmann KE, Goldman L, Young B, et al. Association between cardiac and noncardiac complications in patients undergoing noncardiac surgery: outcomes and effects on length of stay. Am J Med 2003;115:515–20.

[39] Rohan D, Buggy DJ, Crowley S, et al. Increased incidence of postoperative cognitive dysfunction 24 hr after minor surgery in the elderly. Can J Anaesth 2005;52:137–42.

[40] Rudolph JL, Marcantonio ER, Culley DJ, et al. Delirium is associated with early postoperative cognitive dysfunction. Anaesthesia 2008;63:941–7.

[41] Borowicz LM, Goldsborough MA, Selnes OA, et al. Neuropsychologic change after cardiac surgery: a critical review. J Cardiothorac Vasc Anesth 1996;10:105–11 [quiz: 111–2].

[42] Lowery DP, Wesnes K, Brewster N, et al. Subtle deficits of attention after surgery: quantifying indicators of sub syndrome delirium. Int J Geriatr Psychiatry 2010;25:945–52.

[43] McDonagh DL, Mathew JP, White WD, et al. Cognitive function after major noncardiac surgery, apolipoprotein E4 genotype, and biomarkers of brain injury. Anesthesiology 2010;112:852–9.

[44] Yaffe K, Cauley J, Sands L, et al. Apolipoprotein E phenotype and cognitive decline in a prospective study of elderly community women. Arch Neurol 1997;54:1110–4.

[45] Slooter A, Tang M-X, van Duign C, et al. Apolipoprotein E e4 and the risk of dementia with stroke. A population-based investigation. JAMA 1997;277:818–21.

[46] Henderson A, Easteal S, Jorm A, et al. Apolipoprotein E allele e4, dementia, and cognitive decline in a population sample. Lancet 1995;346:1387–90.

[47] Maestre G, Ottman R, Stern Y, et al. Apolipoprotein E and Alzheimer's disease: ethnic variation in genotypic risks. Ann Neurol 1995;37:254–9.

[48] Bird TD. Genetic factors in Alzheimer's disease. N Engl J Med 2005;352:862–4.

[49] Dik M, Jonker C, Bouter L, et al. APOE-e4 is associated with memory decline in cognitively impaired elderly. Neurology 2000;54:1429–97.

[50] Lahoz C, Schaefer E, Cupples L, et al. Apolipoprotein E genotype and cardiovascular disease in the Framingham Heart Study. Atherosclerosis 2001;154:529–37.

[51] Davignon J, Gregg R, Sing C. Apolipoprotein E polymorphism and atherosclerosis. Arteriosclerosis 1988;8:1–21.

[52] Stengard J, Zebra K, Pekkanen J, et al. Apolipoprotein E polymorphism predicts death from coronary heart disease in a longitudinal study of elderly Finnish men. Circulation 1995;91:265–9.

[53] Mahley R, Rall S. Type III hyperlipoproteinemia (dysbetalipoproteinemia): the role of apolipoprotein E in normal and abnormal lipoprotein metabolism. In: Scriver C, Beaudet A, Sly W, et al, editors. The metabolic and molecular bases of inherited disease. New York: McGraw-Hill; 2001. p. 2835–62.

[54] Poirier J, Hess M, May P, et al. Astrocytic apolipoprotein E mRNA and GFAP mRNA in hippocampus after entorhinal cortex lesioning. Brain Res Mol Brain Res 1991;11:97–106.

[55] Boyle J, Zoellner C, Anderson L. A role for apolipoprotein E, apolipoprotein A-1, and low density lipoprotein receptors in cholesterol transport during regeneration and remyelination of rat sciatic nerve. J Clin Invest 1989;83:1015–31.

[56] LeBlanc A, Poduslo J. Regulation of apolipoprotein E gene expression after injury of the rat sciatic nerve. J Neurosci Res 1990;25:162–71.

[57] Mahley R. Apolipoprotein E: cholesterol transport protein with expanding role in cell biology. Science 1988;1988:622–30.

[58] Tardiff BE, Newman MF, Saunders AM, et al. Preliminary report of a genetic basis for cognitive decline after cardiac operations. The Neurologic Outcome Research Group of the Duke Heart Center. Ann Thorac Surg 1997;64:715–20.

[59] Heyer EJ, Wilson DA, Sahlein DH, et al. APOE-epsilon4 predisposes to cognitive dysfunction following uncomplicated carotid endarterectomy. Neurology 2005;65:1759–63.

[60] Lelis RG, Krieger JE, Pereira AC, et al. Apolipoprotein E4 genotype increases the risk of postoperative cognitive dysfunction in patients undergoing coronary artery bypass graft surgery. J Cardiovasc Surg (Torino) 2006;47:451–6.

[61] Abildstrom H, Christiansen M, Siersma VD, et al. Apolipoprotein E genotype and cognitive dysfunction after noncardiac surgery. Anesthesiology 2004;101:855–61.

[62] Leung J, Sands L, Wang Y, et al. Apolipoprotein E e4 allele increases the risk of early postoperative delirium in older patients undergoing noncardiac surgery. Anesthesiology 2007;107:406–11.

[63] Ely EW, Girard TD, Shintani AK, et al. Apolipoprotein E4 polymorphism as a genetic predisposition to delirium in critically ill patients. Crit Care Med 2007;35:112–7.

[64] Parihar MS, Hemnani T. Alzheimer's disease pathogenesis and therapeutic interventions. J Clin Neurosci 2004;11:456–67.

[65] Tsuang DW, Bird TD. Genetics of dementia. Med Clin North Am 2002;86:591–614.

[66] Moretti EW, Morris RW, Podgoreanu M, et al. APOE polymorphism is associated with risk of severe sepsis in surgical patients. Crit Care Med 2005;33:2521–6.

[67] Newman MF, Mathew JP, Grocott HP, et al. Central nervous system injury associated with cardiac surgery. Lancet 2006;368:694–703.

[68] Selnes OA, Goldsborough MA, Borowicz LM, et al. Neurobehavioural sequelae of cardiopulmonary bypass. Lancet 1999;353:1601–6.

[69] Pugsley W, Klinger L, Paschalis C, et al. The impact of microemboli during cardiopulmonary bypass on neuropsychological functioning. Stroke 1994;25:1393–9.

[70] Mathew JP, Shernan SK, White WD, et al. Preliminary report of the effects of complement suppression with pexelizumab on neurocognitive decline after coronary artery bypass graft surgery. Stroke 2004;35:2335–9.

[71] Jensen J, Hedin L, Widell C, et al. Characteristics of heart failure in the elderly—a hospital cohort registry-based study. Int J Cardiol 2008;125:191–6.

[72] Liu YH, Wang DX, Li LH, et al. The effects of cardiopulmonary bypass on the number of cerebral microemboli and the incidence of cognitive dysfunction after coronary artery bypass graft surgery. Anesth Analg 2009;109:1013–22.

[73] Culley DJ, Xie Z, Crosby G. General anesthetic-induced neurotoxicity: an emerging problem for the young and old? Curr Opin Anaesthesiol 2007;20:408–13.

[74] Hole A, Terjesen T, Brevik H. Epidural versus general anaesthesia for total hip arthroplasty in elderly patients. Acta Anaesthesiol Scand 1980;24:279–87.

[75] Berggren D, Gustafson Y, Eriksson B, et al. Postoperative confusion after anesthesia in elderly patients with femoral neck fractures. Anesth Analg 1987;66:497–504.

[76] O'Hara D, Duff A, Berlin J, et al. The effect of anesthetic technique on postoperative outcomes in hip fracture repair. Anesthesiology 2000;92:947–57.

[77] Williams-Russo P, Sharrock N, Mattis S, et al. Randomized trial of hypotensive epidural anesthesia in older adults. Anesthesiology 1999;91:926–35.

[78] Cibelli M, Fidalgo A, Terrando N, et al. Role of interleukin-1 beta in postoperative cognitive dysfunction. Ann Neurol 2010;68:360–8.

[79] Kobbe P, Vodovotz Y, Kaczorowski DJ, et al. Patterns of cytokine release and evolution of remote organ dysfunction after bilateral femur fracture. Shock 2008;30:43–7.

[80] Wang JJ. Group reminiscence therapy for cognitive and affective function of demented elderly in Taiwan. Int J Geriatr Psychiatry 2007;22:1235–40.

[81] Rosczyk HA, Sparkman NL, Johnson RW. Neuroinflammation and cognitive function in aged mice following minor surgery. Exp Gerontol 2008;43:840–6.

[82] Terrando N, Rei Fidalgo A, Vizcaychipi MP, et al. The impact of IL-1 modulation on the development of lipopolysaccharide-induced cognitive dysfunction. Crit Care 2010;14: R88.

[83] Stern Y. What is cognitive reserve? Theory and research application of the reserve concept. J Int Neuropsychol Soc 2002;8:448–60.

[84] Evans DA, Beckett LA, Field TS, et al. Apolipoprotein E epsilon4 and incidence of Alzheimer disease in a community population of older persons. JAMA 1997;277:822–4.

[85] Zhang M. [Prevalence study on dementia and Alzheimer disease]. Zhonghua Yi Xue Za Zhi 1990;70:424–8, 30 [in Chinese].

[86] Letenneur L, Commenges D, Dartigues JF, et al. Incidence of dementia and Alzheimer's disease in elderly community residents of south-western France. Int J Epidemiol 1994;23:1256–61.

[87] Valenzuela MJ, Sachdev P. Brain reserve and cognitive decline: a non-parametric systematic review. Psychol Med 2006;36:1065–73.

[88] Dijkstra JB, Van Boxtel MP, Houx PJ, et al. An operation under general anesthesia as a risk factor for age-related cognitive decline: results from a large cross-sectional population study. J Am Geriatr Soc 1998;46:1258–65.

[89] Abildstrom H, Rasmussen LS, Rentowl P, et al. Cognitive dysfunction 1–2 years after noncardiac surgery in the elderly. ISPOCD group. International Study of Post-Operative Cognitive Dysfunction. Acta Anaesthesiol Scand 2000;44:1246–51.

[90] Billig N, Stockton P, Cohen-Mansfield J. Cognitive and affective changes after cataract surgery in an elderly population. Am J Geriatr Psychiatry 1996;4:29–38.

[91] Gilberstadt H, Aberwald R, Crosbie S, et al. Effect of surgery on psychological and social functioning in elderly patients. Arch Intern Med 1968;122:109–15.

[92] Stockton P, Cohen-Mansfield J, Billig N. Mental status change in older surgical patients. Cognition, depression, and other comorbidity. Am J Geriatr Psychiatry 2000;8:40–6.

[93] Goldstein MZ, Fogel BS, Young BL. Effect of elective surgery under general anesthesia on mental status variables in elderly women and men: 10-month follow-up. Int Psychogeriatr 1996;8:135–49.

[94] Newman MF, Kirchner JL, Phillips-Bute B, et al. Longitudinal assessment of neurocognitive function after coronary-artery bypass surgery. N Engl J Med 2001;344:395–402.

[95] Avidan M, Searleman A, Storandt M, et al. Long-term cognitive decline in elderly people was not attributable to non-cardiac surgery or major illness. Anesthesiology 2009;111:964–70.

[96] Ancelin ML, de Roquefeuil G, Ledesert B, et al. Exposure to anaesthetic agents, cognitive functioning and depressive symptomatology in the elderly. Br J Psychiatry 2001;178:360–6.

[97] Leung J, Sands L, Mullen E, et al. Are preoperative depressive symptoms associated with postoperative delirium in geriatric surgical patients? J Gerontol A Biol Sci Med Sci 2005;60:1563–8.

[98] Leung JM, Sands LP, Vaurio LE, et al. Nitrous oxide does not change the incidence of postoperative delirium or cognitive decline in elderly surgical patients. Br J Anaesth 2006;96:754–60.

[99] Leung JM, Sands LP, Paul S, et al. Does postoperative delirium limit the use of patient-controlled analgesia in older surgical patients? Anesthesiology 2009;111:625–31.

[100] Vaurio L, Sands L, Wang Y, et al. The role of pain and medications on postoperative delirium. Anesth Analg 2006;102:267–73.

Advances in Anesthesia 28 (2010) 285–292

ADVANCES IN ANESTHESIA

INDEX

0737-6146/10/$ – see front matter

doi:10.1016/S0737-6146(10)00022-5